W9-BIC-411

Cardiac Critical Care Nursing

Cardiac Critical Care Nursing

Barbara Homer Yee, R.N., M.S.N.
Clinical Nurse Specialist — Critical Care
  Mt. Auburn Hospital, Cambridge, Massachusetts
Adjunct Clinical Faculty
  Boston University Graduate School of Nursing

Susan Lynn Zorb, R.N., M.S.N., CCRN
Cardiopulmonary Clinical Specialist
  St. Elizabeth's Hospital, Boston, Massachusetts
Adjunct Clinical Faculty
  Boston College Graduate School of Nursing

LITTLE, BROWN AND COMPANY
Boston   Toronto

Library of Congress Cataloging-in-Publication Data

Yee, Barbara Homer.
    Cardiac critical care nursing.

    Includes index.
    1. Cardiovascular disease nursing. 2. Intensive care
nursing. I. Zorb, Susan Lynn. II. Title. [DNLM: 1. Critical
care — nurses' instruction. 2. Emergencies — nursing.
3. Heart Diseases — nursing.
WY 152.5 Y42c]
RC674.Y44   1985   610.73′691   85-16048
ISBN 0-316-96871-4

Copyright © 1986 by Barbara Homer Yee and Susan Lynn Zorb

All rights reserved. No part of this book may be reproduced in any form or by any
electronic or mechanical means including information storage and retrieval systems
without permission in writing from the publisher, except by a reviewer who may quote
brief passages in a review.

Library of Congress Catalog Card No. 85-16048

ISBN 0-316-96871-4

9 8 7 6 5 4 3 2 1

HAL

Published simultaneously in Canada
by Little, Brown & Company (Canada) Limited

Printed in the United States of America

Illustrations by Mark Lefkowitz and Lori A. Messenger

To Hon with Love from Homer T.G.I.O.
  BHY

To Judith Barrett, Mary Ellin Smith, and my
parents, Fred and Cora May Zorb, with thanks
for their support, advice, and encouragement
during the writing of this book. I couldn't have
done it without them.

And to my colleagues at St. Elizabeth's Hospital,
Boston, whose skill and professionalism are vital
to my practice and are reflected in this book.
  SLZ

Preface

This book was written *by* critical care nurses *for* critical care nurses and students of cardiovascular or critical care nursing. Every chapter of *Cardiac Critical Care Nursing*, from assessment to rehabilitation, is devoted to the care of the cardiac patient in the critical care unit.

Care of the cardiac patient has changed dramatically in the past twenty to twenty-five years. Technological advances have improved our ability to monitor, assess, and treat physiological disorders that previously would have resulted in death. Patient management is becoming increasingly more complex, and nurses are assuming more responsibilities for direct patient management. Nursing practice has met the challenge of the past two decades guided by the significant developments made by professional organizations such as the American Association of Critical Care Nurses (AACN). This organization has developed a concept of critical care nursing, principles of practice, and standards of care. These definitions and statements serve to clarify and give direction to the practice of critical care nursing.

Recently, critical care nursing has been defined, by AACN, in terms of three major components: (1) the critically ill patient, (2) the critical care nurse, and (3) the critical care environment. All three components are interdependent and significant. The goals of delivering quality patient care cannot be achieved without qualified staff and a properly equipped environment. To recover from an acute illness, the patient requires care delivered by a nurse who is adequately prepared for the responsibility, in an environment that supports the delivery of care. Thus, all three components are essential and serve as the framework for this text.

Part I, Cardiac Critical Care Nursing, is unique in that it addresses and describes the numerous factors which ensure and maintain the delivery of quality patient care in a critical care unit. Chapter 1 describes the evolution of critical care nursing and the significant accomplishments in the care and management of the cardiac patient over the past twenty-five years. Critical care nursing is defined and described as is the organization and management of a critical care unit. Chapter 1 also addresses the role of the critical care nurse. It includes explanations of the responsibilities of the role, criteria for employment, education, and maintaining standards of care. The members and responsibilities of the multidisciplinary team are also described. Chapter 2, Planning and Delivering Nursing Care, focuses on the critical care environment. It is mainly written for the nurse manager who is in the process of remodeling or building a new unit. However, care delivery systems and documentation are also discussed.

The content of Parts II, III and IV is based on our belief that quality nursing care depends primarily on a sound knowledge base of anatomy, physiology, pathophysiological processes, and assessment skills. This is more evident today than ever before. Without appropriate information the nurse cannot accurately assess, plan, implement, or evaluate care; physiologic data cannot be interpreted; complications cannot be prevented; and pertinent psychological cues cannot help but be missed.

Part II, Assessment of the Cardiac Patient, emphasizes the first step of the nursing process — assessment. This section reviews in-depth anatomy, physiology, and physical examination of the cardiac and respiratory systems. Although physical examination is emphasized, utilization and interpretation of diagnostic tests, such as stress testing and nuclear imaging techniques, are included. This section also includes a chapter on dysrhythmia interpretation and interpretation of a 12-lead electrocardiogram. Since hemodynamic monitoring is such a large part of the management of the critically ill cardiac patient, an entire chapter has been devoted to this topic.

Part III, Alterations in Cardiac Function: In Major Cardiac Disorders, presents in-depth explanations of all the major cardiac disorders encountered in the critical care unit. Pathophysiological processes are explained, as are the nursing and medical interventions. Entire chapters have been devoted to the topics of coronary artery disease, cardiac failure, and mechanical dysfunction of the heart. Each of these chapters focuses on the nursing management of specific disease entities during the acute illness in the critical care unit.

Part IV, Clinical Management of the Cardiac Patient, describes interventions used for the critically ill patient. Cardiac surgery, emergency drugs, pacemakers, intra-aortic balloon pumping, and defibrillation are the major topics addressed.

We are particularly excited about Chapter 15, Cardiac Rehabilitation. This chapter focuses on beginning rehabilitation of the cardiac patient in the critical care unit. A major portion of the chapter is devoted to patient teaching. The principles of teaching, patient assessment, content to be taught, teaching methods, documentation, and evaluation are explained. Barriers to teaching and learning in the critical care unit are presented. Guidelines are offered for rehabilitation programs for the patient with an uncomplicated and complicated myocardial infarction as well as for the cardiac surgical patient.

Each chapter of this book concludes with short answer study questions or case studies that allow the reader to assess their level of comprehension. The study questions and cases may also be used as discussion questions, as a data base for developing nursing care plans, or as a stimulus for further study. These features make the book especially useful for nursing students enrolled in either a critical care or a cardiovascular nursing course, and for nurses in continuing education courses. The book is also intended to serve as a resource for practicing critical care/cardiovascular nurses on critical care units.

ACKNOWLEDGMENTS

Many people deserve thanks and recognition for their contribution toward the development of this text. We would like to first thank our expert contributors for their patience, diligence, and commitment. For their support and encouragement, special thanks are extended to our colleagues at Mt. Auburn Hospital, St. Elizabeth's Hospital, and Boston University School of Nursing. Our deep appreciation and gratitude is extended to our expert typist Laurie Genett. Her devotion, diligence, and high standards transformed many hours of tedious work into a pleasant experience. We are also indebted to our families and friends, particularly those at Little, Brown and Company, for their support, patience, and encouragement.

Contributing Authors

Barbara J. Daly, R.N., M.S.N., CCRN, F.A.A.N.
Assistant Director of Nursing, University Hospitals of Cleveland; Assistant Clinical Professor, School of Nursing, Case Western Reserve University

Kathleen Ahern Gould, R.N., B.A., CCRN
Critical Care Instructor, St. Elizabeth's Hospital, Boston

Alyce Souden Lanoue, R.N., M.S., CCRN
Cardiovascular Research Nurse, Division of Cardiology, Beth Israel Hospital, Boston

Catherine M. McFadyen, R.N., M.S., A.N.P.
Director, Pulmonary Rehabilitation Program, Chronic Care Resource Center, Lemuel Shattuck Hospital, Boston; Adjunct Clinical Associate, Boston College Graduate School of Nursing

Cynthia Moores, R.N., M.S., CCRN
Department Head Nurse, Clinical Nurse Specialist, CCU, Eastern Maine Medical Center, Bangor, Maine

Laura Rossi, R.N., M.S.
Cardiovascular Clinical Nurse Specialist, Brigham and Women's Hospital, Boston; Adjunct Assistant Professor, Boston College Graduate School of Nursing

Janet Secatore, R.N., M.S.
Nurse Specialist, Beth Israel Hospital, Boston

Contents

PART III
Alterations in Cardiac Function: In Major Cardiac Disorders 199

PART IV
Clinical Management of the Cardiac Patient 289

Cardiac Critical
Care Nursing

Notice   The indications and dosages of all drugs in this book have been recommended in the medical literature and conform to the practices of the general medical community. The medications described do not necessarily have specific approval by the Food and Drug Administration for use in the diseases and dosages for which they are recommended. The package insert for each drug should be consulted for use and dosage as approved by the FDA. Because standards for usage change, it is advisable to keep abreast of revised recommendations, particularly those concerning new drugs.

PART I

Cardiac Critical Care Nursing

CHAPTER 1

Introduction to Cardiac Critical Care Nursing

Barbara Homer Yee □ *Susan Lynn Zorb*

INTRODUCTION

Despite a dramatic reduction in mortality over the past decade, cardiovascular disease remains the leading cause of death in the United States and other Western nations. The most prominent of the cardiovascular diseases is coronary artery disease (CAD), which is responsible for as many as 1.5 million heart attacks each year and is estimated to have caused almost 555,000 deaths in 1982. Unfortunately, a large proportion of these victims die before they reach the hospital [4].

The psychological and social adjustments demanded of the victim, family, and community cannot be measured. The cost of medical services, however, is measurable: approximately $72 billion in 1984 [4]. Preventing heart disease through risk factor reduction is a major goal of the American Heart Association (AHA), and it is a less costly method of dealing with CAD.

Care of the cardiac patient has changed tremendously in the past 20 to 25 years. Technological advances have improved our ability to monitor, assess, and treat physiological disorders that previously would have resulted in death. In addition, long-term care of the cardiac patient has improved significantly with the advent of organized cardiac rehabilitation programs. With the help of education, counseling, and exercise programs, the cardiac patient can return to a normal or near-normal lifestyle.

Before 1965 very few hospitals had specialized care units other than the recovery room. As more critical care units opened and patient care needs became more complex, nurses recognized a need for further education and support in their speciality areas. From this need, cardiac nursing and critical care nursing developed. There is probably no other field of nursing that is growing and changing as fast. The challenge of caring for the critically ill cardiac patient is tremendous, as are the rewards.

This chapter will introduce the topic of cardiac critical care nursing. Various aspects of critical care will be discussed, including a philosophy and definition of critical care nursing, standards of care, a multidisciplinary approach to patient care, and characteristics of the patient population and the nursing personnel. To foster an appreciation of the rapid developments in critical care and cardiac nursing over the past 25 years, we first present a historical perspective.

HISTORICAL PERSPECTIVES

The practice of placing the sickest patients together in a location nearest the nurses' station dates back to Florence Nightingale [1] and continues today, both in critical care units (ICUs) and in general units. Specialized care areas were developed in response to particular patient needs. With few exceptions, the earliest special care units were recovery rooms. Then in the late 1950s and early 1960s several events precipitated the creation of special care areas designed specifically for the patient with cardiac disease.

Cardiac catheterization was one of the major innovations in the diagnosis of heart disease. The earliest documented procedure took place in 1929, when Werner Forssman catheterized his own right atrium [33]. This technique was developed and refined in the 1940s and 1950s. In 1959 selective coronary arteriography was introduced by Sones and Shirey [46]. Thereafter, the severity and extent of coronary artery disease could be determined, a development that revolutionized cardiac bypass surgery [33]. Coronary artery bypass grafting is one of the most common surgical procedures performed in the United States today, with almost 170,000 such procedures performed annually [4].

Although many patients benefit from open heart surgery, there are fewer alternatives for the large number of patients with end-stage cardiac disease. A small, select group of such patients may be candidates for cardiac transplantation. The intial transplantation was performed by Barnard in 1967. In early 1968 Stanford University Medical Center initiated a cardiac transplant program, receiving worldwide attention. Since then several hundred patients have undergone cardiac homotransplantation at Stanford [32]. At present a variety of artificial mechanical devices to replace or assist the failing heart are being investigated, but thus far they have had little lasting success.

While special care areas were being developed to provide care for the patient undergoing cardiac surgery, coronary care units (CCUs) were opening to serve the patient with myocardial infarction. According to Whipple [49], the single most important factor leading to the development of CCUs was recognition of the critical 4-minute interval beyond which the brain is progressively destroyed after cessation of cardiac activity. Thus, the purpose of the original CCUs was emergency resuscitation by means of closed-chest cardiac massage, cardiac pacing, and electrical countershock [49].

It was soon recognized that often-fatal dysrhythmias could be prevented with close observation and immediate treatment with drugs, pacemakers, or both. In the late 1950s and early 1960s, temporary and permanent pacemakers were developed and first used in the treatment of patients in complete heart block. Today the annual number of procedures performed for pacemaker insertion, maintenance, or removal (202,000) exceeds the number of coronary artery bypass grafts (CABGs) (170,000) [4].

Hemodynamic monitoring was introduced in the early 1970s, adding another dimension to the care of the cardiac patient. The advent of pulmonary artery catheters permitted continuous measurement and assessment of physiological variables reflecting left atrial and ventricular function. Pulmonary artery catheterization is especially valuable in the assessment and treatment of patients in congestive heart failure or shock. Another technique that has assisted the clinician in the care of the cardiac patient in shock or failure is the intra-aortic balloon pump. This temporary mechanical assist device was first used in 1968 for patients in refractory cardiogenic shock. Over the years the indications for counterpulsation have expanded, and it is now used most frequently for patients with unstable angina or to provide additional cardiac support following cardiac surgery.

In the next decade continued research and technological developments may again alter therapeutic approaches in cardiac care. Percutaneous transluminal coronary angioplasty (PTCA) is a procedure that can reduce coronary artery stenosis without the risk, expense, and recovery period of a CABG. Streptokinase infusion, originally used in the treatment of pulmonary embolism and acute deep vein thrombosis, is now being used in patients with acute myocardial infarction resulting from thrombosis. A new category of drugs, calcium channel blockers, has been approved for use in the treatment of cardiovascular disease. In addition, treatment protocols for patients with refractory dysrhythmias are changing by the development of new antiarrhythmic medications, an implantable automatic defibrillator, and surgical procedures.

The innovations in the care of the cardiac patient over the past 25 years are extraordinary. The success of many of these procedures is directly related to the care delivered in the critical care unit. Specialized care areas staffed and equipped appropriately are devoted to treating patients during the most acute period of an illness. Their continued success depends on the quality and standards of nursing care delivered.

CURRENT STATUS OF CRITICAL CARE UNITS

In 1979 a study was conducted for the American Association of Critical Care Nursing (AACN) to determine the existence and organization of specialized facilities, procedures, and practice involved in the care of the critically ill patient [20]. Hospitals included in the sample were those United States institutions reporting the existence of at least one ICU (69%). The findings that follow were noted by Kinney [36] based on the 49% of eligible hospitals responding.

Most hospitals in the United States with an ICU have one distinct, multipurpose unit (61%). The patient population is a mixture of medical, surgical, and cardiac patients. Approximately 30% of the participating hospitals reported having two ICUs, a combined medical/surgical unit and a CCU. As expected, a correlation between the size of the hospital and the number and types of units was found. Large hospitals (more than 500 beds) may have three or four specialized units, such as cardiac, neonatal, and pediatric. The patient population in an ICU may vary, depending on the size of the hospital, the number of ICUs, the number of beds in the unit, the expertise of surrounding hospitals, the distance to other medical facilities, and other factors.

PHILOSOPHY AND CONCEPT OF CRITICAL CARE NURSING

Philosophy

A philosophy states beliefs and values about patients, their care, the nursing staff, and nursing practice. Each department of nursing has its own philosophy, which is then adapted for use in specific critical care areas. Ideally, the values stated in the philosophy reflect actual practice, and therefore a nurse should examine the philosophy before accepting employment. Exhibit 1.1 presents an example of a philosophy governing a critical care unit.

Concept

Since its inception in 1969, the AACN has grown to be the world's largest specialty organization [10]. Its commitment to quality patient care is evident in its establishment of the National Teaching Institutes, core curriculum, certification examinations, and the like. It is this association that has most clearly defined the concept of critical care nursing. Its model, presented in Figure 1.1, describes the goal of critical care nursing practice as quality patient care, and the method used as the nursing process. The framework is formed by three

EXHIBIT 1.1
Philosophy of the Coronary Care Unit of St. Elizabeth's Hospital

The coronary care unit (CCU) is primarily concerned with providing critically ill patients with prophylactic and supportive care. A highly skilled and caring multidisciplinary team provides close observation and comprehensive critical care for all patients in an atmosphere where dignity and respect are maintained.

Nursing in the CCU requires careful observations of all physiologic and psychologic processes that threaten an individual's well being. Qualities of caring and commitment are vital to maintaining high standards of nursing practice which are necessary for the promotion of the health and well being of all patients.

Adapted from St. Elizabeth's Hospital, Boston, Massachusetts, with permission.

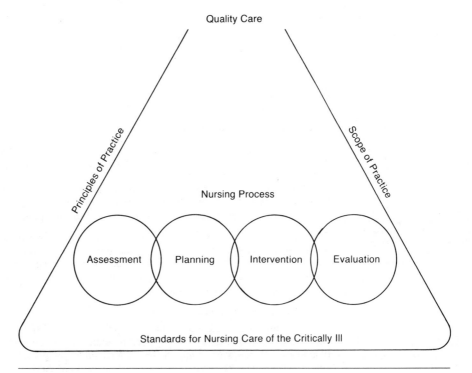

FIGURE 1.1
The concept of critical care nursing as defined by the American Association of Critical Care Nursing. (From Bertram, D. The concept of critical care nursing. *Focus* 9(1):5, 1982. Used with permission.)

components: (a) the scope of practice (Exhibit 1.2), (b) the principles of practice (Exhibit 1.3), and (c) the standards for nursing care. These components serve as the structure within which critical care nursing is practiced [11].

In 1981 the AACN published *Standards for Nursing Care of the Critically Ill.* The work is divided into two sections: the process standards are similar to the American Nurses' Association standards, whereas the structure standards deal with the ICU environment, the education of critical care nurses,

EXHIBIT 1.2
AACN Scope of Practice Statement

Critical care nursing practice is a dynamic process the scope of which is defined in terms of the critically ill patient, the critical care nurse and the environment in which critical care nursing is delivered; all three components are essential elements for the practice of critical care nursing.

The critically ill patient

The critically ill patient is characterized by the presence of real or potential life-threatening health problems and by the requirements for continuous observation and intervention to prevent complications and restore health. The concept of the critically ill patient includes the patient's family and/or significant others.

The critical care nurse

The critical care nurse is a registered professional nurse committed to ensuring that all critically ill patients receive optimal care. This nurse's practice is based on the following:

1. individual professional accountability

2. thorough knowledge of the interrelatedness of body systems and the dynamic nature of the life process

3. recognition and appreciation of the individual's wholeness, uniqueness and significant social and environmental relationships

4. appreciation of the collaborative role of all members of the health care team

To continually refine the practice, the critical care nurse participates in ongoing educational activities. In addition to basic preparation, the critical care nurse acquires an advanced knowledge of psychosocial, physiological and therapeutic components specific to the care of the critically ill. Clinical competency and the ability to effectively interact with patients, families and other members of the health care team are developed. Additionally, an awareness of the responsibility for and environment for safe practice is cultivated.

The critical care nurse utilizes the nursing process as a framework for practice. In caring for the critically ill, the nurse will collect data, identify and determine the priority of the patient's problems/needs, formulate an appropriate plan of nursing care, implement the plan of nursing care according to the priority of the identified problems/needs, and evaluate the process and outcome of nursing care.

The critical care environment

A critical care unit is any geographically designated area which is designed to facilitate the care of the critically ill patient by critical care nurses. It is an area where safety, organizational and ethical standards are maintained for patient welfare. Although critical care nursing usually occurs in a critical care unit, it can occur in any setting that meets the environmental and nursing standards, such as an area which has a psychologically supportive environment for the patients and families, adequately functioning equipment and supplies, readily available emergency equipment, facilities to meet staff needs, and ready access to support departments.

This Scope of Practice statement provides a definition and framework for nursing care of the critically ill. For critical care nursing practice to occur, all three components must be present: the critically ill patient, the critical care nurse and a therapeutic critical care environment. The Standards for Nursing Care of the Critically Ill are viewed as an extension of the Scope of Practice and offer more specific guidance to nurses delivering care to critically ill patients.

From Disch, J. Scope of practice defined. *Focus* 7(3):18, 1980. Used with permission.

EXHIBIT 1.3
AACN Principles of Practice Statement

These Principles of Practice define, promote, and uphold the highest standards of personal conduct among members. A primary responsibility of the critical care nurse is promotion and restoration of health, as well as alleviation of suffering for persons and families facing critical illness. Entrusted with this responsibility, the critical care nurse is accountable for respecting the individuality, wholeness, integrity, dignity, and rights of all humans.

1. The critical care nurse maintains the established standards of critical care nursing practice.

2. The critical care nurse continually updates knowledge necessary for competence.

3. The critical care nurse, as an integral part of the multidisciplinary health care team, coordinates care delivered to patients and supports families within the critical care environment.

4. The critical care nurse recognizes the stresses involved in the critical care environment, and creates a compassionate and humanistic climate by providing support to patients, families, and colleagues. She must also identify psychological and physiological limitations when providing care.

5. The critical care nurse respects the rights of patients, families and colleagues in the promotion or prolongation of life by individualizing each patient situation.

6. The critical care nurse identifies the values of patients, families, colleagues, and self, and incorporates those beliefs and attitudes into situations of ethical dilemmas.

7. The critical care nurse adheres to the Code of Ethics of the American Nurses' Association.

From Bertram, D. The concept of critical care nursing. *Focus* 9(1):5, 1982. Used with permission.

safety issues for both the patient and nurse, management, and research in the ICU. Since their publication the AACN standards have been rapidly incorporated in critical care units. They provide a framework for defining the quality of nursing care delivered to the critically ill patient; they have been used appropriately to facilitate the delivery of consistent nursing care, justify staffing patterns, facilitate orientation of new staff, and assist with quality assurance measurements. Maintaining standards of care is the responsibility of nursing administration.

ADMINISTRATION OF THE CRITICAL CARE UNIT

The critical care unit is generally managed by hospital administrators, a medical director, a nursing supervisor or clinical director, and, at the unit level, the head nurse (HN). The administrative responsibilities of the clinical director and head nurse vary among institutions, depending on the organizational structure of the nursing department. In the past all major decisions regarding the unit were made by the clinical director. The current trend in nursing management is to increase the autonomy of the head nurse, who now frequently handles administrative responsibilities such as hiring and firing. With this management model, the clinical director assumes the leadership role in negotiations with hospital administrators, sets standards of practice, and is responsible for teaching managerial strategies and skills, whether on a one-to-one or a group basis.

Head Nurse

Although numerous titles have evolved over the years to describe this position, most of us are familiar with the title *head nurse*. The leadership style, philosophy of nursing, and standards of practice employed by the HN set the tone for the staff and unit. Because the critical care area generally attracts nurses who are independent and self-directed in their practice, the HN must be a skillful manager who can foster autonomy yet maintain the necessary amount of authority.

The HN is responsible for major decisions regarding hiring and firing of personnel, development and implementation of policies and procedures, maintenance of standards of care, and budgeting for the unit. To make informed decisions the HN must be aware of current health care legislation and its impact on the unit, from both economic and professional practice perspectives. In the ideal situation the responsibility of the HN is combined with an equal amount of authority and power. The HN often has input into all decisions affecting the unit through membership on various committees, such as the critical care unit committee.

Critical Care Unit Committee

The formation of an ICU committee is mandated in the standards for special care units developed by the Joint Commission on Accreditation of Hospitals (JCAH) (Exhibit 1.4). The overall function of this committee is to establish policy and to review and evaluate the quality, safety, and appropriateness of patient care within the unit. The composition of the committee will vary among institutions and depends on the services offered in the unit. In smaller hospitals with one combined medical-surgical unit, representation from several departments — such as medicine, surgery, and nursing — is desirable, in addition to hospital administration. In larger hospitals with multiple units, each ICU may have its own committee. In this situation a combined ICU committee may be formed to oversee the operations of the smaller committees.

Medical Director

A member of the medical staff is appointed director of the unit and is responsible for implementing policies, allocating beds, reviewing and evaluating patient care services, and formulating admission and discharge criteria [34].

Admission and Discharge Criteria

Patients admitted to the ICU are generally those requiring "extraordinary care on a concentrated and continuous basis" [34]. Skilled personnel, lower nurse/patient ratios, access to specialized equipment, and use of a smaller area facilitate the delivery of concentrated nursing care. The criteria governing admission to the unit are generally based on a list of accepted medical diagnoses. The admission criteria must be flexible, however, to allow for unusual circumstances.

The length of stay has traditionally depended on the patient's condition and response to therapy. Today other factors, particularly economic ones, are starting to influence the time allotted for the in-hospital recovery from an illness. Although the average length of stay in a critical care unit is short (four

EXHIBIT 1.4
Joint Commission on Accreditation of Hospitals: Standards for Special Care Units

Principle

Special care units, as appropriate for the hospital, shall be established for patients requiring extraordinary care on a concentrated and continuous basis.

Standards

1. Each special care unit shall be well organized and integrated with other units and departments/services of the hospital. The scope of services provided in each special care unit shall be specified.

2. Each special care unit shall be properly directed and staffed according to the nature of the special patient care needs anticipated and the scope of services offered.

3. All personnel shall be prepared for their responsibilities in the special care unit through appropriate orientation, in-service training, and continuing education programs.

4. The provision of patient care in special care units shall be guided by written policies and procedures.

5. Special care units shall be designed and equipped to facilitate the safe and effective care of patients.

6. As part of the hospital's quality assurance program, the quality and appropriateness of the patient care provided by special care units are monitored and evaluated, and identified problems are resolved.

From The Joint Commission on Accreditation of Hospitals. *Accreditation Manual for Hospitals, 1984.* Chicago, 1983. Used with permission.

to six days) [36], the cost is disproportionately high. In the last few decades, medical technology has expanded exponentially. We now have the ability to monitor, assess, and treat numerous disorders that previously would have resulted in death. This new technology has caused health care costs, especially those in the ICU, to increase at a rate well beyond that of inflation. In 1982 these costs exceeded 10% of the gross national product, an amount larger than the entire defense budget of the United States.

Many attempts are now being made to curtail the costs of health care. The chief effort has come from the federal government in the form of diagnosis-related groups (DRGs) for Medicare and Medicaid reimbursements. DRGs attempt to classify patients according to their major medical diagnoses. Hospitals are reimbursed a predetermined amount for a patient with a particular diagnosis regardless of the patient's actual bill. The goal of this legislation is to encourage hospitals to be more efficient and to reduce expenditures, and thus it will have great impact on the future direction of critical care units. The quality of nursing care delivered has a direct impact on the patient's length of stay and, consequently, on health care cost. Thus, nurses will play a leading role in improving the cost effectiveness of the care they deliver.

JCAH mandates that each unit have criteria for discharge in addition to admission criteria. Many units have developed outcome criteria that guide and facilitate consistency in care from admission to discharge. These criteria should include both physical and emotional considerations for discharge (Exhibit 1.5).

EXHIBIT 1.5
Typical Outcome Criteria for the Coronary Care Unit

Prior to discharge from the coronary care unit, the patient will meet the following criteria:

1. The patient has been hemodynamically stable for 24 hours. The patient's blood pressure is normal without the use of vasopressor agents. The patient is afebrile.

2. The patient has been free of chest pain for 12 hours.

3. The patient demonstrates a stable cardiac rhythm. There has been no evidence of life-threatening dysrhythmias such as ventricular tachycardia, ventricular fibrillation, or frequent multifocal ventricular ectopic beats within the prior 12 hours.

4. The patient and family recognize that transfer from the unit is a positive step in the recovery process.

MAINTAINING STANDARDS OF NURSING CARE

The nurse plays a unique role in the care of the critically ill patient. As the primary care giver, the nurse spends more time per shift with the patient than any other personnel and thus is in a key position to detect changes in the patient's status, implement care, and evaluate the results of various interventions. The nurse also coordinates care. Members of the interdisciplinary team may visit the patient daily but usually do so only for brief periods. Consequently, the nurse provides continuity and information about the patient's status and plan of care. In addition, the nurse frequently develops close relationships with family members and can incorporate the relatives into the patient's daily care.

Selection of Staff

In most hospitals the HN is responsible for hiring all nursing personnel; input may be requested, however, from the clinical director or clinical nurse specialist. The criteria for employment in a particular ICU may vary, depending on the severity and acuteness of illness in the patient population. Most units, however, require one year of general medical-surgical experience. The employment of new graduates in the ICU remains controversial. Although some units do hire new graduates, most authorities believe that some previous nursing experience is necessary. Specialty units, such as neonatal or neurological, may have different or additional requirements. Additional characteristics that the HN may look for in selecting new staff are a sound theoretical base of information; the ability to apply the nursing process to patient care; advanced assessment, observational, communication, and organizational skills; the ability to make appropriate decisions regarding patient care; careful documentation of data; and the ability to work well with others.

The critical care nurse must be committed to the deliverance of quality patient care and to the profession of nursing. Unfortunately, critical care nurses are often viewed as "junior doctors" by other members of the health care team. Recently, through the development of nursing standards, nursing diagnoses, and nursing research, and the influence of professional organizations such as the AACN, critical care nursing has begun to evolve and to make unique contributions to patient care.

Education

In the ICU education must be part of daily practice and is usually the responsibility of the clinical nurse specialist, who works with the HN or preceptor. Upon employment, the new nurse is required to attend a critical care course, which prepares the nurse to function safely in the critical care unit. The length and content of the course vary among institutions, although most programs include such topics as anatomy, physiology, and assessment of major body systems; hemodynamic monitoring; dysrhythmia interpretation; oxygen therapy; electrical safety; infection control; nursing diagnosis; and ethics. Strategies used include lectures, discussions, case studies, conferences, demonstrations, simulations, role playing, patient care rounds, and programmed instruction. Learning is facilitated if the theoretical component of the course is integrated with clinical practice in the critical care unit.

The use of preceptors is extremely helpful in educating the critical care nurse. A preceptor is a senior staff nurse who has developed expertise in critical care nursing practice, has high standards of care, is a good role model, and is willing and able to share this expertise with novice critical care nurses [2]. The orientee works closely with the preceptor, gradually assuming more responsibility for patient care until independence is achieved. A preceptor program provides the orientee with consistency in learning and gives the preceptor the chance to share knowledge and to participate in the professional growth of a new nurse. At the end of the orientation program, the new critical care nurse should be able to care for critically ill patients with minimal assistance.

The novice must recognize that education is an ongoing process in critical care nursing. The nurse must be sufficiently self-directed to remain abreast of new developments in the field. Several critical care nursing journals and texts are available, and educational sessions are provided by the AACN, the AHA, and private universities, hospitals, and teaching institutes.

Clinical Nurse Specialist

The role of the clinical nurse specialist (CNS) has at times been poorly defined and subject to variations in individual interpretation and implementation. The responsibilities of the CNS are clearer now, and the impact on patient care has been appreciated.

In general, the CNS has a single purpose: to improve the quality of patient care [17]. Teaching sessions can be planned formally in a classroom or informally at the bedside. Nursing grand rounds, lecture series, and workshops provide ongoing education for experienced nurses; orientation and preceptor programs may be used for the new staff nurse. In addition to teaching, the CNS may provide direct patient care, conduct or facilitate nursing research, act as a consultant, or assist in the professional development of staff.

THE MULTIDISCIPLINARY TEAM

Caring for the critically ill patient has become increasingly complex in recent years. Although the nurse and physician are the primary care givers in the ICU, the expertise of a variety of other disciplines is often required. Respiratory, physical, and occupational therapists, as well as nutritionists, play a major role in the recovery or rehabilitation of the cardiac patient. Additional services that may be needed are social service and infection control, and technical support services such as x-ray, electrocardiography (ECG), cardiovascular technology, and biomedical engineering. Each discipline has a unique function in the care of the critically ill patient, but they have a common goal: to prevent, monitor, manage, or alleviate physiological, psychological, and social problems related to the acute illness.

Medical Staff

Medical staff in the ICU may include the director, associate directors, attending physicians, and resident staff. The physician is responsible for the diagnosis and treatment of illness and thus is ultimately accountable for the medical care of the patient. Adequate diagnosis and treatment, however, often depend on data obtained by the nurse through observation and measurement. This situation exemplifies the interdependent relationship of the nurse–physician team.

Respiratory Therapist

A well-trained respiratory therapist is an important member of the ICU team. During an acute illness cardiac patients are at great risk of developing respiratory disorders, particularly postoperative patients. Although the exact function of the respiratory therapist may vary among institutions, the major responsibilities are to provide, set up, and maintain all types of respiratory equipment and to assess the patient's respiratory status by collecting data and performing certain tests. In addition, the therapist may administer such procedures as chest physiotherapy, incentive spirometry, and aerosol treatments.

Patients requiring assisted ventilation need more intensive respiratory management. Close observation, frequent assessment of breath sounds, suctioning, turning, and arterial blood gas analysis may be required every hour in certain cases. The therapist may be responsible for all or some of these activities, in addition to adjusting ventilators and weaning patients from ventilators. It is also important that an experienced member of the respiratory therapy department be available on a 24-hour basis to participate in cardiopulmonary resuscitation.

Physical Therapist

Physical therapists also play a major role in the rehabilitative process of both the medical and surgical cardiac patient. The goal of physiotherapy for the medical patient in the CCU is to prevent muscular deconditioning caused by prolonged bedrest and inactivity. In some institutions the physical therapist may also be responsible for assessing, planning, and supervising a progressive exercise program. This program should begin as soon as the patient's condition warrants. In the cardiac surgical intensive care unit (CSICU), physiotherapy is directed toward prevention of respiratory complications related to surgery. Breathing exercises, chest physiotherapy, percussion, and vibration are performed to provide better lung expansion, open atelectatic alveoli, and mobilize secretions. The chronically ill or unconscious patient will also benefit from services provided by the physical therapist, who can supervise range of motion exercises, assess the need for splints or braces, and assist with positioning or transfer of patients.

**Nutritional
Support Staff**

Nutritional support may be provided by a registered dietitian or by nurses and physicians specializing in the nutritional aspects of illness. Any illness alters nutritional needs, but few cardiac patients suffer from prolonged interruptions in their dietary intake or concomitant problems with the gastrointestinal tract. Thus, parenteral nutrition is generally not necessary.

One essential aspect of cardiac care often provided by a dietitian is dietary instruction. The patient and family may require explanations regarding recommended modifications in fat and sodium intake. In addition, if the patient is overweight, a reducing diet may be advised. In many institutions nurses are responsible for this aspect of patient teaching.

**Additional
Consultants**

A variety of additional services may be consulted for the cardiac patient. Attending physicians may request that medical specialists in such fields as hematology, renal function, infectious diseases, respiratory function, and neurology

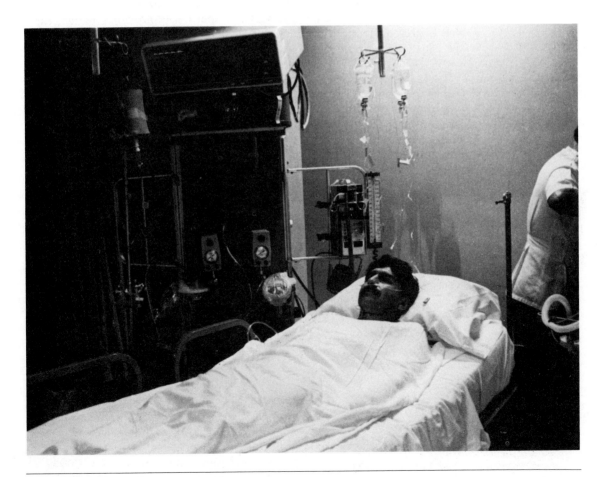

FIGURE 1.2
The critically ill patient requires extensive care by several individuals throughout the day and night. The interruptions are constant.

evaluate the patient and make recommendations. The department of social services may assist with financial problems or transfer to other health care facilities.

Technical Support   Many other individuals are not direct care givers but are indirectly involved with the patient. In the ICU most patients require a daily chest x-ray film and ECG. Cardiovascular technicians may assist with patient care by maintaining certain equipment, such as the intra-aortic balloon pump or hemodynamic monitoring equipment. All electrical equipment that will have direct or indirect contact with the patient must be inspected on a regular basis. Maintaining an electrically safe environment for the patient is a responsibility shared by the nurse and the biomedical engineer.

The large number of persons involved with the critically ill patient on a daily basis creates a continuous flow of traffic that disrupts the patient's ability to sleep, rest, and maintain privacy (Figure 1.2). The only person who observes or appreciates this problem may be the nurse, who is at the bedside on a continuous basis. Consequently, the nurse, in addition to providing patient care, has the responsibility of coordinating the daily activities. Rest periods should be scheduled, and cooperation from other care givers is essential.

SUMMARY

Since its beginning in the early 1960s, critical care nursing has changed dramatically. The nursing profession has successfully implemented the expanded role of the critical care nurse through careful staff selection, orientation programs, and continuing education. A clear definition of the scope and principles of practice, as well as established standards of care, facilitates the delivery of quality nursing care to critically ill patients.

REFERENCES

1. Adler, D. C., and Shoemaker, N. J. *AACN Organization and Management of Critical Care Facilities.* St. Louis: Mosby, 1979.

2. Alspach, J. *The Educational Process in Critical Care Nursing.* St. Louis: Mosby, 1982.

3. American Association of Critical-Care Nurses. *Standards for Nursing Care of the Critically Ill.* Reston, Va.: Reston Publishing Co., 1981.

4. American Heart Association. *Heart Facts.* Dallas: American Heart Association, 1985.

5. American Nurses' Association. *Standards of Cardiovascular Nursing Practice.* Kansas City: American Nurses' Association, 1981.

6. Anderson, C. A., and Basteyns, M. Stress and the critical care nurse reaffirmed. *J. Nurs. Adm.* 11:31, 1981.

7. Argondizzo, N. T., and Reed, P. K. The legacy of coronary care nursing. *Cardiovasc. Nurs.* 11:35, 1975.

8. Barrows, J. Continuing education for the experienced nurse. *Dimens. Crit. Care Nurs.* 2:183, 1983.

9. Berkowitz, D. S. Standards for nursing care of the critically ill. *Focus* 7(6):20, 1980.

10. Bertram, D. L. Testimony for National Commission on Nursing. *Focus* 8(3):4, 1981.

11. Bertram, D. The concept of critical care nursing. *Focus* 9(1):5, 1982.

12. Boller, J. Observations on the development of the critical care nurse. *Focus* 7(6):25, 1980.

13. Braaten, G. The utilization of AACN standards on a chapter level. *Focus* 9(4):21, 1982.

14. Breu, C., and Dracup, K. Survey of critical care nursing practice. III. Responsibilities of intensive care unit staff. *Heart Lung* 11:157, 1982.

15. Breu, C., and Turzan, L. Implementing standards of care through planned change. *Focus* 8(1):24, 1981.

16. Canfield, A. B. Controversy over clinical competencies. *Heart Lung* 11:197, 1982.

17. Clark, S. The clinical nurse specialist in critical care. *Crit. Care Q.* 5:51, 1982.

18. Clough, J. A. Developing and implementing orientation to a critical care unit. *Focus* 9(5):24, 1982.

19. Disch, J. Scope of practice defined. *Focus* 7(3):18, 1980.

20. Disch, J. Survey of critical care nursing practice. I. Characteristics of hospitals with critical care units. *Heart Lung* 10:1017, 1981.

21. Friedman, E. H. Stress and intensive care nursing: a ten year appraisal. *Heart Lung* 11:26, 1982.

22. Gawlinski, A. Quality assurance and standards of care in the critical care setting. *Crit. Care Q.* 5:43, 1982.

23. Goldman, L. The CCU and coronary artery disease mortality. *Primary Cardiol.* 9:84, 1983.

24. Gottschall, M. A., et al. Critical care orientation programs. *Nurs. Management* 14:32, 1983.

25. Grindol, M. A. A critical care staff development program. *Superv. Nurse* 10:31, 1979.

26. Hansell, H. N., and Foster, S. B. Critical care nursing orientation: a comparison of teaching methods. *Heart Lung* 9:1066, 1980.

27. Harrell, J. R. Orienting the experienced critical care nurse. *Superv. Nurse* 11:32, 1980.

28. Hartshorn, J. C. The role of nursing education in critical care. *Superv. Nurse* 12:64, 1981.

29. Henderson, V. V. Implementing the clinical nurse specialist role: a success story. *Nurs. Management* 12:55, 1981.

30. Holloway, N. M. *Nursing the Critically Ill Adult.* Menlo Park, Ca.: Addison-Wesley, 1979.

31. Holmes, A. Survey of critical care nursing practice. V. Type of equipment and responsibilities of personnel with regard to equipment. *Heart Lung* 11:242, 1982.

32. Hurst, J. W., et al. *The Heart.* New York: McGraw-Hill, 1982.

33. Johnson, R. A., Haber, E., and Austen, W. G. *The Practice of Cardiology.* Boston: Little, Brown, 1980.

34. Joint Commission on Accreditation of Hospitals. Special care units. In *Accreditation Manual for Hospitals.* 1984 edition. Chicago: Joint Commission on Accreditation of Hospitals, 1983.

35. Kaldor, P. K. How to develop a critical care nursing course. *Crit. Care Nurs.* 2(3):84, 1982.

36. Kinney, M. Survey of critical care nursing practice. II. Unit characteristics. *Heart Lung* 10:1051, 1981.

37. Lewandowski, L. A., and Kositsky, A. M. Research priorities for critical care nursing: a study by the American Association of Critical-Care Nurses. *Heart Lung* 12:35, 1983.

38. Lindstrom, S. R., and Archibald, E. J. A critical care teaching method. *Superv. Nurse* 11:49, 1980.

39. McIntyre, E. Clinical evaluation of a new critical care nurse. *Focus* 9(5):3, 1982.

40. Morris, K. H., and Schweiger, J. A. Clinical nurse specialist role creation: an achievable goal. *Nurs. Adm. Q.* 4:67, 1979.

41. Pennock, J. L., et al. Cardiac transplantation in perspective for the future. *J. Thorac. Cardiovasc. Surg.* 83:168, 1982.

42. Piazza, D., and Jackson, B. Clinical nurse specialist: issues, power and freedom. *Superv. Nurse* 9:47, 1978.

43. Puntillo, K., and Duncan, J. An alternative learning experience for intensive care unit nurses. *J. Contin. Educ. Nurs.* 11:40. 1980.

44. Pyles, S. H., and Stern, P. N. Discovery of nursing gestalt in critical care nursing: the importance of the gray gorilla syndrome. *Image* 15:51, 1983.

45. Rees, C. Teaching for coronary care unit emergencies. *J. Contin. Educ. Nurs.* 11:39, 1980.

46. Sones, F. M., and Shirey, E. K. Cine coronary arteriography. *Mod. Concepts Cardiovasc. Dis.* 31:375, 1962.

47. Sullivan, S., and Breu, C. Survey of critical care nursing practice. IV. Staffing and training of intensive care personnel. *Heart Lung* 11:237, 1982.

48. Urban, C. Implementation of critical care standards. *Focus* 9(5):30, 1982.

49. Whipple, G. H., et al. *Acute Coronary Care.* Boston: Little, Brown, 1982.

Planning and Delivering Nursing Care

Barbara J. Daly

INTRODUCTION

The nurse manager or head nurse (HN) who is responsible for the delivery of care to critically ill patients must constantly reassess and attempt to improve care delivery systems. We can view the critical care system as consisting of three interacting subsystems — the patient, the care givers, and the environment. Any analysis of the complete critical care system must consider all three. Chapter 1 reviewed elements related to the patient system (characteristics of the population to be served, average length of stay) and elements of the care-giver system (members of the team, roles, education). This chapter will discuss the third subsystem — the environment — and aspects of unit organization that affect the interaction of the three subsystems.

THE ENVIRONMENT

The physical environment of the critical care unit is generally analyzed only after a decision has already been made to build a new unit or remodel an existing one. Our discussion, however, may also be useful to the HN who is anticipating needs or attempting to validate the need for a new unit. We will take the perspective of someone planning a new unit.

Planning

Anyone who has routine or frequent involvement with the unit should be involved in the planning of a new critical care unit, and each person's decision-making authority should parallel his or her degree of unit involvement. Thus, in the case of the cardiac unit, the nurses, cardiologists, and cardiac surgeons should have the greatest input and must be involved from start to finish.

As Bendixen has stated, "the first step in the planning process is to realize that *real* planning will be required" [5] — that is, the planning committee must be formed. Table 2.1 lists the committee personnel, those who make decisions and those who provide consultation. The first three groups in each column should be represented at all meetings of the committee; the others listed can be invited to participate at appropriate times. But care must be taken not to neglect the input of support services. Something as simple as forgetting to plan for space for the laundry cart or a convenient location for a trash chute can create major problems in the eventual day-to-day operation of the unit.

Ideally, the planning process should begin at least 12 to 18 months prior to the intended opening date. All departments should be contacted before construction begins. The sections that follow review, in order, the most common issues to be addressed.

Location

The location of the critical care unit often is not a negotiable item. Even if the location of the unit is predetermined, however, the planning committee should keep the location in mind in order to anticipate problems and identify changes needed in other facilities.

The source of patient admission is probably the most important consideration in determining unit location. If most patients come from the emergency room, the critical care unit (ICU) should be located nearby. If, however, most patients are admitted after surgical procedures, the ICU should be adjacent to the operating room. Other facilities that should be convenient to the ICU in-

TABLE 2.1
Critical Care Unit Planning Committee

Decision Makers	Consultants
Nurses	Architects
Physicians	Hospital engineers
Unit manager or coordinator	Hospital maintenance personnel
Relevant clinical services	General administration personnel
Clinical engineering	Relevant support services
Respiratory therapy	Laundry
Pharmacy	Material management
Social service	Environmental services
Dietetics	

clude, in decreasing order of importance, areas to which the patient must frequently be moved (such as the cardiac catheterization laboratory and the computer tomographic scanning facilities), other intensive care units (in order to permit sharing of services), and important laboratories (for example, blood gas analysis facilities) [12, 26, 37].

Size

Both the number of beds and the actual square footage needed for the ICU must be determined. The following general guidelines can help in the complex process of deciding on the number of beds needed:

1. Ideally, the number of beds in the ICU should constitute 2 to 10% of the total number of beds in the facility [5, 22, 37]. In one report in *Heart and Lung,* the average percentage of ICU beds in the 2,412 hospitals reporting was 6.5 [16].

2. If other ICU, step-down, intermediate-care, or progressive-care beds are available, fewer cardiac ICU beds are needed; if the only alternative to the ICU is general division care, the allotment of ICU beds should be more generous.

3. It is preferable not to exceed ten to fifteen ICU beds per unit [5, 23, 33] because of the difficulties inherent in managing larger units.

4. Occupancy rates for ICUs must be interpreted carefully. Because space must be available for emergency patients, the occupancy rate must be lower than that of general units. As a result, the per-bed operating costs will be much higher than might be desirable. In any ICU with an occupancy rate of 80% or higher, however, it is likely that an unacceptable number of patients are being denied admission — that the "threshold" for admission (how sick the patient must be to be admitted) is too high. The average occupancy rate of all types of ICUs ranges from 54 to 78% [24].

5. The number of days on which all beds are filled should be examined. ICUs typically have a widely fluctuating census. It may be that the average occupancy rate is only 60%, yet the beds are filled — and admissions thus denied — on 50% of the days.

TABLE 2.2
Critical Care Unit Requirements

Feature	Requirement
Space	
Private rooms	175–200 sq. ft./bed
Open ward	125–150 sq. ft./bed
Total	2–3 × bed space
Bedside outlets	
Electrical (110 volt)	6–8
Oxygen	4
Air	1–2
Suction	4–6
Ventilation	10–30 air changes/hr.
Temperature	72°F ± 2° (21–24°C)
Humidity	40–50%

Data from refs. 1, 11, 22, 26, 37.

6. Future trends and developments must be predicted. The answers to the following questions will affect ICU bed demand: (a) Are there any significant changes expected in the number or clinical specialities of referring physicians (e.g., the addition of another cardiac surgeon to the staff)? (b) Are there any community changes that will affect the hospital population (e.g., a nearby hospital closing, the opening of a new dialysis center)? (c) Are there any other major hospital programs planned, such as a transplant program or a trauma service?

Clearly, deciding how many beds are needed entails a balancing of cost and benefit. To build so many ICU beds that the unit is never full and patients never have to be discharged prematurely is unacceptably expensive. If the unit is filled to capacity two or three times a week, however, the level of acuteness being treated in the general divisions is probably higher than desirable. Computer simulation of the effects of variable numbers of beds can be a valuable tool in determining the "ideal" number, and such simulations are recommended if systems consultants are available [11, 42].

Once the number of beds has been determined, the space required can be projected. The space needed depends to some degree on the type of design (private, semiprivate, open ward) and the number of ancillary services desired within the unit (e.g., laboratory space, sleeping room). For initial planning, the figures of 200 square feet per bed and three times the bed space for the total unit may be used. (Table 2.2 gives more specific figures.) Thus, for a ten-bed unit, 2,000 square feet is needed for bed space and 6,000 square feet is needed for the total unit, including beds.

Design

Design characteristics include the shape and type of the patient unit, the number and type of other facilities located within the unit, and the placement of facilities. Shape is often determined by the shape of the building itself. When options are available, the advantages and disadvantages of various shapes

TABLE 2.3
Characteristics of Types of Patient Units

Type of Unit	Advantages	Disadvantages
Private room	Patient privacy	Need for more space per bed
	Ability to isolate patient from noise and other patients	Inflexible dimensions
	Ease of implementing isolation	Visibility problems and increased travel time from nurses' station; thus potential increase in staffing needs
		Possible increased difficulties in managing emergencies in a closed room
Open ward	Need for less space per bed	No patient privacy
	Flexible dimensions	Patient exposure to noise and other patients
	Increased visibility and decreased travel time from bed to bed; thus, possible easing of staffing needs	Difficulties of implementing isolation
	Possibly easier management of emergencies	Possible contribution to ICU psychosis through disturbance of sleep patterns

should be considered. In one of the few studies of this subject, Sturdavant found that a circular unit was preferred to a rectangular one by all nurses and that less time was spent in traveling to and from rooms because distances were shorter [40]. In a survey of ten ICUs, MacDonald and colleagues found that nurses preferred semicircular units to rectangular or L-shaped units [28]. The significant features seemed to be visibility of patients from the nurses' station and ease of access to patient rooms.

The two major types of patient units are private rooms and open wards. Each has advantages and disadvantages, summarized in Table 2.3, that must be evaluated in light of the patient population. For example, in a surgical ICU whose patients are received unconscious directly from the operating room, and where the average length of stay (LOS) is two days, the open-ward design might be best. In a coronary care unit that houses mainly patients with suspected myocardial infarctions, where the priority is quiet observation and rest and the average LOS is five days, the private-room design is undoubtedly preferable. For the mixed medical-surgical unit, a combination of several private rooms and several beds in an open ward might be ideal. Semiprivate rooms and three-walled cubicles represent attempts to preserve the advantages of each type while minimizing the disadvantages. Figures 2.1 through 2.3 show common unit designs. Visiting other hospitals that have units of different designs can also be helpful.

Regardless of the type of patient unit, the bedside components must be planned. These include oxygen, air, vacuum, and electrical outlets. Virtually all critical care units built today use prefabricated modules of some sort: wall consoles, pedestals (extending from floor to waist height), free-standing col-

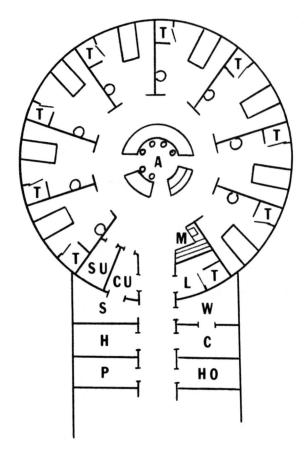

FIGURE 2.1
Circular eight-bed unit. (*T* = toilet; *A* = nurses' station, with central desks and supply shelf; *SU* = soiled utility room; *CU* = clean utility room; *M* = medication area; *L* = nurses' lounge; *S* = storage room; *W* = family waiting room; *H* = head nurse's office; *C* = conference room; *P* = physician director's office; *HO* = house staff sleeping quarters.)

umns (floor to ceiling), and telescoping columns (extending from ceiling to head height). Ceiling and pedestal columns are often chosen for operating and emergency rooms because they allow easy access to the patient from all sides of the stretcher or bed; the wall console provides the easiest access to outlets and is most adaptable in its design.

The wall console or column should be designed primarily by the nurses who will be using the unit. Ideally, a life-size mock-up can be made so that actual dimensions and placement of outlets can be evaluated. A scale drawing is a necessity. The design should be evaluated in terms of the number of each type of outlet needed on each side of the bed, ease of access provided (waist to shoulder height is best), and the space needed to permit brackets for suction bottles and humidifiers. Too many outlets are far better than too few. Recommended numbers of outlets are listed in Table 2.2.

Other services and facilities that should be included in the planning are listed in Table 2.4. Unfortunately, these facilities are often sacrificed to increase bed space, and the nurse manager must be prepared to present a strong case for their necessity. Agreement on the priority of these facilities should be reached early and documented in meeting minutes or by memo. When questions about space utilization arise later, the nurse then can support and clarify his or her position.

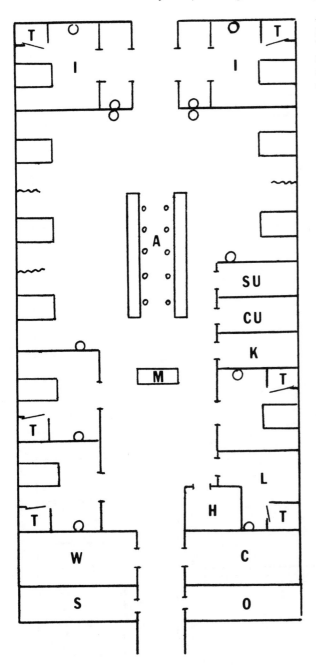

FIGURE 2.2
Ten-bed unit, with three private rooms, two isolation rooms with anteroom (*I*), and five open beds. (*K* = kitchenette; *O* = office or sleeping quarters; other abbreviations as in Figure 2.1.)

The design of the ICU must also provide for infection control. Most important is the provision of adequate hand-washing facilities — the single most effective means of preventing transmission of infection. The unit should contain one sink in each private room, and one sink for every two beds in an open ward. Each sink should have a dispenser for soap and foot pedals or elbow handles. Beds should be at least 7 feet apart [1, 34]. An isolation room with a

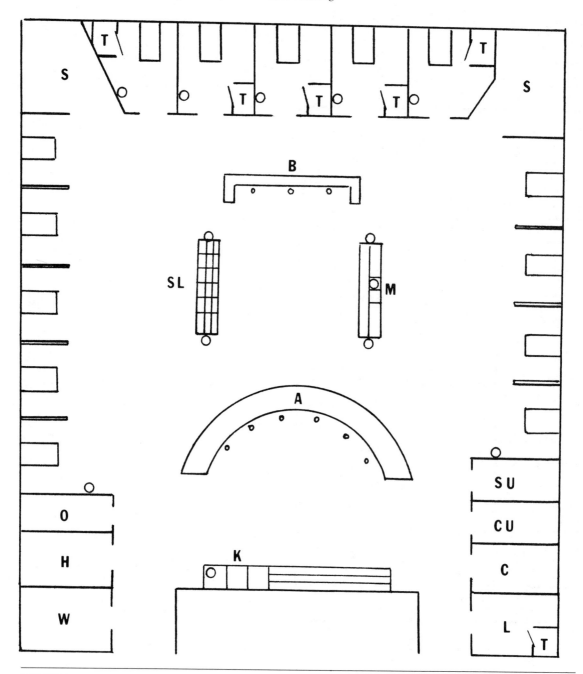

FIGURE 2.3
Fourteen-bed unit, with five private rooms and nine beds separated by half walls.
(*A* = main nurses' station; *B* = second nurses' station; *SL* = supply lockers;
other abbreviations as in Figures 2.1 and 2.2.)

TABLE 2.4
Recommended Critical Care Unit Facilities

Area	Description/rationale
Storage room	Safe and proper maintenance of supplies and expensive equipment requires a separate, secure location for storage. As a rule of thumb, space equivalent to 1 bed (150 sq. ft.) is needed for every 10 beds. This figure does not include storage space within clean and dirty utility rooms.
Separate clean and dirty utility rooms	Separate areas are required to meet JCAH requirements. The clean utility room must be located in a central area, and access to shelves and drawers should not be hindered by storage of large equipment.
Staff locker room/lounge	The staff requires a separate area in which to take breaks and eat meals. If there is a specific area within the unit, personnel have their own area in which to relax yet are still available in an emergency. Providing an area outside the unit will allow the staff to relax more fully. Bathrooms should be included within this area.
Physicians' sleeping room	Bunk beds usually make the best use of available space. Again, if such facilities are not provided, the tired house officer will usually commandeer the nurses' lounge, an empty patient room, or some other inappropriate space to meet this need.
Head nurse's office	Like any manager, the HN requires an appropriate office to function effectively.
Conference room	The ICU, to function as an environment conducive to learning, must have appropriate facilities. The conference room can double as a report room and a family conference room.
Family waiting room	Seating should be provided for approximately two visitors for each bed on the unit. Nearby bathrooms are desirable. The more restrictive the visiting policy, the more important are the waiting room facilities.
Kitchenette	A small food preparation area is needed. It usually includes an ice machine, 2 burners, and cabinet space.
Medication preparation area	The area should be separated so that staff members are not interrupted while preparing medications. It must also be in a central, convenient location, however. In addition to cabinets and locked drawers, a sink is required.
House officer laboratory	Not a requirement; the need for it should be determined early.

JCAH = Joint Commission on Accreditation of Hospitals.

a separate but contiguous anteroom for gowning should be available. The air pressure within the unit should be positive in relation to the outside corridor [37], and there should be more than ten air changes per hour [11, 37].

Other aspects of unit design to be considered by the planning committee include temperature, humidity, lighting, and noise control, all summarized in Table 2.2. Three levels of illumination are necessary: dim for night, medium for daylight, and intense for examination. Noise control is difficult; the most absorbent surfaces are the most difficult to clean and are often impractical for use in ICUs. The ability to isolate patients from noise is one of the biggest advantages of having private rooms. Hallway carpeting does reduce traffic noise, but it is difficult to maintain and is not recommended.

In planning for storage of equipment and supplies, it is useful to construct lists under three headings: routine, emergency, and special procedure. Routine and emergency supplies must be located either at each bedside or in a very central location. The total number of items necessary will usually determine which place is preferable. Items needed only for specific procedures, such as insertion of pulmonary artery catheters, can be kept in the utility room and brought out when needed. The system of supplying the unit will be determined by the hospital's material management system, but use of the exchange cart method rather than individual item restocking is highly recommended.

PROGRAM-DEPENDENT FACILITIES

Thus far our discussion has focused on program-independent facilities: those, such as size of the unit, number of beds, and outlets at each bedside, that are determined by the patient population and general design principles. The next section will address elements of the critical care unit that are, in contrast, integral parts of the patient care programs: patient instrumentation, data management, and care delivery systems.

Patient Instrumentation

Of the many "instruments" used in patient care (such as IV pumps, hypothermia machines, blood warmers, and so on), certainly the most significant is the cardiac monitor.

The head nurse, physician director, and biomedical engineer should meet several times to establish preliminary guidelines for monitor selection. The choice of monitoring systems today is so large and varied that clearly established needs and goals are a prerequisite for sound decision making. The following questions can help in determining these needs [6]:

1. What is the current or projected situation? Relevant factors include the physical layout of the unit, the number of beds, and the location of the nurses' station. The patients should be described in terms of the usual severity of illness, frequency of complications (e.g., dysrhythmias, shock, respiratory arrest), and degree of mobility. The current level of monitoring should be assessed: how many monitors typically are in use, which variables are most frequently monitored, and how often are more monitors or component parts needed? What is the orientation of

nursing care — bedside or central stations? Who uses the monitors — nurses, physicians, technicians?

2. What are the defined unit needs? These may consist of needs for additional or expanded services, such as an increase in the number of monitors or the availability of pressure modules. The primary need may be for a change in type of system, such as the initiation of computerized monitoring. The major need may be simply to improve the quality of monitoring by decreasing the number of false alarms or the frequency of repairs.

3. What are the bedside hardware needs? Will the monitor be mounted on a shelf or wall, or placed on a cart? Which variables are to be monitored — cardiac rate and rhythm, pressure, respiration, temperature? How many of each variable will be monitored at each bedside? Is a recorder necessary? How many channels are needed? What alarms are needed? Are any beds to be equipped for telemetry?

4. What are the central station hardware needs? Is a central station necessary? Which variables are to be displayed? Are alarms or a recorder needed?

Other considerations in choosing bedside monitors are those applicable to the purchase of any equipment — the reliability of the manufacturer's performance record, the kind of guarantee provided, the extent of in-service education offered. The average cost to be budgeted for simple bedside monitors is $10,000 per bed [2].

Computerized Monitoring Systems

Computerized dysrhythmia detection systems have been available for more than a decade. It has been well established that even under the best conditions, human monitor watchers perform much less effectively than do computers [14]. Vigilance, or the watching of even a single display for abnormal events (dysrhythmias), is characteristically imperfect, and accuracy rates of human monitor watchers average 60%; computers average 95 to 100%. Although the minimal acceptable level of vigilance has yet to be determined, there is no question that, as Clipson and Wehrer have stated, "the task of surveillance of waveforms and other patient parameters on a moment-to-moment basis is more suited to the capabilities of a machine than of a human operator" [11].

Capabilities
Computerized systems use two basic methods of recognizing dysrhythmias. The bedside electrocardiographic (ECG) monitor sends analog signals, representing the changing voltage of the patient's ECG tracings, to an analog-to-digital converter. The converter receives the signal and gives the computer a series of discrete digital numbers, representing amplitudes of complexes. The original signals are sampled points of each complex. Given these numbers, the computer uses algorithms, or programmed instruction sequences, to identify dysrhythmias [2, 36, 38].

The waveform feature extraction algorithm measures several features of the QRS complex, such as width and prematurity, compares it with programmed norms, and makes "decisions" as to what to label the complex. The template-matching system samples points of the QRS complex, establishes a basic pattern or template, and simply compares each succeeding beat to the established norm. If the new beat differs on a certain number of points, it is considered abnormal [2, 27].

Many of the newer systems use combinations of the feature extraction and template logics. All of the currently available systems perform best in QRS analysis; P wave and T wave analysis, for recognition of atrial dysrhythmias and ST segment abnormalities, is still not perfected. Most systems are able to identify pacer spikes correctly. (See Chapter 7 for a discussion of ECG complexes.) In addition to the computer itself, systems may include terminals with alphanumeric keyboards used to input data manually, video display units, recorders, and printers to make hard copies of displays.

Choice of Systems

The computerized monitoring systems available differ so widely, and are changing so quickly, that comparisons and choices are difficult to make. It is essential, if computerized monitoring is to be used, that the services of a clinical or biomedical engineer be available. As with bedside monitors, it is useful to prepare for investment in a computerized system by answering a series of questions or listing options. Some of these questions, however, are less straightforward and require an analysis of elements of the care delivery system.

1. Which major functions is the computer expected to perform? In addition to dysrhythmia recognition, computers have recall, edit, and data manipulation functions. The simplest operation involves recording the recognized dysrhythmia and displaying it on demand. The edit option allows the user to change data, for example, to erase the identified dysrhythmia if it is only artifactual. Data manipulation refers to the capacity of the computer to accumulate data, subject data to logical operations, and display data in programmed formats, such as trends over time or columns of data.

2. In addition to dysrhythmias, which variables will the computer monitor? The computer can monitor — that is, observe and record — and alert the user (alarm) to changes in any variable to which it has direct access through the bedside monitor.

3. Who is going to use the computer, and for what purpose? Is the computer basically a sophisticated alarm system, a data collection and storage instrument, or a patient care tool? What level of personnel has access — nurses, secretaries, technicians, physicians? If house officers are not present in the unit (and sometimes even if they are), the nurses will probably be the major users. If so, computer data are more likely to be used by the nurse to evaluate and document therapy and patient status retrospectively than as an ongoing patient management tool. The ability to map trends in variables and manipulate data will probably not be used to any large extent, nor will the recall and edit functions. Surveys done in 1980 and 1981 by *Health Devices* of 192 hospitals

confirm this likelihood: most hospitals reported that trending and data management capabilities were largely unused [2].

Whoever will be using the computer must have input into the system design and configuration. Lack of input from users is one of the chief reasons for subsequent dissatisfaction with the system [4, 27]; it leads to unrealistic expectations of the equipment and mismatch of the equipment with the care delivery system. All new computer systems require in-house advocates — physicians and nurses who are respected peers of the intended users and who are thoroughly familiar with the system and can make the commitment to assist the users in learning to work with it effectively.

If recall, edit, and management functions are to be included and physicians are to be frequent users of the system, a terminal with video display should be available away from the bedside. If both physicians and nurses will use the terminal and more than ten beds are computerized, two terminals will probably be useful to prevent waits for access.

If the computer will be used either in research or to obtain information to be used in making patient care decisions, greater flexibility is required. Exhibit 2.1 lists guidelines for selection of both components and software.

Recently the use of microprocessors has allowed many computer functions to be brought to the bedside. This gives some independence to each bedside unit and provides the option of also having terminals at the bedside, either as separate alphanumeric keyboards or as selector switches on the monitor itself.

The kind of data that serves as input will determine the best location of terminals. If patient data are to be entered manually by the nurse and the orientation of care is to the bedside (common in ICUs), bedside terminals are the obvious choice. If, however, the orientation is more evenly divided between central station and bedside, (as occurs in coronary care units), it may be more useful to have terminals in the nurses' station.

System Efficiency

A familiar and long-used term in computer technology is *GIGO:* garbage in, garbage out. In other words, the quality of computer output is only as good as the input. The expression also reflects the fact that the usefulness of the output will be a direct reflection of the usefulness of the input system. If the system requires duplication of effort in inputting data, if the format of data is not logical and organized, and if the data do not serve a specific purpose, the result will be "garbage."

These points have several ramifications. One is that computerized systems virtually always require more nursing time if they are used properly [27]. They do not replace human functions, they simply perform certain functions more efficiently, more regularly, and more easily. The time they save in doing these automated operations is taken up in required user interactions. If nurses must duplicate computer functions, the increased demands on their time will cause the system to fail.

Second, the format of the data input and output must be consistent with the overall data management system. For example, if the unit uses problem-

EXHIBIT 2.1
Guidelines for Computer Selection

1. Define the long-term goals of the unit
    Change in the number of beds
    Change in the type of patients seen
    Changes in variables being monitored
    Changes in medical procedures
    Changes in nursing procedures
    Changes in patient record documentation

2. Define software needs
    Define which analog waveforms are to be sampled from bedside
    Define which variables are to be sampled automatically
    Define which variables are to be entered manually
    Define all sampling rates
    Define what information is to be stored and the duration of storage
    Define data retrieval
        How is each datum displayed?
        Are analog signals to be reconstructed?
        Are data to be arrayed by computer and displayed in tabular form (which data)?
        Are data to be trended against time (which data)?
        Are data to be trended against other data (which data)?
        Are data to be edited?
        Are data to be manipulated (curve generation, integration, derivation, correlation)?
    Define the level of flexibility required
    Define the level of adaptability required
    Define the level of support required of the computer manufacturer
    Define the level of support required of the system vendor/manufacturer
        Does the manufacturer continuously update algorithms?
        Does updated software become available routinely? automatically? upon request? at what cost?
    Define in-house capabilities
        Is programming to be done?
        What languages are available?
        Does vendor allow or encourage access to its software and hardware?
        Can system software modification be tolerated while patients are being monitored?

3. Decide if computer terminal is needed at bedside
    Define capabilities required of terminal
    Decide who will use terminal
    Determine how often it will be used
    Determine if hard copy generation is required

4. Define central station requirements
    Determine desirability of having a central station
    Determine who will use central station

EXHIBIT 2.1 *(continued)*

Determine need for display of bedside waveforms

Determine if access to all bedsides is required

Define terminal-to-computer link

Define those conditions for which alarms are needed

Define need for hard copy generation

Determine if user-generated routines can be added to the system software

Determine what in-house routines will be generated

Determine what hardware support is required for in-house programming

Determine to whom programmer will report and where programmer will work

5. Documentation

    System hardware

        All documentation required to maintain at system level (block diagrams, wiring diagrams)

        All documentation required to maintain at board level (block diagrams, wiring diagrams, technical manuals)

        All documentation required to maintain at component level (block, wiring, and schematic diagrams, technical manuals, parts list, board layout)

    System software

        Documentation sufficient to locate problems

        Documentation sufficient to access software

        Listing of vendor software

        Listing of computer manufacturer's software

    Patient data

        What data are required for legal records?

        What nursing notes are to be generated?

        What variable and trend strips are to be generated?

        Is system required to generate hospital-formatted documentation?

        Can system standard generation forms be assimilated to hospital medical records?

        What security levels are required?

        Who can access what data?

        How is loss of data to be prevented?

        Can records be generated upon request?

        Can records be generated at standard times without request?

        Where will generated hard copy be kept, and for how long?

After refs. 2 and 6.

oriented charting and the computer is to generate nurses' notes, the program must allow the nurse to enter information according to problem heading, to recall and display recent entries related to that problem, and to print the entries in a form acceptable to the hospital's records authorities.

Third, the computer should be intended to serve a predetermined purpose. A common error is to purchase impressively sophisticated equipment and then try to find a use for it. Decisions related to the purchase of the system and the components should be the last decisions made.

Computers and Data Management

Data management is often considered to be only a function of computerized systems. All critical care units perform data management functions, however, regardless of whether computers are used. The collection and recording of information in organized categories in the individual patient record is a basic, and the most common, form of data management. Data management needs should be determined prior to obtaining instrumentation.

Nurses in the ICU routinely collect quantitative data, such as heart rate and mean arterial pressure. Such data are better suited for computerization than are qualitative data obtained at irregular intervals, such as descriptions of breath sounds. As mentioned earlier, there are two important considerations in employing computers for this type of data management. First, the system should use directly monitored (on-line) data, such as mean arterial pressure, rather than data that must be entered manually or typed onto a keyboard by the nurse. Second, data should be organized into logical categories, such as organ system, problem, and nursing diagnosis.

The second and newer application of computers is in the management of what has been termed "macro-level data," or data related to groups of patients rather than individuals [21]. Such nursing information systems have many potential uses. At the very least, they can be used to store unit statistics, such as average number of admissions, average length of stay, most common time of admission, and acuity level. This information can then be used by the head nurse to assess staffing needs, describe changes in unit operation, justify budgets, and predict trends. The future uses of such systems might include calculation of nursing costs for direct reimbursement of nursing services, comparison with other units for the purpose of evaluating nursing modalities of care, and the development of data bases for research protocol development. Such uses are perhaps the very best for computers: they enable users to work with data that are too cumbersome or complicated to be managed manually.

Care Delivery Systems

As with the other areas we have discussed, our emphasis when we consider care delivery systems will be on the careful, thorough analysis of the *system* and conscious planning based on that analysis.

Many systems are in use in critical care units today. Most are variations of either the traditional team nursing (even if only one "team" is used) or primary nursing models. The nurse manager, in consultation with his or her staff, must consider many variables in choosing the system that best facilitates care delivery. Our discussion here will focus on those factors especially relevant to cardiac critical care units.

Team Nursing

Traditional team nursing generally involves the designation of a shift "leader" (charge nurse, coordinator, or the like). This person makes decisions about the allocation of personnel resources (e.g., makes patient assignments); performs system maintenance functions (e.g., reviews physicians' orders, assigns coverage for lunch breaks); coordinates communication with other areas, such as the emergency room, admitting department, or operating room; supervises the care delivered by others; and assists in the transition from one shift to another by receiving and transmitting reports, checking charts, planning for staffing, and the like. In the ICU this system is often described as "total care": on each shift a nurse is assigned to perform all nursing responsibilities for his or her patients *during that shift* [10]. The major advantage of this system is its efficiency.

Many of these team leader functions can, and should, be performed by individual professional nurses. Nurses can report on their own patients to the next nurse, check their own orders, and arrange coverage with another nurse for lunches and breaks. The belief that all registered nurses require another registered nurse for supervision and accountability is the antithesis of professional critical care nursing.

But these points are not an argument against team nursing. Rather, they must be examined in light of specific unit characteristics. For example, if the unit has a very high level of acuity, with many patients requiring one-to-one nursing care, it is likely that the individual nurses will not be able routinely to check physicians' orders or perform any function away from the bedside. The situation will be especially problematic if the unit does not have a division manager or adequate clerical services.

If the unit has a high rate of patient turnover, with frequent admissions and discharges, someone must coordinate this activity. This person must have not only the information necessary to make efficient and appropriate assignment decisions, but also the authority to do so.

The question of professional nurses requiring supervision is related not to the principle of accountability, but to the pragmatics of proficiency. Although all new graduate nurses require supervision, this period of orientation and dependence on other nurses is prolonged in the ICU because of the technological complexity and level of patient illness. In a 1972 survey conducted of 1,111 hospital nursing directors, 34.5% of respondents believed that new graduates required three to six months of preparation in order to function independently [32]. This need for a prolonged period of supervision has escalated since the time of the survey.

These considerations at the least necessitate having some person on each shift who coordinates and supervises.

Primary Nursing

Primary nursing has been described as both a philosophy and a modality of care delivery [30]. It has been defined as the "assigned, fixed, visible accountability for twenty-four-hour care by one RN for a group of patients throughout their hospital stay" [10]. The major characteristics of primary nursing that differentiate it from team nursing are the direct accountability to the patient, the responsibility over the duration of the patient's stay, and the relationship between the primary nurse and other nurses delivering care to that patient. The major advantages of the system are the comprehensive, individualized quality of care it promotes and the quality of the professional nursing experience it provides to the practitioner.

Primary nursing is not impossible in ICUs, as some believe, but it does require certain modifications. First, the system should be conceived of as providing accountability by one nurse for only one or two patients throughout their time in the ICU. Second, it should be acknowledged that not all ICU patients will benefit from primary care, simply because of their short stay in the unit. For example, the patient who is suspected to have a myocardial infarction but stays only 8 to 12 hours in the ICU before the infarction is ruled out probably will not benefit from entering into the ICU primary care system.

Primary nursing does have a very significant advantage for nurses and patients. By providing for a continuous, rather than a brief, crisis-oriented relationship, it allows the nurse to see and experience the rewards of patient recovery. The potential is lessened for staff members to suffer the "burn-out" caused by caring only for patients in the most acute phase of their illness. Nowhere is the potential for dehumanizing, episodic, crisis-oriented care greater than in critical care areas. By implementing a system in which at least some of the patients with longer stays receive primary nursing, the nurse manager will almost certainly reduce these effects of high technology.

SUMMARY

It is the responsibility of the HN to examine and analyze the interaction of all elements of the critical care system. It has been observed that "too little attention is paid to the fact that a poorly designed and carelessly run ICU can segregate and concentrate the liabilities of the institution, such as congestion, noise, medication errors, electrical hazards, infection exposure, and psychological trauma" [23]. The critical care environment is all too often seen as providing physical overstimulation and emotional understimulation [17], and ICU nurses are all too often viewed as struggling to find their identity.

Careful, detailed, and repeated analysis of the elements of the system and the organizational structure of the unit is the key to addressing these concerns. The major responsibility of the manager is to question. Is the unit structured to allow for efficient delivery of care? Does the structure provide for maximum patient privacy? Is it safe, electronically and biologically? Is the monitoring system adequate? Do needs frequently exceed resources? Is the computer used to its maximum? Are there avenues for input into equipment planning? What are the characteristics of the current delivery system? How is continuity assured? Who is responsible? What aspects of the care delivery system foster episodic care? What measures are used to assess quality? And, most important, what is our future direction?

References

1. Adler, D. C., and Shoemaker, N. J. (eds.). *AACN Organization and Management of Critical Care Facilities.* St. Louis: Mosby, 1979.

2. Arrhythmia monitoring systems: a prima. *Health Dev.* June/July:211, 1982.

3. Badura, F. K. Nurse acceptance of a computerized arrhythmia monitoring system. *Heart Lung* 9:1044, 1980.

4. Beckmann, E., Commack, D. F., and Harris, B. Observations on computers in an intensive care unit. *Heart Lung* 10:1055, 1981.

5. Bendixen, H. H. How to start an intensive care unit. In Kinney, J. M., Bendixen, H. H., and Powers, S. R. (eds.), *Manual of Surgical Intensive Care*. Philadelphia: Saunders, 1977.

6. Braun, R. Personal communication. Department of Clinical Engineering, University Hospitals of Cleveland, Cleveland, Ohio, 1982.

7. Breu, C. S., and Gawlinski, A. A comparative study of the effects of documentation on arrhythmia detection efficiency. *Heart Lung* 10:1058, 1981.

8. Brimm, J. E., and Peters, R. M. Data handling systems. In Kinney, J. M., Bendixen, H. H., and Powers, S. R. (eds.), *Manual of Surgical Intensive Care*. Philadelphia: Saunders, 1977.

9. Brown, A. J. Effects of family visits on the blood pressure and heart rate of patients in the coronary care unit. *Heart Lung* 5:291, 1976.

10. Ciske, K. L. Accountability: the essence of primary nursing. *Am. J. Nurs.* 79:89, 1979.

11. Clipson, C. W., and Wehrer, J. J. *Planning for Cardiac Care: A Guide to the Planning and Design of Cardiac Care Facilities*. Kansas City: Health Administration Press, 1973.

12. *Coronary Care Units*. U.S. Department of Health, Education, and Welfare. Public Health Service, Heart Disease Control Program. P.H.S. Pub. No. 1250, Washington, D.C., 1964.

13. Cross, L. Expanding critical care beds through a surgical observation subunit. *Dimens. Crit. Care Nurs.* 1:174, 1982.

14. Daly, B. J., and Wilson, C. A. The effect of fatigue on the vigilance of nurses monitoring electrocardiograms. *Heart Lung* 12:384, 1983.

15. Dear, M. R., et al. The effect of the intensive care nursing role on job satisfaction and turnover. *Heart Lung* 11:560, 1982.

16. Disch, J. Survey of critical care nursing practice. I. Characteristics of hospitals with critical care units. *Heart Lung* 10:1047, 1981.

17. Gowan, N. J. The perceptual world of the intensive care unit: an overview of some environmental considerations in the helping relationship. *Heart Lung* 8:340, 1979.

18. Happ, B. Should computers be used in the nursing care of patients? *Nurs. Management* 14(7):31, 1983.

19. Harris, R. B. A strong vote for nursing process. *Am. J. Nurs.* 79:1999, 1979.

20. Holloway, N. M. *Nursing the Critically Ill Patient*. Menlo Park, Ca.: Addison-Wesley, 1979.

21. Kiley, M., et al. Computerized nursing information systems (NIMS). *Nurs. Management* 14(7):26, 1983.

22. Kinney, J. M. Design of the intensive care unit. In Berk, J. L., and Sampliner, J. E. (eds.), *Handbook of Critical Care* (2nd ed.). Boston: Little, Brown, 1982.

23. Kinney, J. M., and Walter, C. W. The design of an intensive care unit. In Kinney, J. M., Bendixen, H. H., and Powers, S. R. (eds.), *Manual of Surgical Intensive Care*. Philadelphia: Saunders, 1977.

24. Kinney, M. Survey of critical care nursing practice. II. Unit characteristics. *Heart Lung* 10:1051, 1981.

25. Kirchoff, K. T. Visiting policies for patients with myocardial infarction: a national survey. *Heart Lung* 11:571, 1982.

26. Lindamood, M. O. Getting your input into unit design. *Dimens. Crit. Care Nurs.* 1:36, 1982.

27. Lipschultz, A. Computerized arrhythmia monitoring systems: a review. *J. Clin. Engin.* 7:229, 1982.

28. MacDonald, M. R., et al. ICU nurses rate their work places. *Hospitals* 55:115, 1981.

29. Maher, A. B. A systems approach to nursing the patient with multiple systems failure. *Heart Lung* 10:866, 1981.

30. McAdam, E. Primary nursing demands change. *Nurs. Management* 13(5):50, 1982.

31. Merkel, S. I. Problem-oriented recording in the intensive care unit. *Dimens. Crit. Care Nurs.* 1:232, 1982.

32. Nader, A. F. (ed.). *ICU '72*. Oradell, N.J.: Medical Economics, 1972.

33. National Institution of Health Consensus Development Conference Summary. *Critical Care Medicine*. Vol. 4, No. 6. U.S. Government Printing Office 1983-381-132:3129.

34. Rhoades, C., Adcock, M., and Jovanovich, J. F. Prevention of nosocomial infection in critical care units. *Nurs. Clin. North Am.* 15:803, 1981.

35. Ryan, D. W., et al. Replanning of an intensive therapy unit. *Br. Med. J.* 285:1634, 1982.

36. Sanders, W. J. A consumer's guide to computerized arrhythmia monitors. *JAMA* 248:1745, 1982.

37. Skillman, J. J. *Intensive Care.* Boston: Little, Brown, 1975.

38. Sorkin, J., and Bloomfield, D. A. Computers for critical care. *Heart Lung* 11:287, 1982.

39. Stanley, P. E. Instrument safety. In Zschoche, D. A. (ed.), *Mosby's Comprehensive Review of Critical Care.* St. Louis: Mosby, 1976.

40. Sturdavant, M. *Comparison of Intensive Nursing Service in a Circular and a Rectangular Unit.* Hospital Monograph Series No. 8. Chicago: American Hospital Association, 1960.

41. Uhley, H. Monitoring technicians: the critical interface. *Heart Lung* 9:1009, 1980.

42. Williams, S. V. How many intensive care beds are enough? *Crit. Care Med.* 11:412, 1983.

PART II

Assessment of the Cardiac Patient

CHAPTER 3

Cardiac Anatomy and Physiology

Susan Lynn Zorb

INTRODUCTION

In a normal lifetime an individual's heart beats more than 3 trillion times. From shortly after conception until death, the heart beats in a continuous rhythm, sustaining life. The significance of a disease of the heart goes far beyond the impairment to the organ; it strikes at the very essence of the person's identity. The critical care nurse must be aware of this mystique while caring for the cardiac patient. In addition, the nurse must have a thorough knowledge of the anatomy and physiology of the heart to provide optimal care, help the patient understand what has happened, and assist the patient and family to return to their optimal lifestyle.

ANATOMY

Position of the Heart

The heart, a muscular pump, is located in the mediastinum. Anteriorly it is covered and protected by the sternum and ribs. Two-thirds of the heart lies to the left of the sternum. It is flanked by the lungs laterally and rests on the diaphragm. Tilted slightly forward, the apex is located at the fourth or fifth intercostal space at the midclavicular line (Figure 3.1). In the average adult the heart is approximately 12 cm long and 9 cm wide and weighs 300 to 400 gm. The heart is rotated in the chest; the right ventricle, part of the left ventricle, and the right atrium make up the anterior surface. The inferior (diaphragmatic) surface is composed primarily of the left ventricle and a portion of the right ventricle. The right cardiac border is formed by the superior vena cava and the right atrium, and the left cardiac border by the lateral wall of the left ventricle and the left atrial appendage. The base of the heart, formed by the left atrium

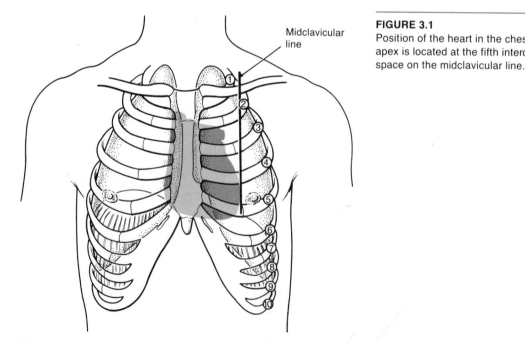

Midclavicular line

FIGURE 3.1
Position of the heart in the chest. The apex is located at the fifth intercostal space on the midclavicular line.

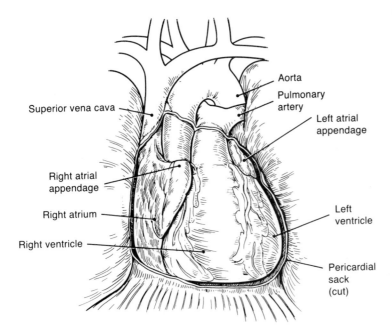

Superior vena cava

Aorta

Pulmonary
artery

Left atrial
appendage

Right atrial
appendage

Right atrium

Left
ventricle

Right ventricle

Pericardial
sack
(cut)

FIGURE 3.2
Cardiac borders. The right ventricle, part of the left ventricle, and the right atrium make up the anterior surface. The right border is formed by the superior vena cava and the right atrium, and the left border by the left ventricle and left atrial appendage.

and a small part of the right atrium, is located at the level of the second rib (Figure 3.2).

The heart is completely enclosed by a fibrous sac, the pericardium, which consists of two layers. The visceral layer, or epicardium, encases the surface of the heart and extends a few centimeters onto the great vessels. It then folds back on itself to form the parietal layer, which is attached to the manubrium, xyphoid process, vertebral column, and diaphragm. These two layers, forming the pericardial sac, have a smooth, serous lining and contain approximately 10 to 30 ml of fluid, which facilitates movement of the heart within the sac. The pericardium also acts as a barrier for infection from the lungs and mediastinum.

Cardiac Chambers

The heart is composed of four chambers (Figure 3.3). The right and left atria are smooth, thin-walled chambers that receive blood from various parts of the body. The right atrium receives unoxygenated blood from the superior and inferior vena cavae, and from the heart via the coronary sinus. The pressure in the right atrium is 2 to 6 mm Hg, with an oxygen (O_2) saturation level of 75%.

The left atrium receives oxygenated blood from the lungs via the pulmonary veins. Normal left atrial pressure is 4 to 12 mm Hg, with an O_2 saturation level of 95 to 98%. The left atrium is directed toward the posterior portion of the chest and is in contact with the esophagus, which may be displaced in left atrial enlargement. The intra-atrial septum divides the right and left atria. In the fetus an opening in the septum called the foramen ovale allows blood to pass from the right side to the left side of the heart, bypassing the lungs. This opening normally closes shortly after birth. If it does not, the person is said to have a patent foramen ovale. Such a patency is one cause of an atrial septal defect (ASD), an opening in the atrial wall. Because left atrial

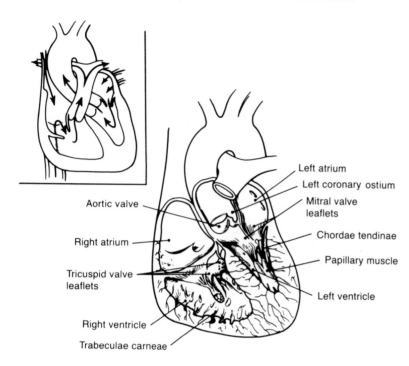

FIGURE 3.3
The internal cardiac structures.

Aortic valve

Right atrium

Tricuspid valve
leaflets

Right ventricle

Trabeculae carneae

Left atrium

Left coronary ostium

Mitral valve
leaflets

Chordae tendinae

Papillary muscle

Left ventricle

pressure is higher than right atrial pressure, a person with an ASD will have shunting of blood from the left atrium to the right. Consequently, oxygenated blood will be recirculated to the lungs rather than into the systemic circulation.

The right and left ventricles are thicker-walled chambers whose primary purpose is to pump blood. The right ventricle receives blood from the right atrium through the tricuspid valve. The right ventricle, the most anterior of all the chambers, is crescent shaped and contracts with a bellows-like action. It is divided into the inflow tract near the tricuspid valve and the infundibulum, or outflow tract, near the pulmonic valve (see Figure 3.3). The anterior and inferior walls are lined with muscle bands called trabeculae carneae, which give a ridge-and-valley appearance to the surface. The most prominent muscle, the moderator band, crosses from the lower interventricular septum to the anterior wall and is the origin of the anterior papillary muscle. The walls of the right ventricle are generally 0.5 cm thick and the pressure is 15 to 30 mm Hg systolic and 0 to 5 mm Hg diastolic, with an O_2 saturation level of 75%.

The left ventricle has the largest muscle mass of any of the cardiac chambers, with a wall thickness of 1.5 cm. It is cone shaped and contracts from the apex toward the base in a squeezing motion. This action is necessary to overcome the high pressure in the aorta. Normal left ventricular pressure is 120 mm Hg systolic and 0 to 10 mm Hg diastolic, with an O_2 saturation level of 95 to 98%. The interventricular septum is functionally a part of the left ventricle. The upper one-third has a smooth wall and contains the small, membranous septum. The lower two-thirds and the rest of the left ventricle, called the free wall, are ridged with trabeculae carneae, from which the papillary muscles originate. The inflow tract is funnel shaped and formed by the mitral valve; the outflow tract is formed by the septal wall, left ventricular free wall, and anterior mitral valve leaflet (see Figure 3.3).

Layers of the Heart

The walls of the heart comprise three layers, each of which serves a different function (Figure 3.4). The innermost layer, the endocardium, is composed of endothelial cells, connective tissue, and elastic fibers that line the chambers of the heart and are continuous with the intima of the blood vessels. This layer provides a smooth surface for blood flow, thereby discouraging clot formation. The myocardium, or muscle tissue, is the middle layer. Its thickness varies in each chamber, with the left ventricle containing the largest myocardial mass. The myocardial fibers perform the actual pumping action of the heart. The epicardium is the outermost layer of the heart as well as the visceral layer of the pericardium. The coronary arteries are embedded in the epicardial layer.

Cardiac Valves

The four valves in the heart act to retain the bood in one chamber until the next chamber or vessel is ready to receive it. Each valve responds to changes in pressure, opening when the pressure in the chamber behind it is greater than the pressure ahead of it and closing in the reverse situation. The valves are divided into two types: the atrioventricular valves, which divide the right and left atria from the right and left ventricles, and the semilunar valves, which divide the right and left ventricles from the pulmonary artery and aorta, respectively. Each type of valve will be discussed separately.

Atrioventricular Valves

The atrioventricular (AV) valves, which separate the atria from the ventricles, have four components: (1) the annulus, the fibrous supporting ring into which the valve inserts; (2) the valve leaflets, or cusps, which are sheets of connective tissue covered by endothelial tissue; (3) the chordae tendineae, which are fibrous cords that attach to the free edges of the leaflets; and (4) the papillary

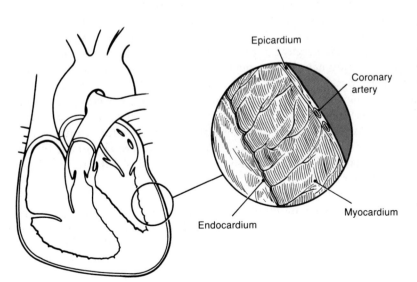

Epicardium

Coronary artery

Endocardium

Myocardium

FIGURE 3.4
The layers of the heart. A coronary artery lies embedded in the epicardial layer. The myocardium is the thick muscular layer. The thin endocardium lines the inner aspect of the chambers.

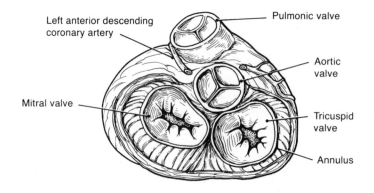

Left anterior descending coronary artery

Pulmonic valve

Aortic valve

Mitral valve

Tricuspid valve

Annulus

FIGURE 3.5
Cardiac valves (superior view). The atrioventricular valves (mitral and tricuspid) separate the atria from the ventricles. The semilunar valves (aortic and pulmonic) separate the ventricles from the aorta and pulmonary arteries, respectively.

muscles, which extend from the ventricular wall to the chordae tendineae (see Figure 3.3). Contraction of the papillary muscles exerts tension on the chordae and prevents the leaflets from bulging backward into the atria during systole. The tricuspid valve on the right side of the heart has three cusps: anterior, posterior, and septal. The mitral valve on the left has two: anterior and posterior. The name *mitral* is derived from the valve's resemblance to a bishop's miter. The junctions of the valve leaflets and the annulus are called the commissures. The anterior leaflet forms part of the left ventricular outflow tract and may be affected by disease of the aortic valve.

Semilunar Valves
The semilunar (SL) valves divide the ventricles from the corresponding arteries. They are composed of the annulus and three cusps, or leaflets (Figure 3.5). The pulmonary valve divides the right ventricular outflow tract from the pulmonary artery. It has three cusps, which are attached to the annulus at the commissures. These cusps are thicker than those of the AV valves and do not require supporting structures. They open during systole and close during diastole. The aortic valve, separating the left ventricular outflow tract from the aorta, is designed and functions in the same manner. The openings, or ostia, for the coronary arteries appear in the aorta just beyond the aortic valve. The cusps of the valve are named according to their anatomical association with the coronary arteries. The left coronary artery arises just above the left coronary cusp, and the right coronary artery just above the right coronary cusp. The third cusp is called the noncoronary cusp, because there is no coronary artery associated with it. The sinuses of Valsalva are small outpouchings of the aorta located just above the valve cusps; they allow for pooling of the blood around the coronary ostia and thus enhance the flow of blood into the coronary arteries during diastole.

Coronary Circulation

Coronary circulation is highly individualized, with each system having a different configuration of major branches and collateral circulation. Table 3.1 lists the major cardiac structures and the arteries that usually supply each structure. Collateral vessels are small vessels that connect branches of the coronary arteries. They are normally present in the coronary circulation, espe-

TABLE 3.1
Area Supplied by Common Arteries

Structure	Usual Arterial Supply	Common Variants
Right atrium	Sinus node artery; branch of RCA (55%)	Sinus node artery; branch of L circumflex (45%)
Left atrium	Major L circumflex	Sinus node artery; branch of L circumflex (45%)
Right ventricle		
Anterior	Major RCA Minor LAD	
Posterior	Major RCA; posterior descending branch of RCA	Posterior descending may branch from L circumflex (10%)
	Minor LAD (ascending portion)	LAD terminates at apex (40%)
Left ventricle		
Posterior (diaphragmatic)	Major L circumflex; posterior descending branch of RCA	Posterior descending may branch from L circumflex (10%)
	Minor LAD (ascending portion)	LAD terminates at apex (40%)
Anterior	LCA; L circumflex and LAD	
Apex	Major LAD	
Intraventricular septum	Major septal branches of LAD; minor posterior descending branch of RCA and AV nodal branch of RCA	Minor posterior descending may branch from L circumflex; AV nodal may branch from L circumflex
LV papillary muscles		
Anterior	Diagonal branch of LAD; other branches of LAD; other branches of L circumflex	Diagonal may branch from circumflex
Posterior	RCA and L circumflex	RCA and LAD
Sinus node	Nodal artery from RCA (55%)	Nodal artery from L circumflex (45%)
AV node	RCA (90%)	L circumflex (10%)
Bundle of His	RCA (90%)	L circumflex (10%)
Right bundle	Major LAD septal branches; minor AV nodal artery	
Left anterior bundle	Major LAD septal branches; minor AV nodal artery	
Left posterior bundle	LAD septal branches; AV nodal artery	

RCA = right coronary artery; L = left; LAD = left anterior descending coronary artery; LCA = left coronary artery; AV = atrioventricular.

From Underhill, S. L., et al. *Cardiac Nursing*. Philadelphia: Lippincott, 1982. Used with permission.

cially in the endocardial surface. They seem to increase in size and number when there is chronic ischemia of the myocardium.

The coronary arteries perform a function vital to life, supplying the blood to the entire myocardium and the conduction tissue. Interruption of blood flow may result in mechanical or electrical disturbances. As previously mentioned, the two major coronary arteries, left and right, arise from the aorta just beyond the aortic valve. These arteries travel over the epicardial surface of the heart, giving off many branches that penetrate into the myocardium (Figure 3.6). The endocardium is the layer most distant from the surface arteries; therefore, its blood supply is the most easily jeopardized. Two-thirds of coronary filling occurs during diastole, when the aortic valve is closed and the sinuses of Valsalva are filled with blood. The myocardial fibers are relaxed at this time, which also promotes flow through the coronary vessels.

Left Coronary Artery

The ostium of the left main coronary artery is located above the left coronary cusp of the aortic valve. The vessel then proceeds between the pulmonary artery and the left atrial appendage, where it divides into two major branches. The left anterior descending (LAD) is the larger division and proceeds down the anterior interventricular sulcus, giving off branches that supply the anterior portion of the interventricular septum and the anterior left and right ventricles (see Figure 3.6). The LAD frequently gives rise to one or more diagonal branches that supply the anterior left ventricular free wall and anterior papil-

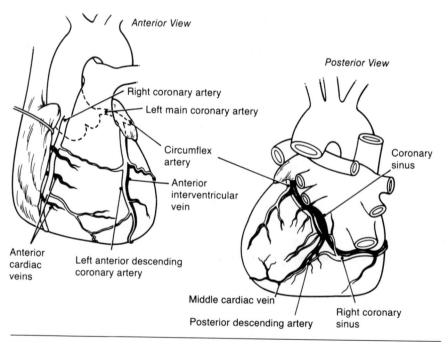

FIGURE 3.6
Coronary circulation: arteries and veins.

lary muscle. In most individuals this vessel curves around the apex to the posterior interventricular sulcus and meets the posterior descending artery (PDA).

The second major branch of the left coronary artery is the circumflex artery, which travels through the left atrioventricular sulcus, giving off branches to the left atrium and the lateral wall of the left ventricle. In 10% of the population, the circumflex artery reaches the crux of the heart, which is the posteriorly located point at which the septa and floor of the atria cross, and forms the PDA, which supplies the posterior wall and septum. Such individuals are said to have a left-dominant system; in this situation the left coronary artery supplies the left ventricle, the AV node, and the septum.

Right Coronary Artery

The right coronary artery (RCA) originates just beyond the right coronary cusp of the aortic valve and travels in the right coronary sulcus, giving off branches to the right atrium and ventricle. In 90% of the population, it crosses the crux and forms the PDA, which supplies the atrioventricular node and bundle of His. Such persons are said to have a right-dominant system. In 55% of the population, a branch of the RCA supplies the sinus node. Branches of the RCA also supply the posterior wall of the left ventricle.

Coronary Capillaries

The coronary arteries branch into arterioles, which further subdivide into capillaries. There is approximately one capillary for each muscle fiber in the normal heart. In the hypertrophied heart, the muscle mass increases but the capillary network appears to remain the same. Each capillary must therefore perfuse a greater mass of myocardial tissue, which reduces the efficiency of oxygen and nutrient exchange.

Coronary Veins

The venous system returns the blood from the myocardium to the right and left atria. It generally parallels the arterial system, with the great cardiac vein following the LAD and the small cardiac vein following the RCA. These veins meet to form the coronary sinus, which traverses the coronary sulcus and empties into the right atrium between the tricuspid valve and the inferior vena cava. The thebesian veins are located in the chamber walls and empty directly into the right and left atria.

The Conduction System

Automaticity, or the ability to generate an impulse spontaneously, is an inherent characteristic of cardiac tissue. Throughout the heart there is specialized conduction tissue whose function is to generate and propagate impulses (Figure 3.7). Conduction tissue comprises three types of cells: p cells, transitional cells, and Purkinje cells. P cells actually initiate the impulse. Transitional cells surround the p cells and slowly conduct the impulse to the Purkinje cells, whose function is to conduct the impulse rapidly to the working myocardial cells. The electrical impulse then stimulates the mechanical events of the heart, or contraction.

The normal site of impulse formation is the sinoatrial (SA) node, located at the junction of the superior vena cava and the right atrium. The SA node is

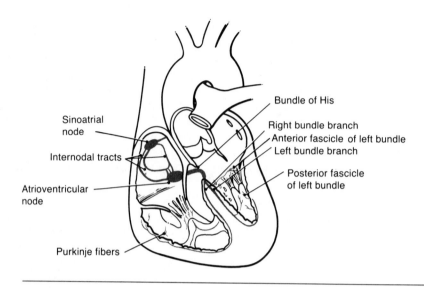

FIGURE 3.7

The conduction system. Specialized bands of tissue that traverse the heart are responsible for initiating an impulse and transmitting it to all cells.

composed of p cells ringed by transitional cells. The impulse travels throughout the atria to the AV node via the internodal tracts, or bundles, composed primarily of Purkinje cells. The AV node is located in the floor of the right atrium near the septal leaflet of the tricuspid valve and the coronary sinus. It is composed of transitional cells and transmits the impulse, after a short delay, into the ventricle via the bundle of His. The area where the AV node and bundle of His meet is called the junctional area; it contains a few p cells that can initiate an impulse.

The bundle of His is made up of Purkinje cells located at the junction of the atrial and ventricular septa below the noncoronary cusp of the aortic valve. It passes from the lower right atrial wall through the membranous septum. Because of its location it is very vulnerable to disease of the aortic valve and to damage during surgical repair of ventricular septal defects. The common bundle divides into two branches just as it enters the ventricular septum. The right bundle branch travels down the right side of the interventricular septum across the moderator muscle band to the anterior papillary muscle. The left bundle branch bifurcates immediately into the anterior fascicle and the posterior fascicle. The slender anterior fascicle travels over the left ventricular surface, crossing the outflow tract to the anterior papillary muscle and the base of the left ventricle. The thick posterior fascicle travels across the inflow tract to the posterior papillary muscle and then onto the posterior wall of the left ventricle. Its size and position make it the least vulnerable to disease of any of the bundle branches.

The heart receives both sympathetic and parasympathetic innervation. The cardiac plexus, which surrounds the aortic root and arch, is made up of both sympathetic and parasympathetic fibers. From here the fibers enter the heart, supplying the SA and AV nodes as well as the atrial and ventricular tissue. The sympathetic fibers are well distributed throughout the entire heart. Sympathetic stimulation results in an increased heart rate, increased conduction speed through the AV node, and more forceful contraction. The parasympathetic fibers, which are part of the vagus nerve, are found primarily in the SA and AV nodes and the atrial tissue. Parasympathetic stimulation decreases the heart rate, slows conduction through the AV node, and decreases the strength of contraction.

PHYSIOLOGY

Cellular Composition of the Heart

The myocardium is composed of long, narrow, branching cells that function as a coordinated unit, or syncytium. The cells are lined by the sarcolemma, a phospholipid and protein membrane that encloses the cellular contents, and are separated from one another by intercalated discs (Figure 3.8). The sarcolemma invaginates into the cell to form the transverse or T tubules. The extracellular fluid fills these channels deep within the cell. Inside the myocardial cell are bands of contractile proteins called myofibrils, which are divided into units called sarcomeres. The cardiac fibers contain numerous mitochondria, the sites of metabolism, to meet the high energy requirements engendered by continual contraction and relaxation. The sarcoplasmic reticulum is an internal channel system that works with the T tubules in the excitation–coupling response. Each myocardial cell has one nucleus containing all the genetic material of the cell.

The sarcomere is the basic functional unit of contraction and gives the myocardial cell its striped, or striated, appearance (see Figure 3.8). The sar-

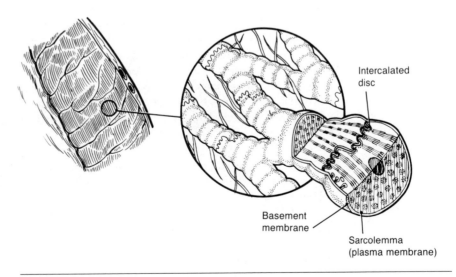

Intercalated disc

Basement membrane

Sarcolemma (plasma membrane)

FIGURE 3.8
The cardiac cell. The branching myocardial cells function as a unit, or syncytium. They are separated by intercalated discs and enclosed by the sarcolemma, a phospholipid and protein membrane.

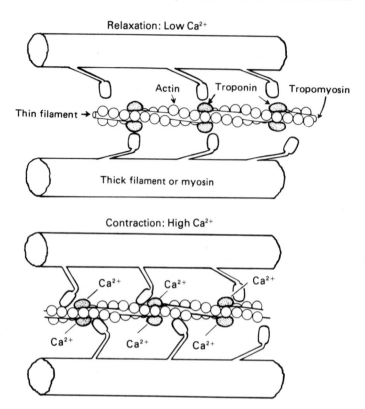

Relaxation: Low Ca²⁺

Thin filament →

Actin   Troponin   Tropomyosin

Thick filament or myosin

Contraction: High Ca²⁺

FIGURE 3.9
Molecular interactions during relaxation and contraction. When intracellular calcium (Ca^{++}) levels rise, troponin combines with Ca^{++} and the tropomyosin–troponin system is altered to allow cross-bridge formation and contraction. (From Underhill, S. L., et al., *Cardiac Nursing*. Philadelphia: Lippincott, 1982. Used with permission.)

comere is bound on both ends by z bands. Attached to these bands are the thin filaments, which are composed of actin, a protein arranged in a double-stranded, intercoiled chain. The protein myosin makes up the thick filament. It is rod shaped, with globular projections, or heads, spiraling off at regular intervals. These heads can join to actin, creating electrochemical cross-bridges between the thick and thin filaments. Myocardial fiber shortening in an isotonic contraction is the result of myosin's binding with actin, flexing, and binding again, which pulls the actin along the myosin filament. In an isometric contraction, tension is created by pulling at the cross-bridge sites without any change in fiber length.

The proteins troponin and tropomyosin are found on the actin filament at periodic intervals (Figure 3.9). Tropomyosin and troponin inhibit cross-bridge formation, which is mediated by calcium (Ca^{++}). In response to a stimulus, Ca^{++} enters the cell via the sarcolemma and T tubules, triggering a release of intracellular Ca^{++} from the sarcoplasmic reticulum. The Ca^{++} binds with troponin, which changes the troponin–tropomyosin complex to allow for cross-bridging between actin and myosin. Contraction results. This is the sequence of the excitation–coupling response. At the completion of contraction, Ca^{++} is actively pumped into the sarcoplasmic reticulum and across the cell membrane out of the cell.

Mechanical Events of the Cardiac Cycle

The primary function of the heart is to pump blood throughout the pulmonary and systemic circulation. This is accomplished by a continually repeating pattern of contraction (systole) and relaxation (diastole) referred to as the cardiac cycle. It is common to discuss the cardiac cycle from the perspective of the left ventricle (LV), bearing in mind that the same process is repeated on the right.

Systole

Ventricular systole begins with the closing of the mitral valve (Figure 3.10) when the ventricle is full of blood. At this time the aortic valve is also closed. The muscle fibers, in response to an electrical stimulus, begin to develop tension and to shorten. Consequently, the pressure in the LV begins to rise. This period is called isovolumetric contraction. When the pressure in the LV exceeds the pressure in the aorta, the aortic valve opens and the period of rapid ejection begins. During this period the LV fibers continue to shorten and two-thirds of the stroke volume is ejected into the aorta. This period of rapid ejection is followed by the period of slow ejection when pressure in the LV begins to decrease. Slow ejection continues until the pressure in the LV drops below the pressure in the aorta and the aortic valve closes, producing the second heart sound. This is the end of ventricular systole.

Diastole

With both the aortic and mitral valves closed, the pressure in the LV drops rapidly as the muscle fibers relax. This period, called isovolumetric relaxation, continues until LV pressure drops below left atrial (LA) pressure. The volume of blood in the LA continues to increase throughout ventricular systole as

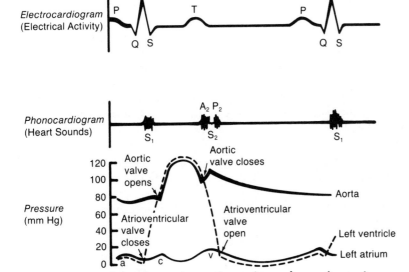

FIGURE 3.10
The cardiac cycle. The mechanical events represented by the left atrial, left ventricular, and aortic pressure waveforms are correlated with the electrical events represented by the electrocardiogram.

blood is received from the pulmonary system. This increase causes LA pressure to rise, which opens the mitral valve, and the period of rapid ventricular filling occurs. The ventricular fibers relax while the chamber continues to fill and enlarge with blood from the atria. Late diastole (diastasis) occurs as blood from the pulmonary system passes through the nearly empty atrium into the LV. It is during this period that there is optimal filling of the coronary arteries. The final period of LV diastole occurs as the LA contracts. Atrial contraction adds an additional 20% to 30% to the end-diastolic volume of the LV. This effect is referred to as atrial kick; it may be lost when synchronized atrial contraction is lost, as in atrial fibrillation. At the end of atrial contraction, the pressure in the LV exceeds the pressure in the LA and the mitral valve closes. This is synonymous with the first heart sound and marks the end of ventricular diastole.

The right ventricular cardiac cycle replicates the events on the left; the right-sided pressures are much lower than the left, however, and there are some slight differences in the timing of the cycle. The pulmonary valve opens just before and closes just after the aortic valve, and the tricuspid valve opens just prior to the mitral valve. As shown in Figure 3.10, there is a slight delay between the electrical events represented by the electrocardiogram and the mechanical events represented by the pressure tracing curves. This differential is referred to as the normal electromechanical delay.

Electrophysiology will be discussed in detail in Chapter 7.

Cardiac Output Determinants

Cardiac output (CO) is the amount of blood (in liters) ejected by the heart in 1 minute. It is the product of heart rate (HR) and stroke volume (SV) and is represented by the formula CO = HR × SV. Stroke volume is the amount of blood ejected with each ventricular contraction. In the average adult, SV is approximately 60 to 100 ml of blood. Factors that affect either HR or SV will alter CO.

The normal CO of 4 to 6 L/min is used as an index of cardiac function. A normal heart is able to increase its output in response to increased demands for O_2 and nutrients, which may occur with exercise, infection, or stress. The impaired heart may not be able to maintain an adequate CO, and signs of failure will be evident (see Chapter 10). The cardiac index (CI) is the CO adjusted for body surface area and is a more accurate way of evaluating cardiac performance. (Chapter 6 presents a complete review of CI.) The term *ejection fraction* (EF) refers to the percentage of left ventricular end-diastolic volume ejected with each stroke. It is normally greater than 60% and is a sensitive index of LV function. A decreased EF indicates that the LV is not contracting efficiently.

The major determinants of CO can be divided into those factors that affect HR and those factors that affect SV.

Heart Rate

Within certain limits, an increase or decrease in HR will increase or decrease cardiac output. These limits are estimated to be between 50 to 170 beats per minute (bpm). At rates greater than 170 bpm, there is inadequate time for diastolic filling of the ventricle; consequently, CO decreases. At rates less than

50 bpm, there is adequate time for filling but the reduced ejections per minute cause a reduction in CO. These limits are approximate and will vary somewhat in each individual — particularly in the patient with minimal cardiac reserve because of disease.

Stroke Volume

The amount of blood ejected with each contraction is determined by three factors: preload, contractility, and afterload. Changes in each of these factors will alter SV, thereby affecting CO.

Preload. Preload refers to the amount of blood in the LV at the end of diastole. It can be estimated at the bedside by measuring the pulmonary capillary wedge pressure (PCWP) or left atrial pressure (see Chapter 6). The Frank-Starling law states that, within limits, the greater the stretch of the myocardial fiber, the more forcefully it will contract. When the end-diastolic volume (preload) increases, the myocardial fibers are stretched, resulting in a more forceful contraction. This action is attributed to the following mechanism: At shorter lengths some of the actin filaments overlap, reducing the total area available for cross-bridge formation and decreasing the force of contraction. When the fibers are stretched, there is more area for cross-bridging to occur and the force of contraction increases. If all other factors remain the same, increasing preload will increase CO. The relationship between preload and CO is illustrated in Figure 3.11. The curves (called Starling curves) are plotted using the patient's

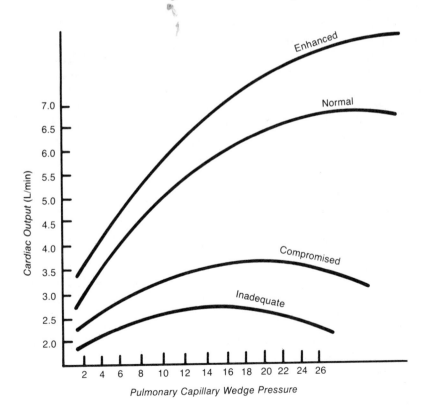

FIGURE 3.11
Starling curves: Normal, enhanced, compromised, and inadequate responses to increases in preload. Starling curves can be plotted at the bedside by using the patient's cardiac output and pulmonary capillary wedge pressure to measure the response to specific interventions.

PCWP and CO. As preload is increased, CO rises until the optimal point is attained. Once the optimal stretch is reached, CO begins to decline with further increases in preload. Preload may be increased by measures that increase venous return to the heart, such as assumption of Trendelenburg's position or the administration of intravenous fluids. It is decreased by such factors as dehydration, hemorrhage, and venous vasodilation.

Contractility.   The myocardial cell has a contractile state that influences CO. It is postulated that biochemical changes in the contractile sites are responsible for changes in contractility. The term *inotropy* refers to the contractile state of the cell. Factors that increase contractility, such as catecholamines, are said to have a positive inotropic effect; factors that decrease contractility, such as acidosis and beta blockers, have a negative inotropic effect. Although its exact role has not yet been defined, Ca^{++} is thought to be an important determinant of the contractile state of the myocardium.

Afterload.   Afterload refers to the amount of pressure the LV must generate to open the aortic valve. This amount is determined primarily by the diastolic pressure in the aorta. Afterload affects the rate of contraction by affecting the force–velocity relationship. The less force the fiber must overcome, the more rapidly and efficiently it can contract. Therefore, a decrease in afterload, resulting from vasodilatation or counterpulsation, will increase CO. An increase in afterload results from such conditions as hypertension, vasoconstriction, and aortic stenosis and will decrease CO.
    Vascular resistance (VR), the force opposing blood flow within the vessels, has a direct effect on afterload. This force is the product of several factors, including the radius of the vessel, the length of the vessel, and the viscosity of the blood. Vessel radius exerts the greatest influence on resistance to flow. A reduction of 1 unit measurement in the radius will produce a fourfold increase in the resistance. VR is frequently calculated clinically to assess the patient's physiological status. Pulmonary (PVR) and systemic (SVR) vascular resistance can be calculated from the following formulas:

$$PVR = \frac{(\overline{PA} - PCW)}{CO} \times 80 \qquad SVR = \frac{(\overline{MAP} - CVP)}{CO} \times 80$$

$\overline{PA}$ = Mean Pulmonary Artery Pressure
CVP = Central Venous Pressure
$\overline{MAP}$ = Mean Arterial Pressure
PCW = Pulmonary Capillary Wedge Pressure
CO = Cardiac Output

Normal SVR is 900 to 1500 dynes/sec/cm²; normal PVR is 45 to 120 dynes/sec/cm². Increased VR increases afterload and therefore decreases CO; decreased VR decreases afterload and increases CO.

Myocardial Oxygen Consumption

Myocardial physiology is best examined in relation to the myocardial O_2 supply/demand ratio. The absolute amounts of O_2 delivered to and consumed by the myocardium are less important than the balance between the two. Myocardial tissue routinely extracts 70% to 75% of the O_2 delivered to it via the coronary arteries. This percentage is quite high when compared with that in skeletal muscle, which normally extracts 35% at rest and up to 75% when exercised. Because myocardial O_2 extraction rates are always high, there is very little reserve for the heart to extract when the O_2 demand increases. Therefore, the only way to increase O_2 supply to the heart is to increase coronary blood flow by coronary artery vasodilatation or to increase the O_2 tension of the blood by the administration of supplemental O_2. In myocardial ischemia the coronary arteries supplying the ischemic section will dilate, thereby increasing the blood supply to that area. If increasing the O_2 supply to an ischemic area is not sufficient to restore the O_2 balance, measures must be taken to reduce O_2 demand. Drugs that affect blood supply and demand are discussed in Chapter 14.

The principal determinants of myocardial O_2 consumption (MVO_2) include myocardial wall tension, HR, and contractile state. A rough index of MVO_2 can be calculated by multiplying the HR by the systolic blood pressure. An increase in this value indicates an increased MVO_2. The aim of therapy in a person with a compromised myocardium is to reduce this value.

Myocardial wall tension refers to the amount of pressure that must be generated to overcome the resistance in the aorta and allow contraction to occur. Laplace's law states that wall tension (T) is proportional to the pressure within the cavity (P) times the radius (R) divided by the mass (M) [3].

$$T = \frac{P \times R}{M}$$

When the ventricle dilates, the radius increases, as does the wall tension. An elevation in afterload raises the pressure in the LV and increases wall tension, and more O_2 is consumed.

Accelerated HRs also cause increased MVO_2. Thus, any factor that causes tachycardia will increase the amount of O_2 the myocardium requires. For example, the person who is anxious or frightened by chest pain may become tachycardic, further compromising myocardial oxygenation. The contractile state of the myocardium is another important determinant of MVO_2. An increase in contractility causes an increase in MVO_2. In a severely compromised patient, a fine balance must be maintained between an optimal CO and an optimal MVO_2; many factors that benefit the former detract from the latter. This dilemma will be further explored in Chapter 9.

SUMMARY

At first glance, the heart appears to be a simple organ consisting of two pumping systems working in synergy. Closer examination reveals a complex machine with efficient mechanisms to maintain its functioning in the most extreme circumstances. The cardiac critical care nurse must understand these mechanisms and their interrelationships to provide optimal care to the critically ill patient.

STUDY QUESTIONS

1. List the components of the conduction system.
2. Name the three major coronary arteries and list the structures of the myocardium supplied by each, including the conduction system.
3. What are the normal pressures in each chamber of the heart?
   RA _____   LA _____
   RV _____   LV _____
4. What are the components of the cardiac valves, and what function does each serve?
5. Define *cardiac output* and list five factors that either decrease or increase it.
6. Define the following terms:
   a. *Isovolumetric contraction*
   b. *Preload*
   c. *Afterload*
   d. *Vascular resistance*
   e. *Ejection fraction*

CASE STUDY

A 56-year-old man has had a myocardial infarction and is in the CCU. In the 6 hours since admission, the following vital signs have been recorded:

	12 Noon	2 PM	4 PM	6 PM
BP S/D M (mm Hg)	90/50 63	96/58 70	110/68 92	100/60 73
HR (bpm)	110	98	80	80
PCW (mm Hg)	6	8	11	16
CVP (mm Hg)	3	5	10	13
CO (L/min)	3.0	4.8	5.5	5.2

1. Calculate his systemic vascular resistance at each of the four times.
2. What is his optimal wedge pressure?
3. Has his MVO_2 increased or decreased since admission?

REFERENCES

1. Andreoli, K. G., et al. *Comprehensive Cardiac Care* (5th ed.). St. Louis: Mosby, 1983.

2. Bates, B. *A Guide to Physical Examination* (2nd ed.). Philadelphia: Lippincott, 1982.

3. Berne, R. M., and Levy, M. N. *Cardiovascular Physiology* (4th ed.). St. Louis: Mosby, 1981.

4. Hurst, J. W., et al. *The Heart Arteries and Veins* (5th ed.). New York: McGraw-Hill, 1982.

5. Jackle, M., and Halligan, M. *Cardiovascular Problems: A Critical Care Nursing Focus.* Bowie, Md.: Brady, 1980.

6. McGurn, W. C. *People With Cardiac Problems: Nursing Concepts.* Philadelphia: Lippincott, 1981.

7. Netter, F. H. *The CIBA Collection of Medical Illustrations. 5: Heart.* New York: CIBA, 1969.

8. Price, S. A., and Wilson, L. M. *Pathophysiology: Clinical Concepts of Disease Processes.* New York: McGraw-Hill, 1978.

9. Rice, V. The heart and calcium antagonists. *Crit. Care Nurs.* 2(4):30, 1982.

10. Rice, V. The role of potassium in health and disease. *Crit. Care Nurs.* 2(3):54, 1982.

11. Sanderson, R. G., and Kurth, C. L. *The Cardiac Patient: A Comprehensive Approach.* Philadelphia: Saunders, 1983.

12. Shepard, N., Vaughan, P., and Rice, V. A guide to arrhythmia interpretation and management. *Crit. Care Nurs.* 2(5):58, 1982.

13. Underhill, S. L., et al. *Cardiac Nursing.* Philadelphia: Lippincott, 1982.

14. Vinsant, M. O., and Spence, M. *Commonsense Approach to Coronary Care.* St. Louis: Mosby, 1981.

15. Wells, S. J. (ed.). *Manual of Cardiovascular Assessment.* Reston, Va.: Reston, 1983.

16. Zschoche, D. A. *Mosby's Comprehensive Review of Critical Care* (2nd ed.). St. Louis: Mosby, 1981.

Assessment of the Cardiac System

Catherine M. McFadyen

INTRODUCTION

A complete assessment of a patient with cardiovascular disease includes both the taking of a health history and a physical examination. This chapter will review the basic elements of a cardiovascular health history and an assessment of the patient in a critical care setting. The critical care nurse must be comfortable with performing a complete cardiovascular examination, evaluating the extremities, neck, and precordium. Highly sophisticated monitoring equipment cannot be relied on as the sole source of clinical data.

There is no single, perfect method of performing a cardiovascular examination. No matter what pattern or sequence is used, however, it should be logical and orderly. The method described here focuses on the peripheral arterial and venous circulation and on a complete examination of the heart.

HISTORY

Often in the rush to attend to a patient's problems at the time of admission to the critical care unit, the health history, or "nursing assessment," is forgotten or set aside for another time. Without a thorough assessment, however, important facts about the patient's perception of illness and general health, as well as the events and symptoms causing the admission, are not obtained.

The health history should be obtained as soon as acute problems have been attended to. A format assessing functional health patterns such as health perception, health management, lifestyle, activity/exercise, nutrition, elimination, sleep/rest, sexuality/reproduction, and coping/stress tolerance patterns can be combined with investigation of the chief complaint, the history of the present illness, pertinent medical history, and family and social history, and a brief review of symptoms. Specifically include (1) previous health problems, such as rheumatic fever, that would cause or contribute to the development of heart disease, (2) modifiable and nonmodifiable risk factors, and (3) the cardinal symptoms of heart disease — angina, dyspnea, fatigue, palpitations, syncope, and edema [1]. When eliciting information from the patient about specific symptoms, whether at the time of the admission or at any point during the hospitalization, have the patient describe the symptoms as to (1) location (have the patient point to the exact point when possible), (2) onset, (3) duration, (4) quantity (use a scale of 1 to 10), (5) quality, (6) precipitating factors, (7) aggravating factors, (8) relieving factors, and (9) associated events or symptoms.

After collecting the data from the physical examination, the nurse develops a realistic problem list, short-term and long-term goals, and a plan for nursing interventions. Evaluation of the effectiveness of the plan is then documented in the daily progress notes.

PHYSICAL EXAMINATION

Once the health history is obtained, the nurse can begin the physical examination. The basic premise of a physical examination is that the examiner, by use of all the senses, can confirm impressions derived from the history and detect variations from the normal state. The examination is divided into the techniques of inspection, palpation, percussion, and auscultation.

Inspection

Inspection is the first technique performed in a physical examination. It involves concentrated observation of specific details of each body system. A thorough visual examination requires good lighting to detect abnormalities such as change in skin color, pulsations, skeletal deformities, and labored breathing.

Palpation

Palpation is often combined with inspection to verify or augment physical findings. Various parts of the examiner's hands are used to collect data. The pads of the fingers are quite sensitive and should be used for those tasks requiring fine discrimination. The skin is thinnest on the dorsum of the fingers and hands, which are used to estimate temperature. Vibrations produced by the movement of air or fluid are best detected with the palmar surfaces of the metacarpal phalangeal joints. Palpation is also employed to evaluate texture, moistness, areas of tenderness, and masses and collections of fluid (as in edema). Masses or other structures can be further examined for position, size, shape, consistency, and mobility by grasping the structure between the fingers.

Percussion

Percussion is a method of examination in which the examiner taps or strikes a part of the body to elicit sounds. As one taps, the underlying structures are set into motion and produce sounds, which are described according to intensity, pitch, duration, and quality. This technique is used to determine the density of underlying structures and to locate the boundaries of various organs and tissues. Percussion penetrates only about 5 to 7 cm and therefore is useful in detecting only superficial lesions. The technique is performed by placing the distal joint of the left middle finger (called the pleximeter) over the surface to be percussed and tapping it sharply with the middle finger of the right hand (called the plexor).

Five percussion notes can be elicited during physical examination; four of these can be heard over the anterior chest (Figure 4.1).

Flatness.   A flat percussion note is produced by tapping over very dense, airless tissue. It is normally heard over large muscles, such as the shoulder or thigh, and is described as a soft, high-pitched sound of short duration.

Dullness.   A dull percussion note can be produced over the liver, heart, and diaphragm. It is described as a soft, high-pitched sound of moderate duration.

Resonance.   A resonant percussion note is the sound heard over the normal lung. It is loud, low in pitch, and of long duration.

Hyperresonance.   Hyperresonance is the only percussion note that is not reproducible on the normal adult. It is an abnormal sound that can be elicited in the presence of trapped air, such as in emphysematous lung tissue. It is very loud, low in pitch, and of long duration.

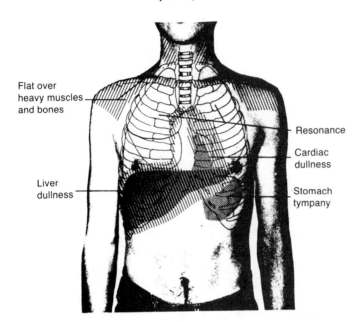

Flat over
heavy muscles
and bones

Resonance

Cardiac
dullness

Liver
dullness

Stomach
tympany

FIGURE 4.1
Percussion notes on the anterior chest.
(From Thompson, J. M., and Bowers, A. C.
Clinical Manual of Health Assessment. St.
Louis: Mosby, 1980. Used with permission.)

Tympany. A tympanic percussion note is characterized by its loud, high-pitched, musical quality. It is elicited over structures that are completely filled with air, such as the stomach or a puffed-out cheek.

Auscultation

Auscultation is the final technique performed during physical examination. Sounds produced by the body can be heard with or without equipment such as a stethoscope or doppler. This technique is valuable in diagnosing abnormalities of the cardiovascular, respiratory, and gastrointestinal systems.

EXAMINATION OF THE EXTREMITIES

Blood Pressure

Taking the blood pressure is the first step in performing a physical examination of the cardiovascular patient. Blood pressures can be measured directly by using an arterial catheter and monitoring equipment, or indirectly with a sphygmomanometer and stethoscope. Indirect routine measurement should be made bilaterally upon admission to the critical care unit (ICU), with the patient in the recumbent position, to provide a baseline.

Special problems can arise in the indirect determination of blood pressure. Obese patients and those individuals with large, muscular upper arms should have their blood pressure determined with an obesity or large-arm cuff. A thigh cuff is not of the same dimensions as a large-arm cuff and should not be used to determine the blood pressure in the arm; erroneous readings will result.

Blood pressure is frequently difficult to auscultate, either because sounds are distant or absent or because the cardiac rhythm is irregular. If sounds are distant or absent, the practitioner should consider three possibilities:

1. Improper placement of the stethoscope over the brachial artery.

2. Venous engorgement of the arm from repeated inflation of the cuff. In this case the cuff should be removed and the patient's arm elevated for 1 to 2 minutes to promote venous return. Then the cuff should be reapplied and quickly inflated with the patient's arm over his or her head, then lowered and auscultated in the usual manner.

3. Hypotension. In this case direct arterial pressure readings will be required. See Chapter 6 for a detailed discussion of direct blood pressure techniques.

Dysrhythmias frequently pose difficulties in obtaining accurate blood pressure readings. Both systolic and diastolic variations commonly occur in patients with atrial fibrillation, atrial flutter, bigeminal rhythms resulting from atrial or ventricular extrasystoles, coupling, frequent irregular ectopic contractions, and atrioventricular dissociation. Under these circumstances several measurements should be obtained and an average taken.

An increased or decreased pulse pressure (the difference between systolic and diastolic readings) can result from many physiological phenomena. Table 4.1 summarizes the common causes of pulse pressure variations. Changes in pulse pressure, especially a sudden decrease, should be recorded and communicated to the physician immediately. The normal pulse pressure is 30 to 40 mm Hg. Pressure differences between the arms have achieved greater diagnostic significance in recent years with the recognition of two conditions: supravalvular aortic stenosis (primarily in children) and the subclavian steal syndrome (in adults). Table 4.2 lists the causes for pressure differences between the right and left arms.

Pulsus paradoxus, considered one of the cardinal signs of cardiac tamponade, is an abnormal fall in the systemic blood pressure during inspiration. Other causes of pulsus paradoxus include pericardial effusion, constrictive pericarditis, restrictive cardiomyopathy, severe chronic obstructive lung disease, and hypovolemia or shock. Pulsus paradoxus can be elicited by inflating the cuff to a level greater than the systolic pressure with the patient breathing normally. As the cuff pressure is slowly released, the Korotkoff sounds become audible during expiration. The difference between the pressure level giving rise to the discernible sound on expiration and the pressure level at which sounds are audible during all phases of respiration is considered an estimate of the degree of arterial paradox. A normal paradox of 5 to 10 mm Hg exists in most individuals. Care must be taken to obtain an accurate reading, particularly in tachycardic patients.

Pulsus alternans refers to the alternating intensity of sound produced with each beat. This phenomenon can be indicative of left-sided heart failure and is best determined by the use of sphygmomanometry. The blood pressure cuff is inflated to about 20 to 30 mm Hg above the systolic reading and slowly lowered to the systolic level. Loud sounds produced by the alternate strong beats will be heard at this level, at approximately half the patient's heart rate. Further deflation of the cuff will uncover the softer sounds of the weak beats, and a regular alternation of loud and soft sounds is produced at the normal heart rate.

TABLE 4.1
Major Causes of Changes in Pulse Pressure

Causes of Increased Pressure

1. Increased stroke volume
   a. Anxiety, exercise
   b. Sinus bradycardia
   c. Aortic insufficiency
   d. Complete heart block

2. Decreased peripheral vascular resistance; decreased aortic distensibility
   a. Anemia
   b. Hyperthyroidism
   c. Fever, exercise
   d. Cirrhosis
   e. Hypertension
   f. Atherosclerosis
   g. Aging
   h. Coarctation of aorta

3. Increased intracranial pressure

Causes of Decreased Pressure

1. Mechanical obstructions
   a. Aortic stenosis
   b. Mitral valve insufficiency
   c. Mitral valve stenosis

2. Peripheral vasoconstriction
   a. Shock, hypovolemia
   b. Vasoconstrictive drugs

3. Decreased stroke volume
   a. Heart failure
   b. Hypovolemia, shock
   c. Cardiac tamponade or construction
   d. Tachycardia $\geq$ 180 bpm

Adapted from Hurst, J. W., et al. *The Heart*. New York: McGraw-Hill, 1978. Used with permission.

Orthostatic readings are frequently required in the cardiac patient to determine the effects of medication administered as well as volume status. Proper technique is essential for accurate evaluation of orthostatic changes. Three positions are usually evaluated: supine, sitting, and standing. In the critical care setting, only supine and sitting positions are usually used, depending on the patient's clinical status. After a change in the patient's position, 2 minutes should be allowed to elapse before the patient's blood pressure is determined again, to avoid erroneous recordings [13, 14].

The nurse must also consider anxiety when assessing an individual's blood pressure. Generally, patients in the critical care unit are overwhelmed by the amount of care and the number of care providers they require. A calm manner and explanations of routine blood pressure measurement techniques will help relieve their anxiety and provide a more accurate determination of their blood pressure.

TABLE 4.2
Pressure Difference Between Right and Left Arm

1. No abnormality (usually 5 mm Hg)

2. Artifactual
   a. Improper cuff placement
   b. Anatomical difference in size of upper extremities
   c. Change in circulatory status between measurement of pressures in right and left arms

3. Congenital heart disease
   a. Supravalvular aortic stenosis
   b. Coarctation of aorta
   c. Patent ductus arteriosus
   d. Aberrant subclavian artery

4. Associated with acquired disease
   a. Dissection of aorta
   b. Aortic arch syndrome
   c. Subclavian steal syndrome
   d. Peripheral occlusive disease

Adapted from Hurst, J. W., et al. *The Heart.* New York: McGraw-Hill, 1978. Used with permission.

After determination of the blood pressure, a carefully organized inspection, palpation, and, when appropriate, auscultation of the extremities and neck will reveal important data concerning the patient's status. Inspection and palpation are usually performed simultaneously by the critical care nurse and therefore will be discussed together in the following sections. For this part of the examination, a good source of illumination is necessary.

Skin

The skin is palpated for temperature and inspected for evidence of perspiration, color, vascularity, hair distribution, and venous patterns. Skin that is warm and dry is a sign of adequate cardiac output. Cool and clammy skin is an indication of increased sympathetic stimulation, which is a compensatory mechanism for decreased cardiac output and a general sign of impending shock. Skin color also provides the examiner with many clues to the cardiovascular status of an individual. Jaundice, most easily detected in the sclera, is usually associated with noncardiac diseases. But jaundice can also be secondary to chronic congestive heart failure (right sided), with liver impairment or hemolysis occurring in the postoperative patient as a result of the destruction of red blood cells by cardiopulmonary bypass, or hemolysis resulting from prosthetic valves [12, 16].

Cyanosis, a slight bluish-gray, slatelike, or dark purple discoloration, is frequently evidenced on the skin and sometimes the mucous membranes. It is usually apparent whenever there is more than 3 to 5 gm of reduced or unoxygenated hemoglobin in the capillaries of the tissues [12]. Normal arterial oxygen (PaO_2) saturation is 95%, and cyanosis appears at a level of 85% or lower. Anemic persons may never appear cyanotic, because even at low PaO_2 levels the reduction in hemoglobin is insufficient to produce cyanosis. Similarly, patients with polycythemia vera may appear cyanotic when the oxygen tensions in their blood is normal or even increased.

There are two categories of systemic cyanosis. Central cyanosis is due to the presence of unsaturated hemoglobin in the arterial and capillary bed. There is generalized pallor or discoloration of the mucous membranes of the buccal mucosa and tip of the tongue. Polycythemia and clubbing are also frequently present. Causes include congenital heart disease with a right-to-left shunt, pulmonary arteriovenous fistula, and advanced pulmonary disease with cor pulmonale. Central cyanosis represents an advanced disturbance in gas exchange.

Peripheral cyanosis occurs in the presence of normal PaO_2 saturation on such portions of the body as the nailbeds, lips, earlobes, and tip of the nose. It is produced by the presence of reduced hemoglobin in the peripheral capillaries and venules and is caused by a reduction in the blood flow through the vascular beds, which allows the capillaries to give up more than the normal amounts of oxygen. Exposure to cold, nervous tension, low cardiac output secondary to valve disease or heart failure, and obstructive peripheral arterial disease are common precipitants of peripheral cyanosis. On examination, the extremities appear cold and have a mottled appearance without the presence of clubbing.

Nails

Splinter hemorrhages and clubbing are frequent signs of cardiovascular dysfunction apparent in the nails. Splinter hemorrhages are thin, brownish, flame-shaped lines in the nail bed (Figure 4.2). These are most often the result of tiny emboli and are associated with subacute bacterial endocarditis. Clubbing is a painless, bilateral condition of the fingernail that results in loss of the normal angle (160 degrees) between the nail and the nail base (Figure 4.3). In early clubbing the angle straightens to 180 degrees and the base is springy when palpated. In late clubbing the angle is 180 degrees and the nail base is swollen. Three common cardiovascular causes of clubbing are cyanotic heart disease, advanced cor pulmonale, and subacute bacterial endocarditis.

Edema

Edema, long thought to be a classic sign of heart failure, is now known to have multiple noncardiac origins. The nurse must have a clear understanding of the causes, definition, and signs of edema.

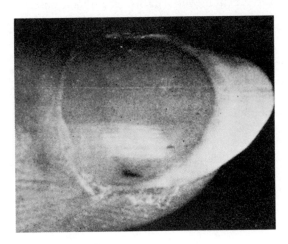

FIGURE 4.2
Splinter hemorrhages. (From Oram, S. *Clinical Heart Disease*. London: William Heinemann, 1971. Used with permission.)

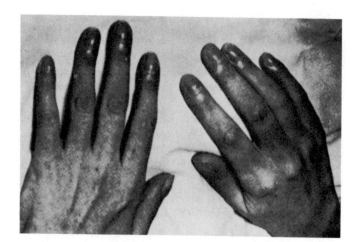

FIGURE 4.3
Clubbing of the nails. (From Oram, S. *Clinical Heart Disease.* London: William Heinemann, 1971. Used with permission.)

Edema is an excessive accumulation of interstitial fluid in the soft tissue or lungs. It can be due to increased capillary permeability, increased systemic venous pressure in right-sided chronic heart failure, obstruction of the lymphatic channels, venous occlusion, reduction in the plasma albumin, or tissue inflammation [12]. It can occur in nondependent as well as dependent areas of the body but is most frequently present in the dorsum of the feet and medial aspect of the ankles.

There are three major points to bear in mind when evaluating a cardiac patient for edematous conditions. First, edema is considered a late sign of congestive heart failure. Second, there are numerous causes of this sign and it is not diagnostic of congestive heart failure. Last, in the adult, 10 to 15 pounds of fluid can accumulate without associated edema, and therefore body weight is a better indicator of fluid retention [11, 12].

There are two types of edema, pitting and nonpitting. The nurse assessing the cardiac patient must distinguish between the two. To demonstrate pitting edema, the thumb should be pressed for 5 seconds into the skin of the patient against a bony surface, such as the subcutaneous aspect of the tibia, fibula, or sacrum. When the thumb is withdrawn, an indentation persists for a short time. The depth of the pit should be estimated and recorded in millimeters, avoiding subjective expressions such as "two" or "three" plus [2, 12].

Nonpitting edema, or brawny edema, is a chronic condition. The subcutaneous tissue and skin become hard or musclelike because of fibrosis or thickening and no longer indent or pit upon pressure. Brawny edema is often associated with peripheral vascular disease caused by arterial occlusion and myxedema.

Arterial Pulses

Palpation of the arterial pulses is the next step in the physical examination of the patient. The arterial pulse is a propagated wave of arterial pressure resulting from left ventricular contraction. With each ventricular systole, blood is rapidly ejected into the aorta. Because the aorta is elastic, the pressure generated from systole is transmitted as a wave through the aorta and its branches.

The forward movement of the blood follows this pressure wave, causing expansion and elongation of the artery, which constitutes the arterial pulse [1].

The examiner places two or three fingers on the artery. The carotid, brachial, radial, femoral, popliteal, dorsalis pedis, and posterior tibial arteries should be assessed bilaterally, compared, and described in terms of the following characteristics:

Rate   rapid or slow

Rhythm   regular or irregular

Size   large, normal, or small

Tension   hard or soft

Quality   bounding, thready

To obtain an accurate evaluation of the rate and rhythm, the carotid or radial pulse is palpated for 1 minute. If an irregular rhythm exists, the pulse should be palpated for another minute and the apical pulse simultaneously determined and recorded as well. Care must be taken when palpating the carotid artery to avoid undue pressure on the carotid sinus and the artery. To avoid excess pressure against the artery, the examiner palpates the artery on the side from which she is standing, not from the opposite side. Only one carotid artery at a time is palpated.

The quality or character of the arterial pulse can provide clues to many cardiac and peripheral vascular diseases. A bounding pulse can be produced by complete heart block, aortic insufficiency, generalized arteriosclerosis of the arterial system, fever, anemia, hepatic failure, thyrotoxicosis, anxiety, and exercise. It is characterized by a wide pulse pressure with a normal or slightly lower diastolic pressure. Upon palpation of the artery, one feels a rapid upstroke, a brief peaking, and a fast downstroke [1, 3].

A weak pulse, known as pulsus parvus, is present in low-output failure caused by aortic and mitral stenosis, acute myocardial infarction, constrictive pericarditis, and shock. Characteristically, there is a narrowed pulse pressure (because of low systolic volume) and associated peripheral vasoconstriction. The pulse feels weak and thready, with a slow, gradual upstroke, a delayed peak, and a prolonged downstroke [1, 3].

Pulsus alternans occur chiefly in elderly persons with myocardial disease and is a cardinal sign of left ventricular failure [2].

A bigeminal pulse (pulsus bigeminus) is a coupling of two beats separated by a pause. It is usually produced by alternating normal and premature contractions. The second beat is weak, because there is reduced diastolic filling time with the premature contraction.

Pulsus paradox may be palpated and is best distinguished from pulsus bigeminus by its regularity.

EXAMINATION OF THE NECK

Examination of the neck includes inspection of the jugular venous pulse (waveform), estimation of the jugular venous pressure, and palpation of the carotid artery. These observations will provide information about the hemodynamics of the right side of the heart. This information is particularly useful during the first minutes or hours after admission to a critical care unit, when invasive monitoring techniques have not yet been instituted. Chapter 6 presents discussion of the physiological components of wave formation.

Satisfactory examination requires the removal of clothing from the patient's neck and upper thorax, good light, and the patient in a semi-Fowler position of 30 to 60 degrees.

Jugular Venous Pulse

Table 4.3 differentiates the findings on physical examination between the jugular venous pulse and carotid arterial pulse in the neck. The venous pulse is best seen at the base of the neck with the patient's head turned slightly away from the examiner. (See Chapter 6 for further discussion of waveform propagation.)

In estimating the right atrial pressure by means of the jugular system, the best estimate can be made from the internal jugular veins. If these are impossible to visualize, the external jugular veins can be used, but they are less reliable. With severe increases in the jugular venous pressure, angles of elevation up to 90 degrees may be needed.

The sternal angle is used as the reference point for measuring venous pressure, because there is a constant relationship between this point and the right atrium. The level of venous pressure is determined by finding the highest point of oscillation in the internal jugular vein. The vertical distance in centimeters between the sternal angle and the point of oscillation is recorded as the venous pressure (Figure 4.4). Pressures more than 3 cm above the sternal angle are considered elevated. A simple scale of normal, mildly, and markedly increased will often suffice for purposes of continuous monitoring and reporting. In addition to cardiovascular factors, exertion, anxiety, premenstrual increases in blood volume, abdominal pressure, and obesity may produce mild elevation in the jugular venous pressure [12].

TABLE 4.3

Differentiation Between Jugular Venous Pulse and Carotid Arterial Pulse on Physical Examination

Jugular Venous Pulse	Carotid Arterial Pulse
Diffuse	Localized
Undulant	Brisk
Low, lateral, under or behind sternocleidomastoid muscle	High and medial to sternocleidomastoid muscle
Disappears or decreases in a sitting position	Unaffected by position
Increases with inspiration	Unaffected by respiration
Obliterated by pressure	Unaffected by pressure

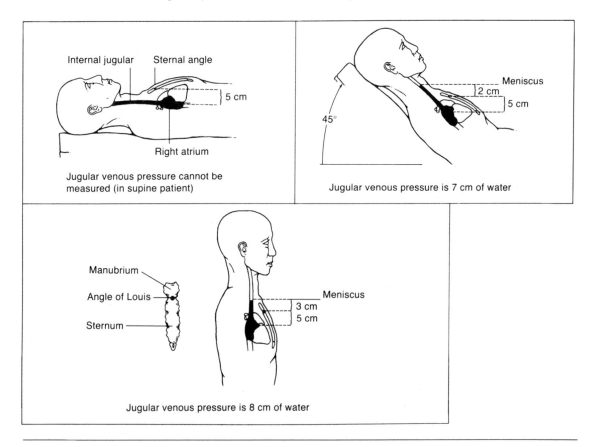

FIGURE 4.4
In all positions the vertical height of the sternal angle remains 5 cm above mid-right-atrial level, making this easily identifiable bony landmark a constant reference point for estimating the jugular venous pressure. With increasing degrees of venous pressure, the patient's head must be elevated to ascertain the mean venous pressure. (From Judge, R. D., Zuidema, G., and Fitzgerald, F. *Clinical Diagnosis* [4th ed.]. Boston: Little, Brown, 1982. Used with permission.)

EXAMINATION OF THE PRECORDIUM

A complete physical examination of the heart includes the four techniques of inspection, palpation, percussion, and auscultation. During the physical examination it is essential to have an understanding of the gross anatomy of the normal heart, its topographic relationship to the anterior chest wall, and the cardiac cycle and its relationship to valvular physiology. Chapter 3 provides a detailed review of cardiac anatomy and physiology.

Inspection and Palpation

To inspect and palpate the precordial area, have the patient lie supine with the head of the bed elevated 30 degrees. Adequate lighting is essential. The examiner stands on the patient's right side. The precordial area is inspected and palpated for abnormal pulsations, lifts, heaves, and thrills. The palmar bases of the fingers are used for palpation. The exact areas to inspect and palpate are displayed in Figure 4.5.

The only normal pulsation on the chest is in the fifth intercostal space at the midclavicular line; it is referred to as the apical impulse or point of maximal impulse (PMI). This impulse, however, is visible in only about half the normal adult population [16]. In the aortic area an abnormal pulsation may indicate dilatation of the ascending aorta; a vibratory thrill is associated with aortic stenosis. In the pulmonary area a diseased pulmonary valve or pulmonary artery can produce a palpable sustained pulsation [1]. Visible pulsations in the third, fourth, and fifth intercostal spaces along the sternal border indicate right ventricular enlargement. A palpable thrill in this area may be an indication of a ventricular septal defect. In the apical area, if the patient has left ventricular enlargement, the PMI is forceful and displaced lateral to the midclavicular line or downward.

The final location to examine is the epigastric area. The descending thoracic aorta is located at the midline and in some individuals is palpable just below the xyphoid process. Abnormally prominent pulsations may indicate an aneurysm; this finding, however, is sometimes confused with right ventricular hypertrophy. Caution should be exercised in palpating a suspected aortic aneurysm because of the danger of dissection.

Percussion

Percussion of the heart is of limited clinical value. It may be used to outline the cardiac borders, but this information is readily obtained from a chest roentgenogram, which is more conclusive and accurate.

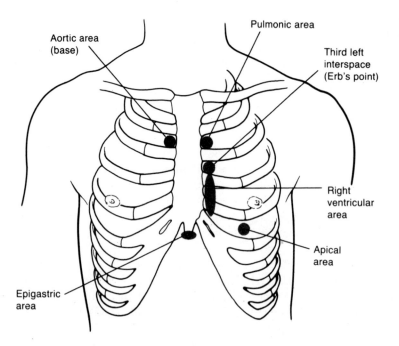

FIGURE 4.5
Five areas for inspection and palpation of the precordium.

Aortic area (base)

Pulmonic area

Third left interspace (Erb's point)

Right ventricular area

Apical area

Epigastric area

Cardiac Cycle and Valvular Mechanics

A thorough understanding of the cardiac cycle is essential to comprehend and appreciate auscultation of the heart. For convenience, the cycle will be reviewed here, with emphasis placed on the mechanical events of the opening and closure of the aortic, pulmonary, mitral, and tricuspid valves. It is the mechanical events of the valves that are reflected in the first and second heart sounds (Figure 4.6).

The cardiac cycle begins with the return of deoxygenated blood from the systemic circulation into the right atrium via the inferior and superior vena cavae, and oxygenated blood into the left atrium via the lungs. Blood flows from the atria through open mitral and tricuspid valves into the relaxed right and left ventricles. As the atria are stimulated to contract, they squeeze the remaining blood into the ventricles. The pressure within the ventricles rises rapidly, causing the mitral and tricuspid valves to snap shut. This closure is referred to as S1 and marks the beginning of ventricular systole.

As the pressure in the ventricles continues to rise, the aortic and pulmonary valves are forced open while blood is ejected through the valves and out into the aorta and pulmonary artery. As the ventricles empty, the pressure falls and the pressure in the aorta and pulmonary artery rises, forcing shut the aortic and pulmonary valves. The shutting of these valves is referred to as S2, or the second heart sound, and begins the period of ventricular diastole.

Blood then flows through the arterial and pulmonary systems. The ventricles continue to relax, and the resultant decreased pressure within allows the tricuspid and mitral valves to open, with subsequent refilling of the ventricles.

Let us clarify the cardiac cycle in terms of valvular mechanisms: Systole

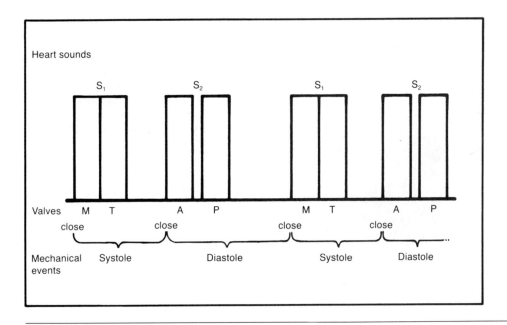

FIGURE 4.6
Systole and diastole are related to the closing of the cardiac valves. (*M* = mitral valve; *A* = aortic valve; *T* = tricuspid valve; *P* = pulmonary valve.)

begins with the closure of the mitral and triscupid valves, known as S1, and ends with the closure of the aortic and pulmonary valves, known as S2. Diastole begins with S2 and ends with the next first sound (see Figure 4.6). A thorough understanding of these mechanical events is absolutely essential for comprehension and appreciation of auscultation of heart sounds.

AUSCULTATION OF THE PRECORDIUM

Auscultating the precordium can provide the nurse with valuable information about the clinical status of a patient. For purposes of simplicity, our discussion will be limited to review of S1, S2, S3, S4, gallops, the diastolic and systolic murmurs of stenosis and regurgitation, and rubs. It is beyond the scope of this book to provide an all-inclusive discussion of cardiac sounds, and the reader is referred to the references given at the end of the chapter for further information.

In an examination of the precordium, traditional landmarks are used for auscultation (Figure 4.7). These landmarks do not necessarily represent the actual location of the valves but, rather, the direction of blood flow through the valves and the point at which the flow can best be heard. As the nurse auscultates the precordium, a logical, methodical, step-by-step process is followed with each examination. There must be a high degree of concentration on each event, a tuning in to a specific feature or sound and a tuning out of other sounds and distractions.

By beginning the process of auscultation at the aortic area, the nurse can determine the timing of the cardiac cycle by identifying the first and second

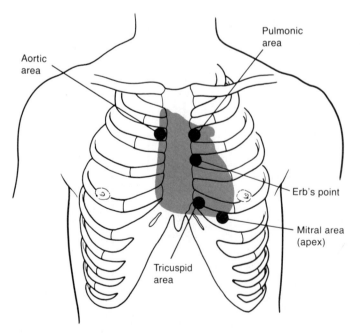

FIGURE 4.7
Areas on the precordium for auscultation. Aortic area: second right intercostal space adjacent to the sternum. Pulmonary area: second left intercostal space adjacent to the sternum. Erb's point: third left intercostal space. Tricuspid area: fifth left intercostal space at the sternal border. Mitral area: fifth left intercostal space at the midclavicular line or apex.

Aortic area

Pulmonic area

Erb's point

Mitral area (apex)

Tricuspid area

heart sounds. This identification of S1 and S2 serves as the basis of further auscultation and determination of systolic and diastolic sounds. On each examination the same procedure is followed, so that a regular pattern is established. The nurse should be positioned at the patient's right side. With the diaphragm of the stethoscope, the nurse should listen at the aortic area; then the stethoscope should be inched over the precordium to the pulmonary area, Erb's point, the tricuspid area, and finally the mitral area. The process is repeated using the bell of the stethoscope. At each site the nurse should do the following:

1. Identify S1 and S2, noting intensity and splitting
2. Identify sounds in systole, noting their timing, intensity, pitch, and location
3. Identify sounds in diastole, noting their timing, intensity, pitch, and location
4. Listen for a pericardial friction rub [1, 2, 12]

The First Heart Sound

The first heart sound, as stated previously, represents the onset of ventricular systole. It is composed of two high-frequency components: mitral valve closure (M1) and tricuspid valve closure (T1). It is loudest at the apex but at times can be louder in the fourth left intercostal space. As noted earlier, the closure of the valves of the left side of the heart precedes closure on the right side of the heart, but the two generally produce one sound. Occasionally the two distinct components of this sound can be identified. When this occurs, the sound is said to be split [23]. The splitting is auscultated in the tricuspid area — the fourth left intercostal space at the sternal border — and usually is considered physiological and not abnormal. The first heart sound is best heard with the diaphragm of the stethoscope.

Factors that alter the intensity of the first heart sound are summarized in Table 4.4.

The Second Heart Sound

The second heart sound marks the onset of ventricular diastole. Like S1, the second sound also has two high-frequency components, representing aortic and pulmonary valve closure, respectively. The aortic component of the second heart sound, referred to as A2, is widely transmitted over the precordium, the neck, and the apex [23] but is identified most easily at the second right intercostal space. The pulmonary component is much softer and heard best at the left sternal border at the second or third intercostal space. Like S1, the second heart sound is auscultated using the diaphragm of the stethoscope.

Splitting of the second sound is much more common than splitting of the first sound. During inspiration there is a decrease in intrathoracic pressure and venous return to the right side of the heart increases. This prolongs right ventricular systole and delays closure of the pulmonary valve. If the delay in this closure is greater than 0.03 sec, the normal splitting of S2 can be recognized and heard at the second left interspace [23]. In adults splitting of the S2 during expiration is considered an abnormal sign.

TABLE 4.4
Factors that Alter the First Heart Sound

1. Louder with
   a. Exercise
   b. Fever
   c. Hyperthyroidism
   d. Anemia
   e. Mitral stenosis
   f. Short PR interval

2. Wide splitting in right bundle branch block

3. Variable intensity with
   a. Atrioventricular dissociation
   b. Atrial fibrillation
   c. Ventricular tachycardia
   d. Ventricular paced rhythms
   e. Pulsus alternans

4. Softer with
   a. First-degree heart block
   b. Aortic insufficiency
   c. Hypertension
   d. Myocardial infarction
   e. Shock
   f. Myocardiopathies
   g. Left bundle branch block
   h. Pericardial fluid accumulation

The extracardiac and cardiac factors that affect the intensity of S2 include the following:

1. Loud aortic component
   a. Systemic hypertension
   b. Severe aortic regurgitation

2. Loud pulmonary component
   a. Pulmonary hypertension
   b. Pulmonary artery dilatation

3. Soft pulmonary component: pulmonary stenosis

The common causes of expiratory splitting of S2 include right bundle branch block, a left ventricular pacemaker, pulmonary stenosis, pulmonary hypertension, atrial septal defect, mitral insufficiency, and ventricular septal defect [23].

The Third Heart Sound

A third heart sound, or S3, occurs during early diastolic ventricular filling soon after S2 (Figure 4.8). The exact cause of S3 has not been determined, but many postulate that it is caused by a sudden deceleration of ventricular filling during diastole in a failing and noncompliant ventricle. When heard in healthy children and young adults, this sound is termed a physiological third heart sound. In adults over the age of 30 years, a third heart sound is considered abnormal and indicative of heart disease [10, 23]. An S3 is frequently associated with

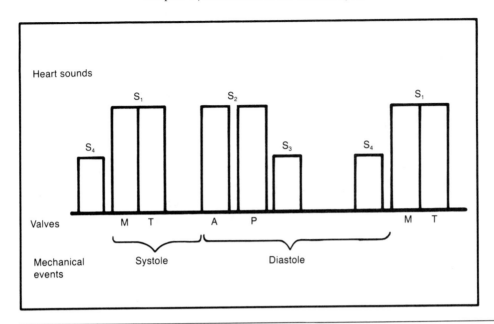

FIGURE 4.8
S_3 occurs in diastole shortly after S_2. S_4 occurs in diastole immediately prior to S_1.
(Abbreviations as in Figure 4.6.)

cardiac decompensation, atrioventricular valve incompetence, and increased end-diastolic pressure, especially in the patient with an acute myocardial infarction [10, 23]. Other common causes of an abnormal S3 include the following:

Elevated left ventricular filling pressure

Elevated left atrial pressure

Elevated pulmonary artery pressure

Anemia

Thyrotoxicosis

Atrioventricular shunts

An S3 is a low-frequency sound heard at the apex or PMI with the bell of the stethoscope pressed lightly against the chest wall. The intensity of S3 is accentuated when the patient is in the left lateral decubitus position.

The Fourth Heart Sound

The fourth heart sound, S4, also occurs during ventricular diastole just prior to the first sound (see Figure 4.8). Controversy concerning the clinical implications of an S4 persists, but most authorities believe the finding is related to a decrease in left ventricular compliance or an increase in ventricular volume [14, 23]. The following are the most common clinical situations in which an S4 is present:

Hypertensive cardiovascular disease

Myocardiopathy

Aortic stenosis

Subaortic stenosis

Myocardial infarction

Angina pectoris

Chronic coronary artery disease

Anemia

Elevated left end-diastolic pressure.

An S4 may be heard in most patients with acute myocardial infarctions and in many patients with coronary artery disease during an acute anginal attack. It often disappears after the acute stage is resolved, thus causing the inexperienced examiner much frustration in determining its presence. S4 is also a low-frequency, low-intensity sound best heard with the bell of the stethoscope.

Care must be taken not to confuse an S4 sound with a split S1 sound. The examiner must remember the timing (diastolic before S2), location, and frequency (low-pitched, heard best with the bell of the stethoscope) of the S4 sound.

Gallops

Frequently when an S3 or S4 sound is present, the resulting sound is referred to as a gallop rhythm because, in combination with the first and second heart sounds, it mimics the gait of a horse. When three distinct sounds are heard, S1, S2, and either S3 or S4, this is called a triple rhythm. Sometimes S3 and S4 diastolic sounds are present together; the result is called a summation gallop or quadruple rhythm results.

HEART MURMURS

Heart murmurs are the result of turbulent blood flow within the heart produced by the following mechanisms [15, 23]:

1. High rates of flow through normal or abnormal valves

2. Forward flow through a constricted or irregular valve

3. Backward flow through an incompetent valve

4. Flow through abnormal passages, such as a septal defect or a patent ductus arteriosus

5. Forward flow into a dilated vessel

Murmurs are described according to their timing in the cardiac cycle (for example, systolic or diastolic), loudness or intensity, duration, location, quality, pitch, radiation, and change during respiration or movement of the patient. By definition, a systolic murmur occurs between S1 and S2. These are further classified into early, mid, and late systolic and pansystolic (holostolic) murmurs, the last occurring throughout systole. A diastolic murmur occurs between S2 and the next S1 and is also classified as early, mid, or late diastolic (Figure 4.9).

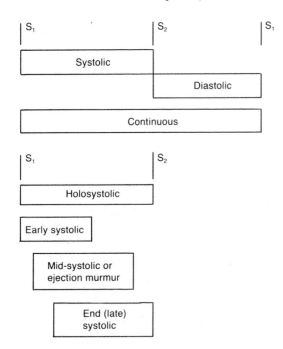

FIGURE 4.9
Murmurs are classified by occurrence in either systole or diastole. (From Tilkian, A. G., and Conover, M. B. *Understanding Heart Sounds and Murmurs*. Philadelphia: Saunders, 1979. Used with permission.)

The loudness of a murmur is graded on a scale of I to VI as follows:

Grade I: Very faint; heard only with special concentration

Grade II: Faint, but heard easily

Grade III: Soft, but louder than grade II

Grade IV: Loud, but of intermediate intensity

Grade V: Very loud; heard with the stethoscope lightly placed on chest

Grade VI: Very loud; heard even when the stethoscope is removed from the chest wall

This scale is subjective; consequently, it is difficult to obtain agreement between examiners [21, 23]. Judgments as to the location and radiation of the murmur are based on topographical landmarks discussed earlier in this section. Some murmurs are localized to small areas, whereas others are heard over large portions of the precordium. Thus, murmurs originating from valve dysfunction are usually but not always best heard in the area to which sounds from that valve are transmitted. Some murmurs also radiate in the direction of the blood flow that produces them. Notation of radiation can assist the examiner in determining the origin of the murmur [5, 6, 12].

To simplify our discussion of murmurs, we will divide them into the two major categories of systolic and diastolic and then further classify them into the subdivisions of stenotic and regurgitant. We can derive the following classification:

1. Systolic Murmurs
   a. Functional
   b. Aortic and/or pulmonic stenosis
   c. Mitral and/or tricuspid insufficiency
   d. Ventricular septal defect
   e. Dilatation of the pulmonary artery
   f. Atrial septal defect
2. Diastolic murmurs
   a. Aortic and/or pulmonic insufficiency
   b. Mitral and/or tricuspid stenosis

Systolic Murmurs

Systolic murmurs occur between S1 and S2, when the mitral and tricuspid valves are closed and the aortic and pulmonary valves are open. Thus, murmurs occurring during ventricular systole are a result of:

1. Increased blood flow across normal valves

2. Abnormal forward blood flow patterns across the aortic and/or pulmonary valves

3. Backward flow of blood through incompetent mitral and/or tricuspid valves

4. Ventricular septal defect [11, 15, 23]

Innocent or functional systolic murmurs are commonly heard in children and young adults and should be differentiated from abnormal murmurs. Functional murmurs occur early in systole. They are brief, of low intensity, and grade II or less; they frequently become inaudible with a position change from supine to sitting and are best heard over the pulmonary area. Functional murmurs are intensified by an increase in cardiac output resulting from anxiety, fever, anemia, pregnancy, liver disease, or thyrotoxicosis.

Systolic Stenotic Murmurs
Aortic or pulmonic stenosis produces a systolic murmur that begins after the first heart sound. As the valves open and blood is forced through a narrowed, ragged, or deformed valve, a harsh or high-frequency vibration is generated and a murmur is produced. Generally the softer, shorter-duration murmur is associated with mild obstruction and the louder, harsher, and longer-duration murmur is associated with more severe obstruction. This relationship can be affected by the presence of emphysema, shock, dysrhythmias, or heart failure, any of which will diminish the murmur intensity of even the most severe obstruction.

Aortic valve murmurs are most audible at the second right intercostal space and radiate to the neck. Pulmonic ejection murmurs are loudest at the third right intercostal space and radiate toward the left shoulder.

Systolic Regurgitant Murmurs
Mitral or tricuspid valve regurgitation or insufficiency produces a systolic murmur that occurs after the first heart sound and lasts throughout systole. It is

due to the backflow of blood from the ventricle through an incompetent or "leaky" valve to the atria during ventricular contraction. As the high pressure within the ventricle forces the blood through the opened aortic and pulmonary valves, it simultaneously forces blood back through the incompetent mitral or tricuspid valve into the atria, producing a regurgitant murmur that lasts throughout systole (holosystolic or pansystolic). The murmur may be musical, blowing, or harsh, is most often high pitched, and is heard best with the diaphragm of the stethoscope [15, 23].

The murmur of mitral regurgitation is auscultated at the apex with the patient turned to the left lateral position, and often radiates to the left axilla or back. The murmur of tricuspid regurgitation is identified along the lower left sternal border and is accentuated by inspiration [16, 23].

Diastolic Murmurs   Normally, diastole is free of murmurs because of the large openings of the mitral and tricuspid valves and the small pressure gradient between the atria and the ventricles, which limits the turbulence of ventricular filling that would be heard as a murmur. Stenosis or obstruction of the mitral or tricuspid valve, insufficiency of the aortic or pulmonary valve, or an increase in atrioventricular blood flow will cause abnormal turbulence, however, and result in a diastolic murmur [23]. Diastolic murmurs occur between S2 and the next S1. These murmurs occur in early, mid, or late diastole and almost always indicate heart disease [11, 15, 16].

Diastolic Stenotic Murmurs
Mitral or tricuspid stenosis is associated with a diastolic murmur that is produced by the flow of blood at greater than normal velocity from the atria into the ventricles through a narrowed mitral or tricuspid orifice. The murmur continues as long as there is a significant pressure gradient between the atria and ventricles. With mild stenosis a significant gradient develops during the rapid filling phase of diastole and decreases as the ventricle fills. This produces a mid-diastolic murmur. With more severe stenosis the murmur becomes of longer duration because ventricular filling is slowed and a significant atrioventricular pressure gradient is present throughout diastole. The sound produced by this murmur is often referred to as a diastolic rumble [21, 23].

The murmur or rumble of mitral stenosis is auscultated at the apex or PMI with the patient turned to the left lateral position. It is a low-frequency sound and therefore auscultated with the bell of the stethoscope placed lightly on the chest. In this position the sound is easily recognized, but it may become inaudible when the stethoscope is moved away from the apex or if the patient is not positioned properly [23].

The murmur of tricuspid stenosis, which is less common than mitral stenosis, is best heard at the lower left sternal border in the xiphoid area using the bell of the stethoscope with the patient recumbent [23].

Diastolic Regurgitant Murmurs
Aortic and pulmonary regurgitant murmurs are produced during early diastole. Aortic valve insufficiency begins with A2 (aortic valve closure) when the

pressure within the aorta exceeds that in the left ventricle. The high aortic pressure causes a backflow of blood through the valve and into the ventricle. As the pressure in the aorta declines, the backflow or regurgitation also diminishes. Thus, this murmur is loud at first then fades in intensity.

The murmur is identified by placing the diaphragm of the stethoscope firmly against the chest wall at the second right intercostal space along the left sternal border. This murmur is often missed if the patient is examined in only the supine or recumbent position, because it is accentuated when the patient is sitting up and leaning forward.

Pulmonary valve insufficiency begins with P2 (pulmonary valve closure), and, as in aortic insufficiency, the murmur is due to a high-pressure gradient that causes a backflow of blood into the right ventricle through an incompetent valve. This murmur also is loud at first and fades in intensity as the pressure gradient decreases [23]. The murmur of pulmonary regurgitation is auscultated with the diaphragm of the stethoscope at the second or third left intercostal space. The frequency, timing, quality, and location of these two murmurs are similar. Differentiation is difficult by auscultation alone, and echocardiography or phonocardiography is often needed for a definitive evaluation [15, 23].

Pericardial Friction Rub

A pericardial friction rub is considered to be an extracardiac sound. It is the characteristic finding in pericarditis, although it is not always present in this condition. A friction rub is described as grating, scratchy, leathery, or like pieces of sandpaper being rubbed together. It is a high-frequency sound heard best with the diaphragm of the stethoscope at the apex or lower left sternal border. It sometimes radiates over the entire precordium, however. The rub can be accentuated by having the patient sit upright and lean forward while holding the breath in expiration. Once heard, the sound is seldom confused with any other cardiac sound.

The technique of auscultation is best learned at the bedside after the nurse has a firm understanding of the anatomy of the heart, the physiology of the cardiac cycle, and the topographical landmarks. It takes time, patience, and a good stethoscope to hear many of the sounds produced by the heart. For a beginning critical care nurse, it is best to start with the obvious. Listen and learn the sounds of the heart on those patients with loud murmurs. Read the notes of co-workers for documentation of murmurs, gallops, and rubs, and then listen to the patient. Eventually, auscultating heart sounds will become easier and less time consuming.

MAJOR DIAGNOSTIC TESTS

Electro-cardiography

For many years the electrocardiogram (ECG) has been a major test for the diagnosis of myocardial infarction, valvular heart disease, ischemic heart disease, atrial and ventricular hypertrophy, conduction defects, dysrhythmias, and a multitude of other cardiovascular problems. It has become a routine part of the cardiovascular examination. ECG interpretation will be discussed in Chapters 7 and 8.

Chest Roentgenography

The chest roentgenogram (x-ray film) has also become a mainstay of clinical assessment of the cardiovascular patient. It assists in the evaulation of the pulmonary vasculature for congestion and also determines heart size, position, and contour, and calcification in the heart muscle, aorta, and coronary arteries. It is also helpful in assessing the placement of invasive catheters and tubes, such as endotracheal tubes.

Phono-cardiography

Phonocardiography is the graphic recording of cardiac sound. It evaluates the timing of heart sounds, especially those that are of low frequency and soft, such as a third or fourth sound or an ejection click. It is not, however, considered a routine laboratory study for the critical care patient.

Echocardiography

Because of its low cost and convenience, the echocardiogram has quickly become a widely used noninvasive diagnostic tool for patients with cardiac problems. It records ultrasound waves that are reflected onto the chest wall from the movement of cardiac structures. The ultrasonic beam plots out the motion of the structures over a period of time [8].

This study is valuable in the assessment of patients with acute or chronic atherosclerotic heart disease and helps in determining the cause of chest pain. In patients with suspected or documented myocardial infarction, echocardiography can often pinpoint the area of involvement when other tests, such as ECG and enzyme studies, are nondiagnostic. In addition, echocardiography can assess ventricular function, mitral valve stenosis and prolapse, idiopathic hypertrophic subaortic stenosis, torn chordae tendineae, vegetations resulting from bacterial endocarditis and atrial tumors, pericardial effusions, aortic stenosis and insufficiency, and postsurgical prosthetic valve function [8].

Patient and family education includes a clear explanation of this procedure, emphasizing its painless noninvasive nature, the ease of operation, and the absence of any need for fasting or additional medications to sedate the patient for the test.

Exercise Testing

Exercise testing, or stress testing, is the observation and recording of an individual's cardiovascular responses during a measured exercise challenge. The objectives of exercise testing include (1) diagnosis of ischemic heart disease, (2) investigation of physiological mechanisms underlying cardiac symptoms (such as angina, functional valve incompetence, and dysrhythmias), (3) detection of latent coronary artery disease, (4) measurement of functional capability for work, sport, or participation in a rehabilitation program, (5) evaluation of response to medical or surgical treatment, (6) monitoring of physical training programs, and (7) determination of prognosis [11, 22].

Exercise tolerance tests are described as maximal or submaximal. A maximal test defines the true state of cardiovascular fitness and exercises the individual until maximal oxygen uptake is attained. A submaximal test is one in which the workload is terminated at a predetermined heart rate, usually 80% to 85% of the maximum age-related heart rate. Most exercise tests in the United States are performed using a treadmill, although bicycle ergometers are also used. Various protocols have been established to administer the exercise test; most common is the multistage test of workloads, starting at zero or stage I, with an increase to the next stage after adequate time for physiological readjustment at each workload. A seventeen-lead, multiple-lead, or bipolar V5 lead ECG tracing is continuously displayed and recorded during the test and throughout the recovery period. A printout of the ECG is obtained every minute to measure heart rate and detect ST segment displacement and dysrhythmias. In addition, frequent blood pressure measurements are obtained and the patient is asked whether he or she is experiencing chest discomfort, dyspnea, or dizziness.

The ST segment response during the test is evaluated to determine the results. In general, ST segment depression of 0.1 mV below the baseline for 0.08 sec is considered indicative of ischemia. The duration of exercise, presence of anginal symptoms, heart rate, and blood pressure response are also important. ST segment elevation and combined ST segment depression and elevation both signify advanced asynergy of the left ventricular wall; the latter also indicates multivessel disease [11]. Unfortunately, certain known factors (potassium and digitalis), and many unknown factors, can affect the ST segment tracings, leading to false-positive results. False-negative results are also known to occur and may be due to the fact that certain areas of the heart are electrically silent. Combining the exercise test with myocardial perfusion imaging enhances diagnostic accuracy [11].

When exercise testing is carried out on patients soon after myocardial infarctions or cardiac surgery, the nursing staff of the cardiac unit often must assume the responsibility of patient education. Many patients have heard of exercise testing from friends or family or in the media but have never experienced the procedure itself. A thorough, careful explanation of the purpose and procedures of the exercise test will help alleviate concerns and clarify misconceptions so that the patient tolerates the test with less anxiety. Information given to the patient includes the following:

1. Location and time of day at which test will be performed, and equipment used during the test

2. Medication changes, such as tapering of beta blockers, and their rationale

3. Appropriate clothing: walking or flat shoes or sneakers (no slippers). Women should wear a bra, a loose-fitting blouse that buttons in the front, or a hospital gown or pajama top, and slacks or pajama pants

4. Diet restrictions: no food for at least 2 hours prior to the test. The preceding meal should be light, without alcohol, coffee, tea, or other caffeinated beverages.

5. Testing protocol of increasing workload by changes in speed and grade of treadmill

6. Assurance of test termination in case of chest discomfort, generalized fatigue, shortness of breath, unsteady gait, dizziness, or light-headedness

General indications for termination of the exercise test include those symptoms just cited as well as a heart rate increase to more than 120 bpm (or

110 bpm if the patient is still receiving beta blockers), ST segment deviation (varies depending on institution protocol), a drop in systolic blood pressure to below the resting level or failure of systolic blood pressure to rise, and significant dysrhythmias.

Other forms of stress testing have been developed for use in the recumbent patient during cardiac catheterization and angiography. In these tests the heart can be stressed by having the patient perform leg exercises with a bicycle device or isometric handgripping exercises by squeezing an ergometer. Another method of recumbent stress testing during cardiac catheterization is the pacing stress test. A pacing catheter is placed in the right atrium and the heart rate is increased by electrical pacing. The advantage of this form of stress test is that hemodynamic measurements can be made during the test via arteriography [11].

Cardiac Catheterization and Arteriography

Until recently, selective arteriography was considered too dangerous for use in the otherwise healthy individual thought to have cardiac disease. Now the safety of the procedure has been demonstrated in patients with both stable and unstable angina and in patients with myocardial infarction [17]. The common clinical indications for cardiac catheterization and arteriography are (1) determination of coronary artery patency, (2) determination of cardiac output, cardiac pressures, and oxygen saturation, (3) visualization of the great vessels and chambers of the heart via injection of contrast dye, (4) installation of pacemaker electrodes, and (5) evaluation of drug efficacy. In addition, coronary arteriography after acute myocardial infarction is becoming more common as interventions such as coronary bypass surgery, streptokinase lysis of an acutely developed thrombus, and transluminal angioplasty become more prevalent. Reasons for performing coronary arteriography after an acute myocardial infarction include recurrent chest pain, suspected mechanical derangements (for example, papillary muscle or ventricular septal rupture), and to provide guidance for future therapy in asymptomatic patients after infarction.

Complications and risks, such as myocardial infarctions, ventricular tachycardia, arterial hemorrhage, and stroke, still exist, however, and the patient must give informed consent prior to the procedure. It is at this time that the critical care nurse can be most helpful to the patient and family. When reinforcing explanations given by the physician, the nurse should know the specific reason the catheterization is being performed; then, after assessing the patient's and family's readiness to learn and their ability to comprehend, the nurse should explain the procedure according to an organized plan. Some areas that may be covered [1, 25] are:

1. Physical surroundings, including equipment, personnel, and the need for periodic darkening of the room
2. The need to withhold meals and fluids for 6 hours prior to the procedure
3. Specific medication ordered
4. Sensations to be expected, such as flushing with dye injection and chest fluttering with passage of the catheter

5. The need to lie still during the procedure

6. Routine postcatheterization procedures, such as frequent checking of vital signs, use of pressure bandages or sandbag at the insertion site, checking of peripheral pulses, bedrest, and the need for fluids administered by mouth or intravenously

7. Reexplanation of specific reasons for catheterization and the risks discussed by the physician

Assessment of the patient's and family's ability to understand this material is essential. Overwhelming a patient with too much information is dangerous to his or her emotional well-being. Not every patient and family has the same learning needs, particularly during a period of high stress. The purpose of explaining the procedure is to reduce this stress, and not to increase the stress inadvertently by giving too much information.

After catheterization the nurse should observe for such complications as vascular spasms, air embolism, pyrogenic reactions, phlebitis and thrombosis, excessive bleeding, and dysrhythmias, including ventricular fibrillation. Assessment after catheterization includes frequent determination of vital signs, including temperature; monitoring for the development of chest pain; observations for bleeding from the insertion site; and palpation of pulses distal to the insertion site, with comparison to the opposite pulse. Blood pressures are taken in the arm or extremity opposite the insertion site until the risk of bleeding has passed [1, 10]. Fluid intake must be monitored carefully after catheterization to prevent dehydration and ensure removal of the dye from the body. If the patient is unable to tolerate a high fluid intake by mouth, fluids should be administered intravenously.

Nuclear Imaging

The rapid growth and validation of nuclear imaging techniques during the past decade now permit noninvasive evaluation of cardiac function and myocardial perfusion. In addition, completely mobile units that can be taken to the bedside in critical care units have made performance of nuclear imaging a frequent, if not yet a routine, procedure. Three types of radionuclide imaging will be reviewed, and then the nursing implications and responsibilities will be discussed.

Pyrophosphate Scanning

Originally used in nuclear medicine for bone scans in the early 1970s, technetium 99m pyrophosphate was also shown to be taken up by injured myocardial tissue and thus to produce a "hot spot" image [25]. The scan is most helpful when the ECG is unable to confirm a diagnosis of myocardial infarction, especially in patients with a complete left bundle branch block or in those with previous myocardial infarctions. It is also useful when enzyme determinations are unreliable, as in postoperative cardiac patients or those in whom intramuscular injections have caused elevations in cardiac enzyme levels [25].

The procedure is performed by injecting the isotope in a peripheral vein and then scanning the patient 2 to 3 hours later. The timing of this scan is crucial: it will show no abnormalities for the first 12 hours after a myocardial infarction and then again after six or seven days. Thus, the scan should be conducted during the peak activity period 36 to 72 hours after a myocardial infarction [24, 25].

Thallium 201 Scanning

A second agent used in nuclear imaging is thallium 201. It is an intracellular ion that is actively transported into normal cells. When a cell becomes ischemic, it does not take up the thallium and therefore produces a "cold spot," indicating old infarcts or acute alterations in blood flow [24].

Scanning with thallium 201 can help differentiate ischemic muscle from normal and infarcted muscle. For example, if a patient experiences angina or chest pain, the isotope can be injected during the pain. The thallium will spread to normal tissue but will not be taken up by the ischemic tissue. If the patient is then rescanned when the pain has subsided and there is no ischemia, the previous "cold spots" will be filled in if the chest pain was indeed ischemia but will remain "cold" and will not take up the isotope if the tissue is infarcted [25].

It is for this reason that the thallium 201 exercise test has been developed to detect myocardial ischemia during physical stress. The exercise test is conducted according to standard protocol. Thallium is injected 1 minute prior to the cessation of the test, while the patient continues to exercise if possible. Then the scan is obtained and the presence of "cold spots" noted. Approximately 3 to 4 hours after the initial imaging is completed, a repeat scan is obtained and assessed for redistribution of blood flow or disappearance of the "cold spots." If a patient experiences chest pain or anginal symptoms that are not relieved by rest, nitroglycerin can be administered without affecting the results of the scan [19, 24].

Thallium scanning with exercise is most useful in evaluating lesions of borderline significance found on arteriography and in detecting areas of ischemia in patients with left bundle branch block, a situation in which the standard exercise test is inaccurate [19].

Gated Blood Pool Scan and First-Pass Studies

The gated blood pool scan and first-pass study are the most common type of nuclear imaging performed at the bedside in the critical care unit.

Gated blood pool studies are used to evaluate left ventricular function. The patient's blood is tagged with technetium 99m. The detecting equipment, scintillation camera, and computer are synchronized with the patient's ECG, specifically the R wave. With each R wave a pulse is sent to the computer, and a rapid sequence of images during systole and diastole is obtained and an isotope count is taken. The left ventricular ejection fraction is measured by comparing the count of tagged cells in the left ventricle at the end of diastole with the count at the end of systole [24].

First-pass studies are done at the time of injection of the technetium 99m for the gated blood pool scan. A rapid sequence of images is obtained with the gamma camera and computer as the bolus passes through the right side of the heart, lungs, and left side of the heart. The first-pass study is used to evaluate and measure the right and left ventricular ejection fraction and left-to-right shunts [24, 25].

Nursing Responsibilities

The most important responsibilities for the critical care nurse in the area of cardiovascular nuclear medicine are patient education and reduction of anxiety. With the increasing consumer exposure to the hazards of nuclear substances, patients are often concerned about the risk of cancer from injection of the isotopes. Patients should be reassured that both thallium 201 and technetium 99m pyrophosphate deliver less radiation than a gallbladder series [24]. In addition, the patient and family should be informed of the reasons for the procedure, the equipment and personnel involved, the time needed (approximately 45 to 60 min), injections to be administered, the need to lie quietly in a flat position, and the positioning on the table. A patient who is to undergo a thallium 201 exercise test should be made aware of treadmill and monitoring devices, exercise protocol, and the need to abstain from food for 6 to 12 hours prior to the test. As with any exercise test, the patient should also be reassured that the test can be stopped in case of chest pain, leg pain, severe shortness of breath, overall fatigue, or abnormal changes in the blood pressure or heart rhythm [24].

Electro-physiological Testing

Intracardiac electrophysiological studies are a new development in the field of diagnostic cardiology. Simply stated, electrophysiological testing is a programmed electrical stimulation of the heart combined with intracardiac electrograms. Its major diagnostic value is in evaluating the efficacy of pharmacological therapy in patients with recurrent sustained ventricular tachycardia or chronic ventricular tachyarrhythmias by reproducing the dysrhythmia under safe and controlled conditions.

Patients undergo electrophysiological study unsedated or mildly sedated. Multiple electrode catheters are inserted percutaneously or by cutdown and are positioned in the heart under fluoroscopic guidance, usually at the right ventricular apex. An electrical stimulation by a single, double, triple, or, occasionally, quadruple impulse is delivered to the myocardium by a specifically designed programmable stimulator to reproduce the patient's dysrhythmia.

This procedure is based on the assumption that the dysrhythmia initiated by the programmed electrical stimulation is identical to the clinical dysrhythmia. Drugs are then administered that will render the dysrhythmia noninducible, permitting selection of pharmacological therapy to be based on objective data rather than empirical (trial and error) choice. A control study is conducted prior to drug administration, and an additional study after the administration of each drug to be evaluated. Studies have demonstrated that suppression of life-threatening ventricular tachyarrhythmias that were electrically inducible prior to drug therapy is highly predictive of freedom from recurrent episodes. Provocative electrophysiological testing, however, carries risks of morbidity and mortality, although the reported incidences are small. Complications resulting from vascular catheterization, such as venous bleeding, phlebitis, and arterial emboli, can occur. These risks and the risk/benefit ratio must be clearly explained to the patient by the physician and reviewed and reinforced by the nurse.

In addition to measuring individual drug efficacy, electrophysiological testing can assist in the evaluation of combination drug regimens, the determination of long-term drug therapy, and the prediction of unsuccessful regimens. New horizons exist for the use of electrophysiological studies in developing treatment protocols for nonsustained ventricular tachycardia and ventricular fibrillation and in patients who have suffered cardiac arrest or are at high risk of sudden cardiac death.

SUMMARY

The development of a complete and accurate data base is essential for developing a successful plan of care for each individual. This chapter has reviewed the physical examination procedures to be used in the patient with known or suspected cardiovascular disease. It has outlined a logical and systematic approach to obtaining data on the physical status of a patient admitted to a cardiac critical care unit.

The new critical care nurse must fully appreciate that skill in the technique of cardiovascular examination is obtained best at the bedside. It is through continued practice of the techniques described that expertise in physical assessment will be obtained.

STUDY QUESTIONS

1. List the nine characteristics of chest pain that should be evaluated by the critical care nurse.
2. List three possibilities the nurse should consider if a blood pressure is difficult to auscultate.
3. Define *pulsus paradoxus*.
4. Explain the procedure for determining the presence of a paradoxical pulse.
5. Which of the following is *not* true about edema?
   a. It is a late sign of congestive heart failure.
   b. It is a diagnostic sign of congestive heart failure.
   c. In the adult, 10 to 15 pounds of fluid can accumulate without associated edema.
6. Distinguish between pitting edema and nonpitting edema.
7. List three possible causes of a bounding pulse.
8. Explain the differences evident on physical examination between the jugular venous pulse and carotid arterial pulse.
9. Describe the procedure for estimating the central venous pressure on physical examination.
10. Explain the relationship of the first and second heart sounds to the cardiac cycle and valvular mechanics.
11. Describe the areas of the chest that should be auscultated for determination of heart sounds.
12. True or False: An S3 is best heard with the diaphragm of the stethoscope at the lower left sternal border.
13. List three possible causes of an S3.

14. True or False: An S4 is related to left ventricular noncompliance.

15. What is the clinical significance of an S4?

16. Explain how to differentiate between splitting of S1 and an S4.

17. List three causes of a diastolic murmur.

18. Are functional murmurs associated with systole or diastole?

19. True or False: Aortic stenosis and tricuspid insufficiency are systolic murmurs.

20. Pericardial friction rubs are characteristic of _____.

21. Cyanosis is usually evident whenever there is more than _____ gm of reduced or unoxygenated hemoglobin.

22. True or False: Pulsus alternans is a cardinal sign of left ventricular failure.

23. Define *clubbing*.

24. Orthostatic blood pressure should be evaluated _____ min after position change.

25. True or False: An S4 is an early systolic heart sound.

CASE STUDIES

CASE 1

A 45-year-old male banker was admitted to the coronary care unit two days ago to rule out myocardial infarction. Since admission he has continued to experience chest pain without ECG abnormalities or enzyme changes. He is very anxious about his hospitalization and is extremely upset because of an upcoming thallium 201 scan.

1. What measures should be taken to help alleviate this man's anxiety?

2. Explain the rationale for using the thallium scan to rule out myocardial infarction.

The thallium scan does not indicate an infarct. The patient has been scheduled for a cardiac catheterization with selective arteriography in two days.

1. Outline a teaching plan for the patient, explaining the catheterization procedure.

2. List the nursing observations and actions to be conducted after catheterization.

CASE 2

A 78-year-old woman was admitted to the coronary care unit after a car accident, complaining of chest pain and dyspnea. The chest roentgenogram in the emergency room revealed multiple fractures of the left third, fourth, and fifth ribs, left ventricular hypertrophy, and bilateral infiltration consistent with congestive heart failure. The ECG showed ischemic T wave changes from previous readings. The medical history reveals chronic congestive heart failure and hypertension.

1. List the physical findings that might be expected on examination.

2. Based on this patient's history and present status, what, if any, changes would you make in your assessment technique?

REFERENCES

1. Andreoli, K. G., et al. *Comprehensive Cardiac Care* (4th ed.). St. Louis: Mosby, 1979.

2. Bates, B. *A Guide to Physical Examination* (3rd ed.). Philadelphia: Lippincott, 1983.

3. Boozer, M., and Craven, R. F. Nursing care of the patient with chronic occlusive peripheral artery disease. *Cardiovasc. Nurs.* 15:13, 1981.

4. Criscitielllo, M. G. Clues to the diagnosis of treatable heart disease. In S. Proger and M. Barza (eds.), *Diagnostic Imperative*. New York: Thieme-Stratton, 1981.

5. DeGowin, E., and DeGowin, R. *Bedside Diagnostic Examination* (3rd ed.). New York: Macmillan, 1976.

6. Delp, M., and Manning, R. T. *Major's Physical Diagnosis: An Introduction to the Clinical Process.* Philadelphia: Saunders, 1981.

7. Gillis, D. A., and Alyn, I. B. *Patient Assessment and Management by the Nurse Practitioner.* St. Louis: Saunders, 1976.

8. Henrick, A., and Stephandides, L. Common diagnostic uses of echocardiography. *Cardiovasc. Nurs.* 14:5, 1978.

9. Horowitz, L., Josephson, M., and Kastor, J. Intracardiac electrophysiologic studies as a method for the optimization of drug therapy in chronic ventricular arrhythmia. *Prog. Cardiovasc. Dis.* 23:81, 1980.

10. Hudak, C. M., Lohr, T., and Gallo, B. M. *Critical Care Nursing* (2nd ed.). Philadelphia: Lippincott, 1977.

11. Hurst, J. W. (ed.). *The Heart.* New York: McGraw-Hill, 1978.

12. Judge, R. D., and Zuidema, G. D. (eds.). *Methods of Clinical Examination: An Introduction to the Clinical Process* (3rd ed.). Boston: Little, Brown, 1974.

13. Kennedy, G., and Crawford, M. Proper position and timing of orthostatic blood pressure and heart rate measurments post–nitrate administration. Abstracts of the 53rd Scientific Sessions. *Circulation* 62 (Suppl. 3):184, 1980.

14. Kennedy, G., and Crawford, M. Optimal position and timing of blood pressure and heart rate measurements to detect orthostatic changes in patients with ischemic heart disease. *J. Cardiac Rehabil.* 4:219, 1984.

15. Leonard, J., et al. Auscultation. *Examination of the Heart*, Part 4. Dallas: American Heart Association, 1974.

16. Malasanos, L., et al. *Health Assessment* (2nd ed.). St. Louis: Mosby, 1981.

17. Mautnes, R. K., and Phillips, J. H. Coronary arteriography prior to hospital discharge after first myocardial infarction. *Heart Lung* 12:17, 1983.

18. Merrill, S. A., and Froelicher, V. F. Exercise testing. *Cardiovasc. Nurs.* 13:23, 1977.

19. Panatelo, N., et al. Thallium myocardial scintigraphy and its use in the assessment of coronary artery disease. *Heart Lung* 10:66, 1981.

20. Prior, J., Silberstein, J., and Stang, J. *Physical Diagnosis* (6th ed.). St. Louis: Mosby, 1981.

21. Sherman, J. L., and Fields, S. K. *Guide to Patient Evaluation.* New York: Medical Examination, 1978.

22. Sivarajan, E. S., and Bruce, R. A. Early exercise testing after myocardial infarction. *Cardiovasc. Nurs.* 17:1, 1981.

23. Tilkian, A. G., and Conover, M. B. *Understanding Heart Sounds and Murmurs.* Philadelphia: Saunders, 1979.

24. Walsh, C., and Graham, M. Nursing implications in cardiovascular nuclear medicine. *Cardiovasc. Nurs.* 19:1, 1983.

25. Zeluff, G., Cashion, W. R., Jr., and Jackson, D. Evaluation of the coronary arteries and myocardium by radionuclide imaging. *Heart Lung* 9:334, 1980.

CHAPTER 5

Assessment of the Respiratory System

Barbara Homer Yee

INTRODUCTION

The cardiac patient with an acute illness is at great risk of developing a variety of pulmonary complications. Because of the interdependent functions of the cardiac and respiratory systems, disorders in one system will frequently precipitate disorders in the other. For example, the patient with acute left-sided congestive heart failure evidences many respiratory symptoms, such as dyspnea, orthopnea, and crackles (rales), which can eventually develop into gross pulmonary edema. In addition, the physical immobility and recumbent position associated with an acute illness predispose the patient in the critical care unit (ICU) to pulmonary embolus formation, hypoventilation, atelectasis and stasis of secretions. Also, the patient may be sedated, in pain, inadequately hydrated, or nutritionally deficient, or may have a history of smoking, any of which can further inhibit normal respiratory functioning in a patient already at high risk.

Primary prevention of pulmonary complications is an essential goal for all patients in the ICU. If pulmonary disorders do develop, however, accurate assessment and diagnosis, combined with effective interventions, can minimize the consequences to the patient. Assessment is performed continually throughout the patient's stay in the ICU and involves the collection of data from both physical examination and laboratory tests.

This chapter will provide background knowledge and explain the skills needed by the critical care nurse (CCN) to assess the respiratory system accurately. The chapter is divided into three major sections: (1) history and physical examination, (2) arterial blood gas interpretation, and (3) bedside evaluation of pulmonary function. Brief explanations of pathophysiological processes will be included throughout.

HISTORY AND PHYSICAL EXAMINATION

History

The patient with cardiac disease may be admitted directly into the coronary care unit (CCU) or to a general medical or surgical unit. The first priority upon admission is to treat any immediate physical problems, such as chest pain, dysrhythmias, or dyspnea. Once the patient's condition stabilizes, a complete history is taken and a physical examination conducted, usually by the physician. The health history includes information regarding the chief complaint, a descriptive account of the present illness, a history of past illnesses, a family health history, and a review of systems. Previous hospitalizations or surgical procedures for pulmonary problems, or a history of respiratory disease such as tuberculosis, pneumonia, asthma, emphysema, or bronchitis, would be revealed during the review of the respiratory system. Signs and symptoms of respiratory diseases, such as cough, hemoptysis, sputum production, cyanosis, difficulty or pain with breathing, wheezing, and exertional dyspnea, should be evaluated, not only on admission but throughout the hospital stay. Each symptom must be assessed as to onset, location, duration, quality, quantity, time of day of occurrence, precipitating or relieving factors, and any associated symptoms. The patient's occupation, work environment, date of the last chest roentgenogram, and smoking history are also ascertained. Once the health history is taken the physical examination is begun.

Physical Examination

The respiratory status of the patient in the ICU is assessed on a continual basis. During an acute illness, the patient's condition may change rapidly; thus, the nurse must constantly observe the patient for subtle changes. Observation of a sign such as simple hemoptysis in the patient receiving anticoagulants, or shallow breathing in the patient who is being weaned from a respirator, can significantly alter the plan of care and, possibly, the outcome.

Four techniques are used during physical examination: inspection, palpation, percussion, and auscultation. In the ICU inspection and auscultation are used more frequently than palpation and percussion. Some of the information obtained with the latter techniques is more accurately diagnosed with a chest roentgenogram. Thus, clinicians rely heavily on daily chest films to confirm pulmonary changes in the acutely ill patient.

Our discussion of physical examination will emphasize those techniques used most frequently with acutely ill patients in the ICU. The nurse must be proficient in all techniques used in physical examination. Skill is developed through continued practice and expert verification of abnormal findings. The nurse must improve and refine the senses of sight, touch, and hearing to collect data accurately.

Topographical Anatomy

Before beginning the assessment process, the nurse must have a clear mental image of the underlying structures in the chest and be able to describe the exact location of any abnormalities found. Topographical, or surface, landmarks on the chest consist of imaginary lines drawn on the thorax and several prominent points on the thoracic cage.

Anterior Thorax

Surface landmarks on the anterior chest consist of three imaginary vertical lines drawn from specific anatomical points on the thoracic cage (Figure 5.1A). The midsternal line divides the sternum and chest in half. The midclavicular lines (right and left) are drawn from the midpoint of the clavicles and divide the anterior chest into quarters. Parallel to these lines is the anterior axillary line, which is drawn from the anterior axillary fold. In addition to these imaginary lines, various external landmarks can be identified from protuberant points on the skeletal cage.

The anatomical landmarks used most frequently during physical examination of the respiratory system are the suprasternal notch, manubriosternal junction, xiphoid process, costal margin, sternal border, ribs, and intercostal spaces (see Figure 5.1A). Two points on the sternum are of particular importance. The point of intersection between the manubrium and the body of the sternum is called the manubriosternal junction, or angle of Louis. This junction protrudes slightly, is easily palpated, and identifies the point of articulation of the second rib. Rib palpation and identification begins at this point and proceeds downward in an oblique line several centimeters lateral to the sternal edge. More medial palpation may result in errors in rib identification because of the close approximation of the costal cartilages of ribs 6 through 10, which

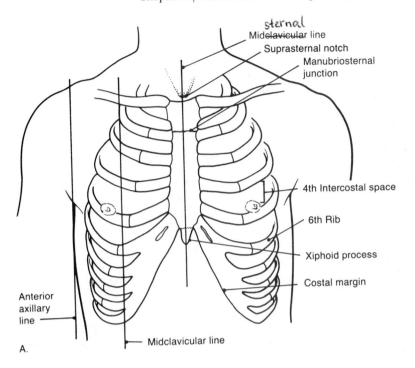

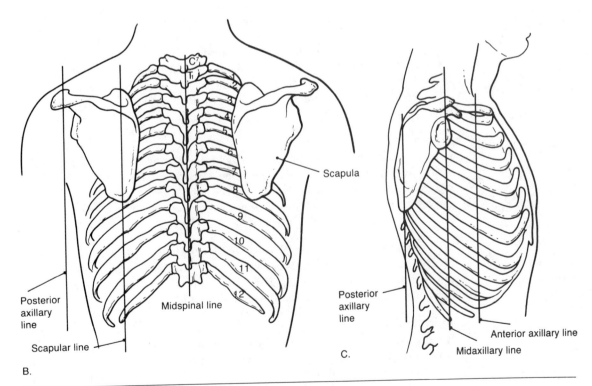

FIGURE 5.1
Surface landmarks on the (A) anterior thorax, (B) posterior thorax, and (C) lateral thorax.

are not distinguishable from ribs on palpation. The eleventh and twelfth ribs can be palpated only laterally and posteriorly, respectively. Individual rib identification is necessary when taking an electrocardiogram (ECG), auscultating heart and lung sounds, and describing the location of various abnormalities. The other important point on the sternum is the xiphoid process, which must be identified and avoided when performing cardiopulmonary resuscitation to prevent laceration of the liver.

Posterior Thorax

Surface landmarks on the posterior chest (Figure 5.1B) consist of three lines, the scapula, and the most prominent spinous processes. The chest is divided in half by the midspinal line (also called the vertebral line), which is drawn vertically along the spinous processes. The scapular line is drawn from the inferior angle of the scapula and runs parallel to the midspinal line. The posterior axillary line extends downward from the axillary fold.

Surface landmarks on the posterior chest are few and slightly more difficult to identify than those on the anterior chest, because they are not as prominent. The optimal position of the patient for examination of the posterior chest is sitting upright, leaning forward with the head bent slightly and the arms folded over the chest. In this position the scapulae move laterally and the vertebral column is more prominent. In the neck area the first prominent landmark is the spinous process of the seventh cervical (C7) vertebra. In some individuals two vertebrae appear equally prominent; these are C7 and the first thoracic vertebra (T1). The spinous processes of T4 through T12 angle obliquely downward; thus, each lies over the body of the vertebra below it rather than its own (see Figure 5.1B). Anatomically, the spinous process of T6, for example, is located below the seventh rib and lies over the body of T7. Other landmarks on the posterior chest include the inferior angle of the scapula, which lies approximately at the level of the eighth rib or interspace, the ribs, and the interspaces.

Lateral Thorax

Landmarks on the lateral thorax are drawn in relation to the axilla with the arm extended upward. The locations of the anterior and posterior axillary lines have been described previously. The midaxillary line is drawn vertically from the apex of the axilla and is located approximately midway between the anterior and posterior axillary lines (Figure 5.1C).

Underlying Thoracic Structures

To interpret the findings of a physical examination accurately, the nurse must be able to visualize the location of the underlying organs and lung borders during both inspiration and expiration. The surface landmarks and imaginary lines previously described assist the examiner in identifying these borders.

Anterior Thorax

Anteriorly, the lungs are divided, by fissures, into three lobes on the right and two on the left. Differentiating the various lung lobules is particularly important when describing abnormal breath sounds. The right upper lobe is divided from the right middle lobe by the horizontal fissure, which is located opposite the fourth rib, or approximately at the nipple line in males. The oblique fissure divides the middle lobe from the right lower lobe; it curves diagonally below the armpit across the sixth rib. The left upper lobe occupies almost the entire anterior chest. It is divided from the left lower lobe by the oblique fissure, which has a location analogous to that of the right oblique fissure (Figure 5.2A).

The apex of each lung rises about 1.5 inches above the inner third of the clavicle. The inferior borders of the lungs rest on the diaphragm and extend down to the sixth rib at the midclavicular line and the eighth rib at the midaxillary line [1]. The medial surface of each lung is concave to allow room for the mediastinal structures. The left lung is more concave because of the position of the heart. The average heart is approximately 9 cm, or 3.5 inches, wide at the widest point [41]. About two-thirds of the heart extends to the left of the midsternal line at the level of the third to the sixth ribs. With this information the examiner can accurately outline the cardiac silhouette and the medial border of the left lung.

The major structure in the upper mediastinal area is the trachea. It extends vertically from the larynx into the thorax, where it divides into the two bronchi at the carina. This bifurcation occurs just below the manubriosternal junction anteriorly and at the spinous process of T4 posteriorly. The right main stem bronchus is shorter, wider, and more nearly vertical than the left. This anatomical difference is clinically significant: aspirated foreign objects or endotracheal tubes that are inserted too far tend to enter the right main stem bronchus rather than the left.

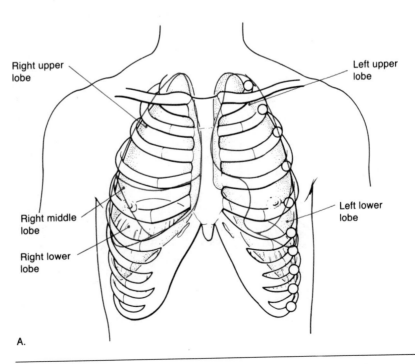

A.

FIGURE 5.2
Lung lobules on the (A) anterior thorax, (B) posterior thorax, and (C) lateral thorax.

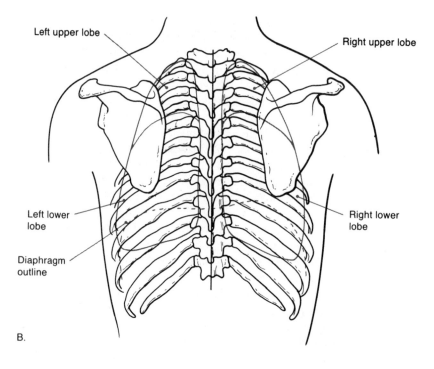

Left upper lobe

Right upper lobe

Left lower lobe

Right lower lobe

Diaphragm outline

B.

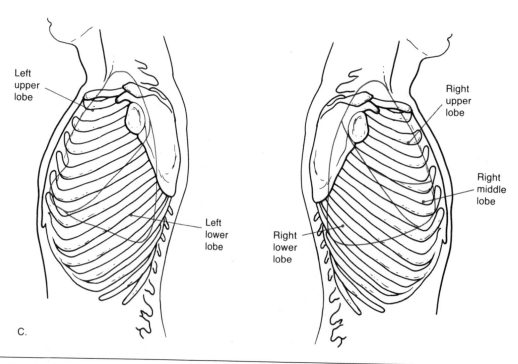

Left upper lobe

Right upper lobe

Left lower lobe

Right middle lobe

Right lower lobe

C.

FIGURE 5.2   *(continued)*

Posterior Thorax

On the posterior thorax the lungs are divided into the upper and lower lobes by an oblique, or major, fissure that can be drawn from the third thoracic spinous process obliquely downward and laterally. Thus, the lower lobes appear to occupy almost two-thirds of the posterior thorax (Figure 5.2B). The lung apices extend up to T1, with the lower borders extending to T10 on expiration and T12 on deep inspiration. Additional structures that should be noted on the posterior thorax are the level of the diaphragm and the inferior angle of the scapula.

Lateral Thorax

The lung lobules of the lateral chest are shown in Figure 5.2C. The lungs extend from the apex of the axilla to the sixth rib at the midclavicular line and slope back and down to approximately the level of the eighth rib along the posterior axillary line. The lower lobes occupy almost half of the lateral thorax and are divided from the upper lobes by a line drawn from the spinous process of T3 on the posterior thorax to the sixth rib at the midclavicular line. The right upper lobe is divided from the right middle lobe by a horizontal line at the level of the fourth rib (see Figure 5.2C).

Procedures of the Physical Examination

Inspection

During inspection of the patient's respiratory status, the color of the skin, lips, and nailbeds is assessed for signs of cyanosis, pallor, or flushing. In addition, the patient's nailbeds are observed for signs of clubbing. Nurses are accustomed to examining the nailbeds to detect cyanosis, a late and unreliable sign of hypoxemia; it is better to look at the tongue and oral mucous membranes, because these structures are less susceptible to changes in blood flow [40]. Peripheral cyanosis often occurs in the acutely ill patient and results from vasoconstriction, which may be due to hypothermia, vasoactive medications, or other factors.

The patient's breathing pattern should be assessed for rate, depth, and evidence of respiratory distress. Although normal respirations are regular, quiet, and occur 12 to 20 times per minute, patients often display normal variations outside these limits. One should note also the depth of respirations as well as the time it takes to inspire and expire. Inspiration (I) is generally shorter than expiration (E), and the two are recorded as a ratio; the normal I/E ratio is 1:1.5 or 1:2. Prolonged or shortened inspiration or expiration may be an early sign of respiratory dysfunction. Other signs of respiratory distress may be evident when observing the head, neck, and thorax: flared nostrils, gasping, facial expressions of anxiety, elevation of the clavicles or shoulders with inspiration, retractions of the sternum, retractions or bulging of the intercostal spaces, abnormal posturing, and use of accessory muscles.

The patient's respiratory pattern must be evaluated in relation to position and activity. Orthopnea, or difficult breathing in a recumbent position, is evident with various cardiac and pulmonary disorders. The condition may be improved or relieved if the head of the bed is elevated or the patient sits upright or stands. Relief in the upright position results from an increased vital capacity, a decreased venous return, and a decrease in hydrostatic pressure in the upper portion of the lungs [16]. Exertional dyspnea is also associated with various cardiac and respiratory disorders. During an acute illness, even mild increases in activity, such as washing, shaving, or walking, can cause dyspnea. In such a case, it is important to note the amount of activity that precipitates dyspnea. This will give an indication of the severity of the problem and can serve as baseline data to evaluate the patient's improving or worsening condition.

After assessing the patient's color and breathing pattern, one examines the chest for symmetry, shape, and the presence of skeletal deformities. The normal chest moves symmetrically with inspiration. Asymmetrical movement may be observed in such conditions as fractured ribs, injuries of the chest wall, scoliosis, and kyphosis. Other skeletal deformities that may alter the shape of the chest are pectus excavatum (funnel chest), pectus carinatum (pigeon chest), and the typical barrel chest of the patient with chronic obstructive pulmonary disease (Figure 5.3). A barrel chest is easily identified by the increased antero-posterior diameter.

The posterior thorax is also inspected for symmetry of movement and skeletal deformities. The spine, normally straight, may be curved because of scoliosis, kyphosis, or other orthopedic abnormalities.

The patient should be observed and evaluated for a cough and sputum production. The color, consistency, odor, and amount of sputum should be noted.

Palpation

Palpation is often combined with inspection to verify or augment physical findings. Palpation of the chest requires discrimination through touch, to detect structural abnormalities and symmetry of expansion and to feel vibrations transmitted from the lungs to the chest wall. The nurse begins palpating the

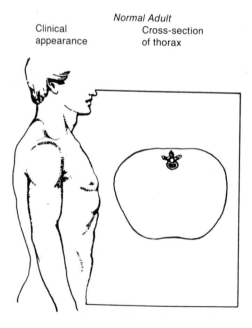

Clinical
appearance

Normal Adult
Cross-section
of thorax

FIGURE 5.3
Normal chest configurations and thoracic deformities. (From Harper, R. W. *A Guide to Respiratory Care.* Philadelphia: Lippincott, 1981. Used with permission.)

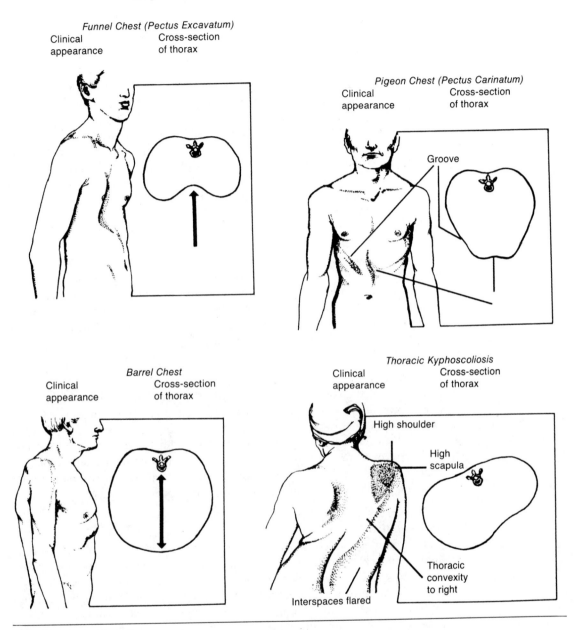

Funnel Chest (Pectus Excavatum)
Clinical appearance   Cross-section of thorax

Pigeon Chest (Pectus Carinatum)
Clinical appearance   Cross-section of thorax
Groove

Barrel Chest
Clinical appearance   Cross-section of thorax

Thoracic Kyphoscoliosis
Clinical appearance   Cross-section of thorax
High shoulder
High scapula
Thoracic convexity to right
Interspaces flared

FIGURE 5.3 *(continued)*

chest in a systematic manner to evaluate the temperature, turgor, and moistness of the skin, any area of pain or tenderness, and any masses. Next, the position of the trachea is evaluated. The trachea is located by palpating the suprasternal notch. With slight depression of the finger through the suprasternal notch, the tracheal rings can be felt and the midline position of the trachea assessed. Tracheal deviation can result from several conditions. A pleural effusion, spontaneous pneumothorax, or tumor will cause tracheal deviation to the opposite side. Conversely, conditions such as atelectasis and fibrosis will pull the trachea and mediastinum toward the affected side. If tracheal deviation is detected on physical examination a chest roentgenogram should be obtained to determine the cause of the shift.

Thoracic expansion is assessed for symmetry and depth. On the anterior chest, the examiner's hands are placed over the anterolateral chest with the thumbs extended along the costal margin, joining at the xiphoid process. The patient is instructed to take a deep breath while the nurse feels, observes, and compares both sides for depth and symmetry of movement. This procedure is repeated posteriorly, with the nurse's hands placed around the posterolateral chest at the level of the tenth rib. Any asymmetrical chest movement is abnormal and may indicate pneumothorax, atelectasis, pneumonia, or splinting resulting from pain. Depth of lung expansion should also be evaluated, especially to detect limited expansion on inspiration, which can alter oxygen and carbon dioxide exchange.

Any patient who has sustained an injury, invasion, or operation of the thorax is examined for crepitus. Crepitus, also called subcutaneous emphysema, is caused by air leaking from the lungs into the subcutaneous tissues. On palpation, cracking or popping will be heard and felt. This condition may occur as a consequence of chest tube or central line catheter placement, a broken rib, or air leakage around a tracheostomy.

Percussion

Percussion of the chest is used to identify the lung boundaries and such abnormal conditions within the lung as fluid accumulation. Changes in the percussion notes from resonant to dull or hyperresonant give clues that the normal air-filled lung has been replaced by fluid or solid matter. Dullness replaces resonance over areas of the lung that are consolidated or atelectatic or that contain pleural fluid, as with effusions. Hyperresonance is associated with air trapping, which occurs in emphysema or with a pneumothorax.

Auscultation

Auscultation is frequently performed on the critically ill patient to assess the quality and character of breath sounds, the effectiveness of suctioning and chest physiotherapy, and the position of endotracheal tubes.

The optimal position of the patient for auscultation is sitting upright and undressed to the waist; the optimal environment is warm and quiet. If the patient cannot sit upright, the posterior chest can be auscultated with the patient on his side. Abnormalities may be heard in the dependent lung, however, that are related to positioning rather than to a pathophysiological condition. When the patient is on his side, expansion on inspiration is decreased, gravitational stress predisposes the airway to collapse at low lung volumes [25], and there is increased blood flow to dependent regions of the lung. Controlling environmental noise may necessitate temporarily shutting off oxygen, suction, and the audio pulse of the cardiac monitor, as well as closing the door and eliminating conversation.

The nurse auscultates the anterior, posterior, and lateral chest at about 5 cm intervals from top to bottom, comparing one side of the chest with the other, while the patient breathes deeply through the mouth.

Although the exact origin and mechanism of breath sounds are unclear, the sounds are thought to be produced by the movement of gases through the airways, which creates vibrations either within the gas or from the walls of the airways. Normal breath sounds vary in quality over different portions of the lung; these various sounds previously were called bronchial, bronchovesicular, and vesicular. Although the terminology and characteristics of normal breath sounds are clearly described in the literature, pulmonologists generally agree that the terminology has been confusing, and findings have varied among examiners [26]. In addition, experimentation with advanced instrumentation has altered earlier beliefs about the cause of breath sounds [13]. In response to these problems and changes, the Joint Committee on Pulmonary Nomenclature, which includes members from the American Thoracic Society and the American College of Chest Physicians, has recommended changes in pulmonary nomenclature (Table 5.1) [42].

Breath sounds heard over the larger airways are to be called *bronchial.* These sounds are heard over the trachea, in the midline of the upper anterior chest both to the right and to the left of the sternum, and in the right anterior chest, as well as on the back between the scapulae [26]. Sounds that travel the shortest distance are heard as the loudest; thus, bronchial breath sounds are described as loud, harsh, and high pitched. Expiration is generally louder and longer than inspiration, with a brief pause between these phases. Breath sounds heard at a distance from the large airways are best described as *normal* (previously called vesicular) [42]. They are heard over most of the lung fields and are described as soft and low pitched. Inspiration is longer and louder than expiration. Normal breath sounds are best heard when the patient is taking deep breaths and may be diminished if the patient is hypoventilating or has a thick chest wall.

In abnormal situations breath sound transmission is altered. Sounds are enhanced when air spaces are filled with fluid or consolidated, conditions that occur in pneumonia, pulmonary edema, and partial atelectasis. The result is the production of bronchial sounds over areas where normal sounds should be heard.

TABLE 5.1
Revised Terminology for Breath Sounds

Old Terminology	New Terminology	Clinical Association
Bronchial; bronchovesicular	Bronchial	Large airways
Vesicular	Normal	Lower lung tissue
Rale	Crackle	Pulmonary edema, pneumonia, atelectasis
Rhonchus	Rhonchus	Sputum production
Wheeze	Wheeze	Airway narrowing

Decreased or absent breath sounds may result when air flow is interfered with, such as by an obstructed bronchus or misplaced endotracheal tube, and when air or fluid fills the pleural cavity, as in pneumothorax and pleural effusion.

Adventitious sounds are abnormal breath sounds that are superimposed on normal sounds. They previously were called rales, rhonchi, and wheezes, with further subdivisions to describe varying quality. Rales, for example, were described as fine, medium, or coarse and as wet, dry, or crepitant. The Joint Committee on Pulmonary Nomenclature [42] recommends that adventitious sounds be defined by their acoustic properties, with two main categories: discontinuous and continuous sounds.

Discontinuous sounds are intermittent, crackling, or bubbling and are called *crackles* (rather than rales). These are heard best on inspiration and are of short duration. They are further subdivided into coarse sounds, which are louder, longer, and lower pitched, and fine sounds, which are softer, shorter, and higher pitched. At present it is uncertain whether the crackle sound results from air pressure equalization in the air spaces, from the bursting of a film of surface material as a collapsed segment of the airway opens, or from a combination of the two sources [26]. Crackles are commonly found in patients with pulmonary edema, airway obstruction, interstitial fibrosis, atelectasis, and pneumonia.

Continuous sounds have a musical quality and a longer duration than discontinous sounds. High-pitched sounds, called *wheezes*, are thought to result from air passing through a narrowed airway. Wheezes are most commonly associated with asthma. Low-pitched continuous sounds are called *rhonchi*. They are often associated with chronic sputum production, as occurs in chronic obstructive pulmonary disease.

Another adventitious sound heard in the chest, but one not classified as continuous or discontinuous, is a pleural friction rub. This sound is produced by inflammation within the pleura and is described as rough, grating, scratching, or creaking. It is heard best over the anterolateral chest, during both inspiration and expiration, but may disappear after a few breaths. This sound is unaffected by coughing and can be differentiated from a pericardial friction rub because it disappears with breath holding.

The findings from the history taking and physical examination can be used to assess the patient's condition, plan the necessary interventions, prevent complications, and guide the selection of various laboratory tests necessary to make accurate diagnoses. One particular laboratory test that is used very frequently in the ICU is arterial blood gases.

ARTERIAL BLOOD GAS INTERPRETATION

Arterial blood gases (ABGs) are ordered in a variety of clinical situations. The information obtained from this simple laboratory test is invaluable in the assessment, diagnosis, and treatment of the critically ill patient. Blood gases reveal information regarding the acid-base status of the patient and the adequacy of tissue oxygenation. Acid-base balance is determined by evaluating the pH, arterial carbon dioxide tension ($PaCO_2$), and bicarbonate (HCO_3^-) level. Tissue oxygenation is determined by evaluating the arterial oxygen tension (PaO_2) and the O_2 saturation.

The most common indications for blood gas sampling are (1) pulmonary disorders such as chronic obstructive lung disease, respiratory failure, respiratory distress syndrome, and atelectasis; (2) cardiac disorders such as myocardial infarction, congestive heart failure, and pulmonary edema; (3) metabolic problems such as diabetic ketoacidosis; (4) any critical illness or postoperative state, and (5) any form of oxygen therapy or mechanical ventilation. In addition, blood gas analysis may be used to evaluate the effectiveness of a particular intervention or change in therapy.

A blood gas sample is obtained by withdrawing approximately 2 to 5 cc of blood from an artery, either from a preexisting arterial line or by percutaneous puncture. A heparinized syringe is used to prevent clotting. The specimen is immediately immersed in ice to reduce the metabolic activity of the blood cells and to prevent oxygen consumption within the syringe [24]. Information that should be noted on the accompanying laboratory requisition form includes the patient's temperature, the inspired oxygen concentration (FIO_2), and, if the patient is receiving ventilatory assistance, the respiratory rate and tidal volume.

Any patient who requires frequent ABG analysis should have an arterial catheter inserted to minimize the discomfort and potential complications associated with repeated direct arterial puncture. The arteries most commonly used to obtain an ABG sample are the radial, brachial, and femoral, with the last being the least preferred site, for several reasons. First, there is a high incidence of atherosclerotic plaques in the femoral area, and these have the potential to break off and travel to any area of the body. Second, the femoral artery is a large vessel and therefore has a greater potential for causing retroperitoneal bleeding that may go undetected. Third, the potential detriment to distal circulation is great.

Arterial spasm, emboli, and hematoma or aneurysm formation are additional complications that may result from arterial puncture. Hematoma or aneurysm formation at the puncture site may be prevented by applying firm pressure over the area for approximately 5 to 10 minutes after puncture. If arterial spasm is suspected, a warm, moist towel applied over the artery for 5 minutes may relieve the spasm.

The nursing responsibilities associated with ABG analysis vary among institutions but may include (1) assessing the patient's condition and determining the necessity for and frequency of ABG sampling, (2) obtaining the specimen, (3) interpreting the results in conjunction with other clinical findings, (4) planning and implementing the appropriate interventions, and (5) evaluating the effectiveness of the interventions.

ABG results should be interpreted systematically. First, the PaO_2 and percentage of O_2 saturation should be evaluated to determine the adequacy of oxygenation. Then the pH, PCO_2 and HCO_3^- level should be examined to determine the acid-base balance of the patient. Normal values are listed in Table 5.2. The procedure for systematic analysis of acid-base disorders is outlined in Exhibit 5.1, along with some important points to remember for ABG analysis. Once the blood gas is evaluated and a diagnosis made, therapy should

TABLE 5.2
Normal Blood Gas Values

Blood Gas	Arterial Blood	Mixed Venous Blood
pH	7.35–7.45 (7.40)	7.31–7.41 (7.36)
PCO_2	35–45 mm Hg	41–51 mm Hg
HCO_3^-	22–26 mEq/L	22–26 mEq/L
PaO_2	80–100 mm Hg	35–45 mm Hg
% sat.	$\geq$ 95%	70–75%

be initiated, if necessary, and evaluated. The goal of ABG analysis is to treat the primary or underlying problem, not interpret the results.

Evaluating Oxygenation

Before we discuss the method of evaluating oxygenation from ABG values, we will present a brief review of the principles of O_2 transport.

After O_2 has been inspired and diffuses the aveolar–capillary membrane, it must be carried to the tissues to be used in metabolic processes. Tissue oxygenation depends on three factors: (1) the arterial O_2 content of the blood (PaO_2), (2) total blood flow (cardiac output), and (3) the amount of hemoglobin (Hgb).

The normal O_2 carrying capacity of the blood is approximately 20 ml per 100 ml of blood. Almost all of this O_2, 98%, is bound to Hgb and is reported in the arterial blood gas result as the percentage of saturation (% sat.), also called So_2 or O_2 sat. The remainder of the O_2 is dissolved in solution (0.3 ml per 100 cc of blood) and is reflected in a blood gas result as the PaO_2, also called PO_2. It is the dissolved portion of oxygen that determines the PO_2 and affects the amount of oxygen that combines with Hgb. The relationship between the PO_2 and the O_2 sat. is illustrated in the oxyhemoglobin dissociation curve, which will be discussed in more detail later in this chapter. When the PO_2 is within normal limits, about 97% of the Hgb becomes saturated with O_2. Assuming that a patient has a normal cardiac output and Hgb count, tissue oxygenation is generally considered adequate if the O_2 sat. is at least 90%.

PO_2

The PO_2 represents the pressure of the oxygen dissolved in solution and is normally between 80 and 100 mm Hg. When evaluating a patient's PO_2, one must take the following factors into consideration: (1) the FIO_2 at the time the sample was drawn, (2) the expected PO_2, (3) the patient's age, and (4) the altitude. The FIO_2 of room air is 21%. In the absence of underlying abnormalities, any increase in the percentage of O_2 delivered will result in an increase in the PO_2. Thus, the expected PO_2 at any FIO_2 can be estimated by multiplying the delivered FIO_2 by 5 [14]. For example, a patient receiving 35% O_2 should have a PO_2 of approximately 175, that is, 35% $\times$ 5 = 175. Comparing the expected PO_2 with the actual PO_2 provides an indicator of the extent of underlying abnormality. Generally, the greater the difference, the more severe

EXHIBIT 5.1
Systematic Analysis of Acid-Base Balance

Important Points

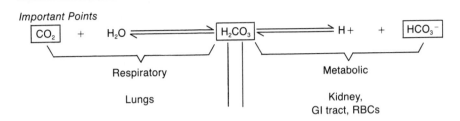

$$CO_2 \; + \; H_2O \rightleftharpoons H_2CO_3 \rightleftharpoons H+ \; + \; HCO_3^-$$

Respiratory

Lungs

Metabolic

Kidney,
GI tract, RBCs

Respiratory

	pH	PCO$_2$
Acidosis	↓	↑
Alkalosis	↑	↓

Metabolic

	pH	HCO$_3^-$
Acidosis	↓	↓
Alkalosis	↑	↑

Normal Values

pH 7.35–7.45   PCO$_2$ 35–45 mm Hg   HCO$_3^-$ 22–26 mm Hg

Analysis

Step 1: Examine the pH: is it normal, acidotic, or alkalotic?

A pH < 7.35 indicates acidemia.

A pH > 7.45 indicates alkalosis.

A normal pH with an abnormal HCO$_3^-$ level + PCO$_2$ indicates a compensated acid-base disorder.

Step 2: Examine the PaCO$_2$: is it normal, elevated, or decreased?

↑ PaCO$_2$ with ↓ pH indicates respiratory acidosis.

↓ PaCO$_2$ with ↑ pH indicates respiratory alkalosis.

↑ PaCO$_2$ with a pH > 7.40 indicates compensation for metabolic alkalosis.

↓ PaCO$_2$ with a pH < 7.40 indicates compensation for metabolic acidosis.

Step 3: Examine the HCO$_3^-$ level: is it normal, elevated, or decreased?

↑ HCO$_3^-$ with ↑ pH indicates a metabolic alkalosis.

↓ HCO$_3^-$ with ↓ pH indicates a metabolic acidosis.

↑ HCO$_3^-$ with a pH < 7.40 indicates compensation for a respiratory acidosis.

↓ HCO$_3^-$ with a pH > 7.40 indicates compensation for a respiratory alkalosis.

Step 4: Determine the cause of the acid-base disorder by examining the patient's history and present physiological status.

Step 5: Institute the appropriate therapy.

Step 6: Evaluate the effectiveness of therapy by repeating an ABG analysis.

Adapted from Vinsant, M., and Spence, M. *Commonsense Approach to Coronary Care.* St. Louis: Mosby, 1981. Used with permission.

the problem. If the actual PO_2 is approximately equal to the expected PO_2, then gas exchange is near normal.

Age must also be considered when evaluating a patient's PO_2. The value of 80 to 100 mm Hg is considered normal for children and adults through middle age. Older persons, more than 60 years of age, generally have lower PO_2 levels. To estimate the normal PO_2 for persons over the age of 60, some authors recommend subtracting 1 mm Hg from the minimal 80 mm Hg for every year over 60 [36]. Thus, the estimated PO_2 for a 70-year-old man would be 80 mm Hg − 10 years = 70 mm Hg.

Altitude also affects the PO_2 and, consequently, the O_2 sat.; the change is not apparent, however, unless the elevation exceeds approximately 5,000 feet. With ascent to high altitudes, there is a decrease in the total atmospheric pressure and in the partial pressure of oxygen inhaled. At sea level the inspired O_2 tension is 150 mm Hg, at 5,000 feet it is 125 mm Hg, and at 10,000 feet it is 100 mm Hg. Although these changes represent a relatively large decrease in arterial O_2 tension, the effect on arterial O_2 saturation is much less because of the shape of the oxyhemoglobin dissociation curve. Thus, following adaptation to an elevation of 14,000 feet, the arterial O_2 saturation is still 85% [16].

Hypoxemia

Hypoxemia is defined as a low arterial O_2 level (PaO_2) and is categorized into three types, according to severity [18]. *Mild hypoxemia* is associated with a PO_2 of 60 to 75 mm Hg. Patients with mild hypoxemia are often asymptomatic, because the blood is still approximately 90% saturated. In *moderate hypoxemia* the PO_2 is between 40 and 60 mm Hg and is associated with confusion, anxiety, restlessness, dyspnea, tachycardia, and hypertension. *Severe hypoxemia*, in which the PO_2 is below 40, may result in hypotension, dysrhythmias, cyanosis, coma, or cardiac arrest. Hypoxemia is a common problem in the critical care area, and thus its causes warrant further discussion. The four physiological causes of hypoxemia are depicted in Figure 5.4.

Hypoventilation.   Hypoventilation is defined by the presence of an increased $PaCO_2$, or hypercapnia. The lungs are not able to eliminate the CO_2 produced by the body, and as the alveolar CO_2 tension increases, the alveolar PO_2 decreases, resulting in a decreased arterial PO_2 (see Figure 5.4B). Hypoventilation can result from a variety of conditions, including (1) injury to or depression of the respiratory center by increased intracranial pressure, oversedation, anesthesia, or other causes; (2) interference with neuromuscular impulses, as occurs in Guillain-Barré syndrome and myasthenia gravis; (3) airway obstruction; and (4) decreased compliance of the lungs or reduced chest wall mobility related to a flail chest, or splinting caused by pain or obesity. The treatment of hypoventilation is related to the particular cause and may range from administering analgesics, to encouraging coughing and deep breathing for the patient who is splinting because of incisional pain, to providing assisted mechanical ventilation for the patient with myasthenia gravis.

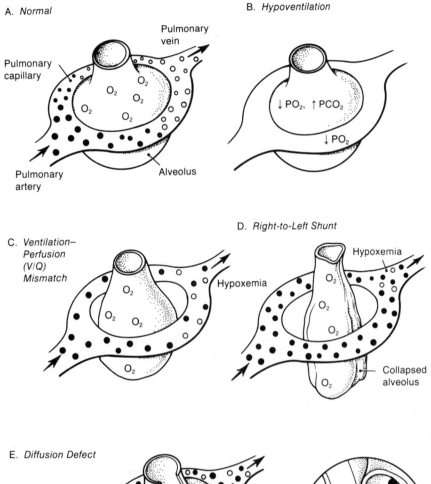

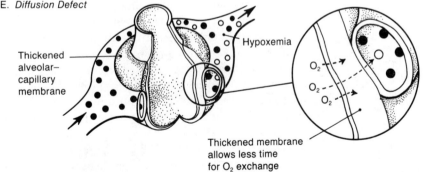

FIGURE 5.4
The four physiological causes of hypoxemia. (A) A normal alveolar–capillary unit.
Unoxygenated blood (*filled circles*) in the pulmonary capillary obtains O_2 from the alveolus.
Oxygenated blood (*open circles*) leaves via the pulmonary veins. (B) Hypoventilation
results in an increased PCO_2 and decreased PO_2. (C) Ventilation–perfusion mismatch
resulting from poor alveolar ventilation; hypoxemia results. (D) Right-to-left shunt.
Hypoxemia results from many disorders, all of which lead to collapsed alveoli. (E) Diffusion
defect. The diffusion of O_2 across the alveolar–capillary membrane is decreased when the
membrane is thickened or filled with fluid.

Ventilation–perfusion mismatch.   The transfer of O_2 and CO_2 across the alveolar–capillary membrane depends on the movement of gases into and out of the alveoli (ventilation) and adequate blood flow (perfusion) through the pulmonary capillaries. Imbalances or mismatches in the ventilation/perfusion ratio (V/Q ratio) are one of the most common causes of arterial hypoxemia. Alveolar ventilation averages about 4.2 L per minute, and pulmonary capillary blood flow averages about 5.0 L per minute; therefore, the normal V/Q ratio is 4.2:5.0, or 0.8. Because either ventilation or perfusion can be affected by disease, V/Q ratios can be greater or less than 0.8; only low or diminished V/Q ratios contribute to arterial hypoxemia, however. Low V/Q ratios result when alveoli are poorly ventilated but perfused adequately. This condition is illustrated in Figure 5.4C. Some of the common clinical disorders that result in poor or decreased alveolar ventilation are pulmonary edema, pneumonia, atelectasis, and bronchitis. High V/Q ratios occur when portions of the lungs are underperfused but adequately ventilated, as in the presence of pulmonary emboli or low cardiac output. Patients with low cardiac output still experience tissue hypoxia, but it is related to reduced O_2 delivery rather than to decreased alveolar or arterial PO_2.

Right-to-left shunt.   A right-to-left shunt occurs when venous blood that has not been oxygenated mixes with arterial blood. A physiological shunt consists of two components, an anatomical shunt and an intrapulmonary (also called capillary) shunt [34]. A normal anatomical shunt occurs in all individuals when unoxygenated blood from the bronchial, thebesian, and pleural veins enters the left side of the heart, bypassing the pulmonary capillaries. This blood makes up about 2% to 5% of the cardiac output but has minimal effect on arterial PO_2. Abnormal anatomical shunts occur with congenital heart defects such as atrial and ventricular septal defects. Such conditions may cause right-to-left or left-to-right shunting.

Intrapulmonary shunting will cause varying degrees of hypoxemia, depending on the surface area affected. In this situation perfusion is normal but the alveoli cannot participate in gas exchange because they are underventilated, obstructed, collapsed, or filled with fluid or secretions. Such a condition is also called an absolute or true shunt. Intrapulmonary shunting can occur with pulmonary edema, atelectasis, pneumonia, alveolar collapse, or airway obstruction. The effect on arterial PO_2 is illustrated in Figure 5.4D.

Diffusion defects.   The diffusion of gases across the alveolar–capillary membrane is affected by the pressure gradient, the thickness of the membrane, the total surface area, and the diffusion coefficients of the gases. Diffusion defects occur in patients with pulmonary edema, interstitial fibrosis, and sarcoidosis. In addition, the surface area may be decreased by such surgical procedures as lobectomy. Patients with mild to moderate diffusion defects usually have a normal PO_2 at rest but exhibit hypoxemia with exercise. Patients with severe defects exhibit hypoxemia even at rest (Figure 5.4E).

Alveolar–arterial oxygen difference.   Calculation of the alveolar–arterial O_2 difference, A-aDO_2 or P(A-a)O_2 or the A-a gradient, is frequently employed in the critical care unit to differentiate shunting from other causes of hypoxemia, to assess a patient's ability to be weaned from a respirator, and to evaluate the patient's condition. On room air, the normal A-aDO$_2$ is 5 to 15 mm Hg. With hypoventilation, hypoxemia appears, but the A-aDO$_2$ is normal. The gradient is elevated when hypoxemia is related to V/Q imbalances, diffusion defects, or right-to-left shunting. Patients with V/Q imbalances or diffusion defects demonstrate a normal PO$_2$ and A-aDO$_2$ after the administration of 100% O$_2$. Patients with right-to-left shunts, however, continue to have an elevated A-aDO$_2$ even after inspiring 100% O$_2$, because there is normal perfusion to underventilated alveoli [40]. Table 5.3 illustrates the differences in the PO$_2$, PCO$_2$, and A-aDO$_2$ on room air and 100% O$_2$ for the four causes of hypoxemia [4]. The procedure and equation for calculation of the A-aDO$_2$ is given in Exhibit 5.2.

TABLE 5.3
Physiological Bases of Hypoxemia

	FIO$_2$ 21% (Room Air)			FIO$_2$ 100% (20 min)	
	PO$_2$ (mm Hg)	PCO$_2$ (mm Hg)	A-aDO$_2$ (mm Hg)	PO$_2$ (mm Hg)	A-aDO$_2$ (mm Hg)
Normal	80–100	35–45	5–20	550–650	10–100
Hypoventilation	Low	High	Normal	Normal	Normal
V/Q imbalance	Low	Low, normal, high	Elevated	Normal	Normal
Diffusion block	Low	Low, normal	Elevated	Normal	Normal
Right-to-left shunt	Low	Low, normal	Elevated	Elevated	Elevated

Adapted from Burton, J. Arterial blood gases. I. *Crit. Care Update* 9(8):25, 1982. Used with permission.

EXHIBIT 5.2
Calculation of Alveolar–Arterial Oxygen Difference (A-aDO$_2$)

1. Administer 100% O$_2$ for 15 minutes.

2. Draw an ABG sample and send it for analysis.

3. Measure the patient's temperature and determine the water vapor pressure at that temperature. (See step 4.)

4. Calculate the alveolar oxygen tension (PAO$_2$) according to the equation

    $$PAO_2 = PB - PH_2O - PaCO_2{}^a$$

    where   PB = barometric pressure (760 mm Hg at sea level),
    PH$_2$O = water vapor pressure (47 at 37°C), and
    PaCO$_2$ = arterial carbon dioxide tension (normally 40 mm Hg).

5. Calculate the A-aDO$_2$ according to the equation

    $$A\text{-}aDO_2 = PAO_2 - PaO_2$$
    (normal value in 100% O$_2$, 10–100 mm Hg)

^{a}To calculate A-aDO$_2$ in room air (FIO$_2$ = 21%), the equation must be altered as follows:

$$PAO_2 = 0.21 (PB - PH_2O) - PaCO_2$$
(normal value, 5–15 mm Hg)

Hyperoxemia

Supplemental O_2 is commonly used in the ICU for the management of patients with hypoxemia, but the nurse must also be aware of the detrimental effects of high concentrations of O_2 on lung tissue. Hyperoxemia, or an elevated PO_2, results when too much O_2 is delivered. Recall that a PO_2 of 100 mm Hg is associated with a Hgb saturation level of approximately 98%. Therefore, any additional O_2 is of no benefit to the patient and may actually be detrimental.

Oxygen toxicity is related to two factors, the amount of O_2 delivered and the duration of exposure. The pulmonary changes associated with O_2 toxicity are alveolar and interstitial edema, alveolar hemorrhage, capillary endothelial cell damage, and alveolar membrane thickening. Cellular dysfunction leads to a decreased production of surfactant, atelectasis, and pulmonary edema, which reduces pulmonary compliance and creates severe hypoxemia because of intra-pulmonary shunting [14].

Every attempt should be made in the clinical area to prevent O_2 toxicity. Regardless of the method of O_2 delivery, clinicians should always use the low-est FIO_2 that will provide adequate tissue oxygenation. Although the normal saturation level is greater than 95%, tissue oxygenation is generally considered adequate so long as the percentage of saturation is more than 90; such a level corresponds to a PO_2 of approximately 60 mm Hg. Unfortunately, many crit-ically ill patients do not respond to O_2 therapy and may require higher con-centrations of O_2 to prevent hypoxemia. Attempts should be made, however, to keep the O_2 concentration inspired by the respirator-assisted patient below 50%. Additional therapeutic measures that may improve O_2 exchange and decrease the necessity for high concentrations of O_2 are chest physiotherapy, diuretics, and the addition of positive end-expiratory pressure (PEEP).

O_2 Saturation

The physiological relationship between the PO_2 and the oxyhemoglobin satu-ration level is illustrated in Figure 5.5. The top of the curve is relatively flat, which illustrates that a large drop in partial pressure, from 100 mm Hg to 70 mm Hg, lowers the Hgb saturation only from 97.5% to 92.7%. This small change in Hgb saturation has almost no effect on tissue oxygenation. As the PO_2 decreases below 60, the downward slope of the curve steepens, represent-ing a substantial decrease in Hgb saturation.

Several factors alter the affinity of Hgb for O_2 and thus the position of the oxyhemoglobin dissociation curve. Fever, acidosis, and hypercapnia are common in critically ill patients and cause a shift of the curve to the right. A shift in this direction indicates that Hgb has a decreased affinity for O_2 and thus releases O_2 to the tissues more readily. The curve is also shifted to the right by increased levels of 2,3-dephosphoglycerate (2,3-DPG). This inorganic phosphate, found in the red blood cell, is found in increased amounts with hypoxemia and anemia. Low levels of 2,3-DPG shift the curve to the left, as do alkalosis, hypocapnia, and decreased temperature. In these situations the affinity of Hgb for O_2 is increased, resulting in decreased dissociation at the cellular level (see Figure 5.5).

Although the normal saturation level of arterial blood is 95% or greater, the adequacy of oxygenation in each patient cannot be evaluated without ad-

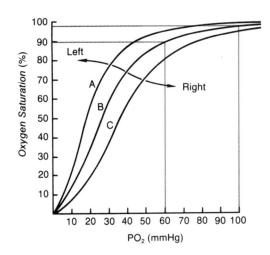

FIGURE 5.5
The oxyhemoglobin dissociation curve (B). The curve shifts to the right (C) with acidosis, fever, hypercapnia, and increased levels of 2,3-DPG. It shifts to the left (A) with decreased levels of 2,3-DPG, alkalosis, hypocapnia, and hypothermia.

ditional information. The patient's history, physiological state, metabolic needs, cardiac output, hemoglobin level, and age must all be considered. Another test that is commonly used in the ICU when evaluating oxygenation is the difference between arterial and venous oxygen content (A-VDO$_2$).

A-VDO$_2$. The arterial–venous oxygen content difference represents the amount of O$_2$ extracted by the tissues and is used as an estimate of cardiac output. The A-VDO$_2$ is derived from blood gas values from samples of arterial and mixed venous blood drawn and analyzed simultaneously. The normal values are listed in Table 5.2. A mixed venous sample is aspirated from a catheter in the pulmonary artery, where venous blood from all parts of the body is optimally mixed before being oxygenated [44]. The O$_2$ content of arterial blood is approximately 20 ml per 100 ml of blood; this is the amount of oxygen being delivered to the tissues. The oxygen content of venous blood is approximately 15 ml per 100 ml of blood. Thus, only 5 ml of O$_2$ in each 100 ml is extracted for utilization by the tissues. The formula for calculating either arterial or venous O$_2$ content is:

grams of Hgb × 1.34 × % sat.

where 1.34 represents the amount of O$_2$, in milliliters, that each gram of Hgb can store when fully saturated. Therefore, the arterial O$_2$ content in a patient with a Hgb concentration of 15 gm and an O$_2$ sat. of 95% is 15 gm Hgb × 1.34 ml O$_2$/Hgb × 95% = 19.1 ml O$_2$ per ml blood. The same equation is then used to calculate the venous O$_2$ content. If the O$_2$ sat. of venous blood is 70% (normal value, 70% to 75%), then the venous O$_2$ content is 14.1 ml. The A-VDO$_2$ is then calculated by subtracting the venous O$_2$ content from the arterial O$_2$ content (i.e., A-VDO$_2$ = 19.1 − 14.1 = 5 ml O$_2$ per 100 ml blood). An increase in the A-VDO$_2$ indicates that either tissue oxygen extraction has increased or cardiac output has decreased. Conversely, a decrease in the A-VDO$_2$ represents an increase in cardiac output.

The preceding discussion focused on the ABG values of PO$_2$ and O$_2$ sat. as indicators of tissue oxygenation. When they are evaluated in conjunction with the patient's cardiac output, Hgb concentration, and additional pulmonary measurements, the clinician can easily diagnose pathophysiological conditions and plan interventions accordingly. ABG studies are also frequently used to evaluate the patient's acid-base status.

Evaluating Acid-Base Balance

Basic Concepts of Acid-Base Balance

Hydrogen ions (H^+) greatly influence enzyme function and therefore most metabolic reactions in the body. Accordingly, the hydrogen-ion concentration (pH) of extracellular fluid is one of the most closely regulated chemical quantities in the body [43]. Acids are continuously liberated as metabolic by-products, yet the pH is kept within a narrow range of 7.35 to 7.45. The normal pH is maintained by the body's buffer systems, which prevent large changes in pH by chemically combining acids with other ions.

The most important buffer system is the bicarbonate buffer system, in which CO_2, a major end-product of metabolism, combines with water (H_2O) to form carbonic acid (H_2CO_3). Carbonic acid then dissociates into bicarbonate (HCO_3^-) and hydrogen ions (H^+). These chemical reactions are reversible and are illustrated in Figure 5.6. The law of mass action states that an increase in the concentration of any substance on one side of a reaction forces the reaction in the opposite direction [43]. Therefore, if the amount of either acid, free H^+, or CO_2 were increased, that substance would immediately combine and drive the reaction in the opposite direction. The normal pH of 7.35 to 7.45 is maintained by keeping a constant 20:1 ratio between the amounts of HCO_3^- and H_2CO_3 (see Figure 5.6). Acidemia, a pH below 7.35, results when the amount of acid increases or the amount of base decreases. Alkameia, a pH greater than 7.45, results when the amount of acid decreases or the amount of base increases.

The concentration of CO_2 in the bicarbonate buffer system is closely regulated by the lungs, and the concentration of HCO_3 is regulated by the kidneys. Thus, the respiratory system serves as a compensatory mechanism for metabolic acid-base imbalance and the renal system compensates for respiratory imbalances. Acid-base imbalances can be caused by primary disturbances in the respiratory system, such as a large pneumothorax, or by those in the renal system, such as acute renal failure. There are also numerous secondary causes of acid-base imbalances, such as electrolyte imbalance, overdose of sedatives, and neuromuscular dysfunction. In most individuals the diagnosis of respiratory acidosis or alkalosis, metabolic acidosis or alkalosis, or a mixed disorder can be made by evaluating the pH, HCO_3^-, and PCO_2. To determine the cause of the problem, however, the patient's history and present illness and other variables must be known.

Clinical Indications of Acidosis and Alkalosis

Because blood gas values are not always available, the nurse in the ICU should be familiar with the clinical indications of acid-base imbalances. Detecting subtle changes in the patient's behavior facilitates prompt diagnosis and treatment.

The early symptoms of acidosis are related to depression of the central nervous system. Tachypnea, complaints of headache, confusion, or lethargy

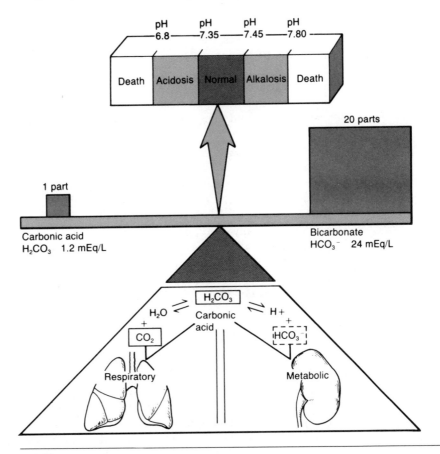

FIGURE 5.6
Acid-base balance is maintained by keeping a constant 20:1 ratio between the amounts of HCO_3^- and H_2CO_3. (See text for discussion.)

may be evident. As the condition worsens, dysrhythmias, dehydration, Kussmaul respiration, or coma may ensue.

The major effect of alkalosis is overexcitability of both the peripheral and central nervous systems. The patient may complain of dizziness, numbness or tingling in the fingers and toes, sweating, and develop dysrhythmias. In the more advanced stages, muscle weakness or spasm may occur. In the acute care setting, acid-base abnormalities are treated promptly before severe symptoms can develop.

Respiratory Acidosis
Respiratory acidosis results from an increase in PCO_2. The underlying mechanism is hypoventilation. Elimination of CO_2 by the lungs is directly related to the rate and depth of respiration. In hypoventilation, the PCO_2 rises to above 45 mm Hg, causing an automatic decrease in pH. Representative blood gas values in a patient with respiratory acidosis are a pH of 7.27, a PCO_2 of 55 mm Hg, and an HCO_3^- level of 24 mEq/L. Generally, a change of 10 mm Hg

in the PCO_2 is associated with a change in the pH of 0.08 in the opposite direction [22]. The causes of respiratory acidosis include oversedation with analgesics or other agents, neuromuscular disorders, trauma or injury to the chest, obstructive lung disease, and any other condition causing hypoventilation. Treatment is directed toward eliminating the precipitating factor. The goal of treatment is to increase ventilation, which should then correct the primary acidosis and return the pH to within normal limits.

Respiratory Alkalosis

Respiratory alkalosis occurs when exhalation of CO_2 from the lungs is increased. Such a condition results from hyperventilation. As the PCO_2 decreases, the pH increases. Representative blood gas values of a patient with respiratory alkalosis are a pH of 7.53, a PCO_2 of 25 mm Hg, and HCO_3^- level of 25 mEq/L. Any condition or disorder that causes hyperventilation will result in respiratory alkalosis. Some of the more common causes are anxiety, pain, pneumothorax, pulmonary embolism, brain injury, and overventilation with a controlled mechanical ventilator. Once the cause of the problem is identified, therapy is initiated to correct the alkalosis and restore the pH to normal.

Metabolic Acidosis

Metabolic acidosis results from either a loss of HCO_3^- or an increase in the amount of fixed acids. Sample blood gas values in metabolic acidosis are a pH of 7.10, a PCO_2 of 40 mm Hg, and a HCO_3^- level of 12 mEq/L. Disorders that increase the amount of fixed acids are ketoacidosis related to diabetes or starvation, lactic acidosis resulting from shock or cardiac arrest, renal failure, and poisonings. Metabolic acidosis can also result from a loss of bicarbonate, which can be caused by persistent diarrhea, and from treatment with acetazolamide or ammonium chloride [2]. The management of metabolic acidosis first involves identifying and treating the cause. If the pH is below 7.20 to 7.25, however, sodium bicarbonate is generally administered.

Metabolic Alkalosis

Metabolic alkalosis results from an increase in the HCO_3^- level. Such an increase can occur in two ways: through either an increase in the base bicarbonate level or a loss of fixed acids. Representative blood gas values in metabolic alkalosis are a pH of 7.58, a PCO_2 of 40 mm Hg, and a HCO_3^- level of 36 mEq/L. This condition often results when chloride ions (Cl^-) or potassium ions (K^+) are lost from body fluids because of vomiting, gastric suctioning, or excess diuresis. Alkalosis can also result from an increased ingestion of bases, as in excessive antacid intake. Treatment, again, is directed toward alleviating the cause.

Combined Disturbances

In certain situations patients may experience more than one primary acid-base abnormality at the same time. These conditions are called combined or mixed acid-base disturbances and are commonly encountered in the patient who has had a prolonged cardiopulmonary arrest. Blood gas analysis generally reveals a profound acidosis, as indicated by a pH of, for example, 7.10, which is caused by both a respiratory and a metabolic acidosis. The metabolic acidosis results from an accumulation of lactic acid, which is produced when metabolism occurs without adequate O_2. In addition, without ventilation, CO_2 is retained, resulting in a respiratory acidosis. Patients with respiratory or renal failure may also experience combined disturbances. Blood gas results, in these instances, may be more difficult to interpret.

Compensation

As previously mentioned, the maintenance of a normal pH is essential for normal cellular metabolism. If a primary acid-base abnormality is not corrected, the body's compensatory mechanisms will attempt to restore the pH to normal. In compensation, then, the pH is returned to the normal range by altering the system not primarily affected.

The kidneys compensate for a respiratory disorder by excreting or retaining HCO_3^-. A constant relationship exists between pH and HCO_3^-: As HCO_3^- decreases, so does the pH, and as HCO_3^- rises, so does the pH. Thus, if the kidneys excrete HCO_3^-, the pH will automatically drop. This is the mechanism involved in a compensated respiratory alkalosis. Conversely, if the kidneys retain HCO_3^-, the pH will increase, as in the case of a compensated respiratory acidosis (Table 5.4). Renal compensation occurs slowly over several days. Initially, blood gas values may reveal partial compensation, indicated by abnormal pH, PCO_2, and HCO_3^- values. Full compensation will take two to four days and is indicated by a normal pH coupled with abnormal PCO_2 and HCO_3^- values.

The respiratory system compensates for a metabolic disorder by retaining (through hypoventilation) or "blowing off" (through hyperventilation) CO_2. Respiratory compensation occurs faster, beginning within 1 to 2 hours after the onset of a metabolic imbalance. Here there is a constant relationship between pH and PCO_2, but this relationship is inverse: As the PCO_2 decreases,

TABLE 5.4
Representative Blood Gas Values in Uncompensated and Compensated Acid-Base Imbalances

Condition	pH	PCO₂ (mm Hg)	HCO₃⁻ (mEq/L)
Respiratory acidosis			
Uncompensated	7.27	55	24
Compensated	7.38	55	34
Respiratory alkalosis			
Uncompensated	7.53	25	25
Compensated	7.42	25	18
Metabolic acidosis			
Uncompensated	7.10	40	12
Compensated	7.38	22	12
Metabolic alkalosis			
Uncompensated	7.58	40	36
Compensated	7.42	58	36

pH increases, and as the PCO_2 increases, pH decreases. These relationships result from shifts in the bicarbonate buffer equation that alter the base-to-acid ratio.

Compensation for a metabolic acidosis results from hyperventilation. In severe cases, however, full compensation may not occur, because CO_2 excretion via the lungs is limited. In metabolic alkalosis, compensation results from hypoventilation, which increases the PCO_2 and decreases the pH (see Table 5.4). Again, in severe cases complete compensation is unusual. Once the PCO_2 rises to approximately 50 to 60 mm Hg, other ventilatory stimuli take over to prevent further increases in the PCO_2.

All the compensatory mechanisms function to return the pH to within normal limits. The detrimental effects of an acid-base disorder are directly related to the abnormal pH, not to the abnormal HCO_3^- or PCO_2 levels. The body generally does not overcompensate; thus, if the pH is 7.25, compensatory mechanisms may increase the pH to 7.40 and no further. This fact allows the clinician to determine the primary acid-base disturbance when a compensated blood gas sample is analyzed. Consider the following blood gas values: pH, 7.43; PCO_2, 53 mm Hg; HCO_3^-, 33 mEq/L. In this case the pH is normal, yet the PCO_2 and HCO_3 levels are both increased. One must decide which abnormal value, the increased PCO_2 or the HCO_3^-, is responsible for the primary process and which is the compensatory process. When analyzing compensated blood gas samples, 7.40 is used as the normal pH. Any value less than 7.40 is considered acidotic, and any pH greater than 7.40 is considered alkalotic. In this example, the pH of 7.43 indicates that the primary process is alkalosis, but is it respiratory or metabolic? This question is answered by recalling the relationships between pH and PCO_2, and pH and HCO_3^-. The relationship between pH and PCO_2 is inverse; that between pH and HCO_3^- is always in the same direction. In the example, then, the HCO_3^- level of 33 mEq/L would result in an alkalotic pH. With a metabolic alkalosis, the respiratory system compensates by retaining CO_2. As the CO_2 level rises, the pH will decrease. Thus, the primary process is a metabolic alkalosis with respiratory compensation.

BEDSIDE EVALUATION OF PULMONARY FUNCTION

Physical examination and ABG measurement are invaluable in the respiratory assessment of the critically ill patient. Chest roentgenography and various measurements of pulmonary ventilation, however, may also be useful.

Chest Roentgenograms

Chest roentgenograms are obtained from cardiac patients in the ICU for a variety of reasons. On admission to the hospital or ICU, a chest film may be used as part of the preoperative evaluation or to establish a baseline for subsequent comparison. The major use for this diagnostic test, however, is to evaluate the cardiac and pulmonary structures of the chest. Various cardiac and pulmonary disorders, such as pneumothorax, pleural effusions, infiltrates, pulmonary edema, cardiac hypertrophy, and atelectasis, may be evident on a chest roentgenogram and not on physical examination. Another major use of chest films in the ICU is to determine proper placement of various tubes and catheters, such as central or pulmonary artery catheters, cardiac pacing wires, and endotracheal, chest, and nasogastric tubes. In these cases a film should be obtained immediately after insertion and daily thereafter. Serial chest roentgenograms are frequently obtained of the cardiac surgical patient postoperatively to assess the mediastinum, which may widen if blood accumulates in the chest. Films made with portable equipment are obtained because it may be extremely difficult and dangerous to transport the ICU patient to the x-ray department. Unfortunately, the quality of the film obtained with a portable machine is generally inferior. The quality may be improved, however, by sitting the patient upright and, if possible, moving or removing equipment on the chest.

Ventilatory Volumes

Ventilation refers to the movement of air into and out of the lungs. Effective ventilation requires patent airways, compliant lungs, efficient musculoskeletal movement, and an adequate supply of air. The purpose of ventilation is to bring adequate amounts of air to the alveoli for gas exchange. Not all the air inspired with each breath participates in gas exchange, however.

Tidal Volume

Tidal volume (VT) is defined as the volume of air moved in and out of the lungs with each breath. The average VT for an adult is between 450 and 600 ml, or approximately 10 to 15 ml per kilogram. If the respiratory rate is constant, then decreases in VT are associated with hypocapnia. VT is divided into two categories to distinguish between the volume of air used for gas exchange and that wasted. That portion of ventilation that fills the tracheobronchial tree is called anatomical dead space (VD) or dead space ventilation, because it does not participate in gas exchange. This volume equals approximately 150 ml, or 1 ml per pound of body weight. Alveoli ventilation (VA) is that portion of ventilation that reaches the alveoli and participates in gas exchange. The formula to calculate VA is given in Exhibit 5.3. Although VA is easily calculated at the bedside, a more meaningful measurement is the ratio between dead space and tidal volume (VD/VT ratio).

VD/VT Ratio

This variable is used to assess a patient's ability to sustain prolonged spontaneous ventilation and may also provide diagnostic information about pathophysiological disorders [15]. The ratio is calculated from the PCO_2 of samples of arterial blood and mixed expired CO_2 (see Exhibit 5.3). The normal ratio ranges from 0.2 to 0.4 [24]. Ratios exceeding 0.6 indicate that the patient may have difficulty maintaining spontaneous ventilation.

Minute Ventilation

Minute ventilation (VE) is the total volume of air inhaled in 1 minute. It is the product of tidal volume and the respiratory rate: $VE = TV \times RR$. This test is easily performed at the bedside and may be used to evaluate a patient's ability to be weaned from a ventilator. The normal range of values is from 5 to 7 L per minute. Increases in VE may result from hypoxia, hypercapnia, and

EXHIBIT 5.3
Abbreviations, Normal Values, and Formulas for Ventilatory Volumes

VT	Tidal volume (450–600 cc or 10–15 cc/kg)
VD	Anatomical dead space (150 cc or 1 ml/lb)
VA	Alveolar ventilation (4,200 ml/min)
f or RR	Frequency or respiratory rate (12/min)
VD/VT ratio	Ratio of dead space to tidal volume (0.2–0.4)
VE	Minute ventilation (5–7 L/min)
VC	Vital capacity (70 cc/kg)
IRV	Inspiratory reserve volume (3,100 ml)
ERV	Expiratory reserve volume (1,200 ml)
IF	Inspiratory force (-60 to -100 cm H_2O)

$$VA = (VT - VD)RR$$

$$VD/VT = \frac{PaCO_2 - PECO_2}{PaCO_2}$$

where a = arterial, E = expired

$$VE = VT \times RR$$

$$VT = \frac{VE}{RR}$$

$$VC = IRV + VT + ERV$$

acidosis [15]. VE is also used to measure tidal volume more accurately. Because VT varies with each breath, it is more accurate to average the VT over 1 minute. We do so by dividing the VE by the respiratory rate (see Exhibit 5.3).

Vital Capacity
Vital capacity (VC) is defined as the maximal volume of air exhaled following a maximal inspiration. It is the sum of three lung volumes: the inspiratory reserve volume (IRV), tidal volume, and the expiratory reserve volume (ERV). Individual variations in VC are determined by age, sex, and height. The normal VC is approximately 70 ml per kilogram of body weight; adequate blood gas exchange can generally be maintained so long as the VC is above 15 ml per kilogram, however. Any disease or disorder that reduces pulmonary compliance will decrease VC.

Inspiratory Force

Inspiratory force or negative inspiratory force is a measurement of ventilatory reserve and muscle strength. It is often used to assess a patient's ability to be weaned from a mechanical ventilator. An inspiratory force meter is connected to the patient's airway. The patient is instructed to take a deep breath against an occluded airway; in the unconscious patient, inspiratory force is measured on a normal inspiration. Normal inspiratory force is approximately -60 to -100 cm H_2O. Patients with an inspiratory force exceeding -20 to -25 cm H_2O are generally able to maintain adequate ventilation. Measurements below

-20 cm H_2O indicate reduced respiratory strength, necessitating respiratory support. Such reduced strength may be caused by neuromuscular disorders, drugs, or chemicals.

SUMMARY

Thorough, accurate, and frequent assessment of the respiratory system of the critically ill patient is essential. Physical assessment, combined with data from various measurements, will allow the nurse to detect changes early and prevent physiological deterioration. Documentation and careful evaluation of trends, rather than isolated measurements, serves as the basis for planning, implementing, and evaluating therapeutic interventions.

STUDY QUESTIONS

1. List four reasons why the critically ill cardiac patient is at risk for pulmonary complications.
2. What specific information about the respiratory system should be obtained when completing a health history?
3. During inspection of the respiratory system, what should the nurse look for?
4. Define *orthopnea,* and list three physiological reasons why the condition is improved in the upright position.
5. List three possible causes of asymmetrical chest movement on inspiration.
6. What causes subcutaneous emphysema and with what conditions is this usually associated?
7. What percussion notes are associated with the following conditions?
   a. Normal lung tissue
   b. Emphysema
   c. Pleural effusion
   d. Atelectasis
8. Describe the proper procedure for auscultation of the respiratory system.
9. What type of breath sounds are heard over the following areas or in the following conditions?
   a. Trachea
   b. Normal lung tissue
   c. Consolidation
   d. Pneumothorax
   e. Pulmonary edema
10. Describe a pleural friction rub. Where is this best heard, and how can it be distinguished from a pericardial friction rub?
11. What are the two primary reasons for obtaining an ABG sample?
12. What five values are reported on an ABG sample, and what are the normal values?
13. List five possible complications associated with direct arterial puncture.
14. What factors should be considered when evaluating your patient's PO_2?

15. List four pulmonary changes associated with O_2 toxicity.

16. How does the bicarbonate buffer system influence pH?

17. List the acid-base disorder described by each of the following sets of ABG values:

pH	PCO$_2$ (mm Hg)	HCO$_3^-$ (mEq/L)	Disorder	
a. 7.30	55	25	_____	_____
b. 7.20	36	11	_____	_____
c. 7.45	50	30	_____	_____
d. 7.58	42	35	_____	_____
e. 7.52	24	24	_____	_____

18. List three signs and symptoms associated with acidosis, and three indicative of alkalosis.

19. What information can be obtained from a chest roentgenogram?

20. List the normal values for the following respiratory variables:
    a. Tidal volume
    b. Minute ventilation
    c. Vital capacity
    d. Inspiratory force

CASE STUDIES

CASE 1

A 60-year-old man has been admitted to the hospital for a triple coronary artery bypass graft. He is mildly overweight and has smoked two packages of cigarettes a day for 20 years.

You are assigned to care for the patient on his first postoperative day. The night shift has reported that the patient is still groggy and has not received medication for pain. Vital signs are temperature 98°F, pulse 76 beats/minute, and respiratory rate 10 breaths/minute; blood pressure is 100/70 mm Hg. Breath sounds are diminished at the bases bilaterally. The patient is receiving 40% O_2 via face mask, and ABG samples reveal a pH of 7.28, a PCO$_2$ of 55 mm Hg, a PO$_2$ of 70 mm Hg, HCO$_3^-$ level of 24 mEq/L, and a % sat. of 92%.

1. What is your interpretation of these blood gas values?

2. On the basis of these data, what factors could be contributing to or causing these ABG results?

3. What would your goal be for this patient, and what nursing interventions could improve this patient's ABG values?

4. How would you evaluate your interventions?

5. What ABG values would you expect to result with effective nursing care?

CASE 2

A 50-year-old woman admitted from the emergency room to the coronary care unit complains of severe retrosternal chest pain radiating to her left shoulder and arm. On admission she appears anxious and diaphoretic, and vital signs reveal a blood pressure of 140/90 mm Hg, pulse of 120 per minute, and respiratory rate of 28 per minute. Blood gas samples were drawn and revealed a PO$_2$ of 70 mm Hg, a PCO$_2$ of 25 mm Hg, an HCO$_3^-$ level of 24 mEq/L, a pH of 7.47, and a % sat. of 92%.

1. What is your interpretation of these ABG values?

2. What is the primary cause of the acid-base disorder in this patient?

3. Explain the physiological basis for these pH and % sat. values.

4. Does this patient need supplemental O_2? Explain the rationale for your answer.

5. What would be the primary nursing interventions for this ABG abnormality?

REFERENCES

1. Bates, B. *A Guide to Physical Examination* (3rd ed.). Philadelphia: Lippincott, 1983.

2. Broughton, J. O. Assessment Skills for the Nurse: Respiratory System, Understanding Blood Gases. In C. M. Hudak et al. (eds.), *Critical Care Nursing* (3rd ed.). Philadelphia: Lippincott, 1982.

3. Bull, S. Vascular pressures and critical care management. *Nurs. Clin. North Am.* 16:225, 1981.

4. Burton, J. Arterial blood gases. I. *Crit. Care Update* 9(8):25, 1982.

5. Burton, J. Arterial blood gases. II. *Crit. Care Update* 9(9):27, 1982.

6. Burton, J. Acid-base balance. III. *Crit. Care Update* 9(10):23, 1982.

7. Burton, J. Compensation of acid-base disturbances. IV. *Crit. Care Update* 9(11):15, 1982.

8. Cardin, S. Acid-base balance in the patient with respiratory disease. *Nurs. Clin. North Am.* 15:593, 1980.

9. Cohen, S. Blood-gas and acid-base concepts in respiratory care. *Am. J. Nurs.* 76(6):1, 1976.

10. D'Agostino, J. S. Set your mind at ease on oxygen toxicity. *Nurs. '83* 13(7):55, 1983.

11. Durham, N. Looking for complications of abdominal surgery. *Nurs. '75* 5(2):24, 1975.

12. Flenley, D. C. Blood gas and acid-base interpretation. *Basics RD* 10(1):1, 1981.

13. Forgacs, P. The functional basis of pulmonary sounds. *Chest* 73:339, 1978.

14. Harper, R. W. *A Guide to Respiratory Care.* Philadelphia: Lippincott, 1981.

15. Hunter, P. M. Bedside monitoring of respiratory function. *Nurs. Clin. North Am.* 16:211, 1981.

16. Hurst, J. W., et al. *The Heart.* New York: McGraw-Hill, 1982.

17. Jenkinson, S. G. Oxygen toxicity in acute respiratory failure. *Respir. Care* 28:614, 1983.

18. Kenner, C. V., Guzzetta, C. E., and Dossey, B. M. *Critical Care Nursing.* Boston: Little, Brown, 1981.

19. Kirilloff, L. H., and Maszkievicz, R. C. Guide to respiratory care in critically ill adults. *Am. J. Nurs.* 79:2005, 1979.

20. Levitzky, M. G. *Pulmonary Physiology.* New York: McGraw-Hill, 1982.

21. Malasanos, L., et al. *Health Assessment* (2nd ed.). St. Louis: Mosby, 1981.

22. McIntyre, K. M., and Lewis, A. J. *Advanced Cardiac Life Support.* Dallas: American Heart Association, 1981.

23. Mechner, F. Patient assessment: examination of the chest and lungs. *Am. J. Nurs.* 76(9):1, 1976.

24. Morrison, M. L. *Respiratory Intensive Care Nursing.* (2nd ed.). Boston: Little, Brown, 1979.

25. Murphy, R. L. Auscultation of the lung: past lessons, future possibilities. *Thorax* 36:99, 1981.

26. Murphy, R. L., and Holford, S. K. Lung sounds. *Basics RD* 8(4):1, 1980.

27. Neilsen, L. Assessing patients' respiratory problems. *Am. J. Nurs.* 80:2192, 1980.

28. Neilsen, L. Interpreting arterial blood gases. *Am. J. Nurs.* 80:2197, 1980.

29. Nett, L., and Petty, T. I. Oxygen toxicity. *Am. J. Nurs.* 73:1556, 1973.

30. Petty, T. L. Acid base and electrolyte disturbances in respiratory failure. In T. L. Petty (ed.)., *Intensive and Rehabilitative Respiratory Care* (3rd ed.). Philadelphia: Lea & Febiger, 1982.

31. Petty, T. L., and Bailey, D. A new versatile blood gas syringe. *Heart Lung* 10:672, 1981.

32. Robertson, K. J., and Guzzetta, C. E. Arterial blood-gas interpretations in the respiratory intensive care unit. *Heart Lung* 5:256, 1976.

33. Rokosky, J. S. Assessment of the individual with altered respiratory function. *Nurs. Clin. North Am.* 16:195, 1981.

34. Sanderson, R. G., and Kurth, C. L. *The Cardiac Patient* (2nd ed.). Philadelphia: Saunders, 1983.

35. Shapiro, B. A., Harrison, R. A., and Trout, C. A. *Clinical Application of Respiratory Care* (2nd ed.). Chicago: Year Book, 1979.

36. Shrake, K. The ABC's of ABG's. *Nurs. '79* 9(9):26, 1979.

37. Summer, S. M. Refining your technique for drawing arterial blood gases. *Nurs. '80* 10(4):65, 1980.

38. Thompson, J. M., and Bowers, A. C. *Clinical Manual of Health Assessment*. St. Louis: Mosby, 1980.

39. Tobey, J. A commonsense approach to arterial blood gases. *Crit. Care Q.* 2:67, 1979.

40. Traver, G. A. *Respiratory Nursing: The Science and the Art*. New York: Wiley, 1982.

41. Underhill, S. L., et al. *Cardiac Nursing*. Philadelphia: Lippincott, 1982.

42. Updated Nomenclature for Membership Reaction. *Am. Thorac. Soc. News* 3(4):5, 1977.

43. Vander, A. J., Sherman, J. H., and Luciano, D. S. *Human Physiology: The Mechanisms of Body Function* (2nd ed.). New York: McGraw-Hill, 1975.

44. Vinsant, M. O., and Lemberg, L. Arterial blood gases in the coronary care unit. III. *Heart Lung* 6:881, 1977.

45. Vinsant, M. O., and Spence, M. I. *Commonsense Approach to Coronary Care* (3rd ed.). St. Louise: Mosby, 1981.

46. Wade, J. F. *Comprehensive Respiratory Care* (3rd ed.). St. Louis: Mosby, 1982.

CHAPTER 6

Hemodynamic Assessment and Monitoring

Barbara Homer Yee □ *Susan Lynn Zorb*

INTRODUCTION

Advances in invasive hemodynamic monitoring techniques have significantly altered the care of the critically ill patient. Specialized catheters and electronic monitoring equipment allow the clinician to obtain additional information regarding the patient's cardiovascular status. These techniques permit the nurse to assess changes in the patient's physiological status more closely and to intervene before complications develop.

In the critical care unit, four techniques are frequently used to obtain direct measurements of various cardiac pressures. Arterial pressure monitoring can yield valuable information regarding blood pressure, cardiac function, and vascular resistance. Central venous pressure (CVP) measurements are useful in assessing the pressure in the right atrium. Information regarding left ventricular function can be obtained with the use of pulmonary artery (PA) catheters. Left atrial catheters provide a direct measurement of the pressure in the left atrium (LA) and are frequently used by cardiac surgeons.

Once a catheter is inserted by the physician, it must be connected immediately to a pressure transducer monitoring system. Therefore, all the necessary equipment must be assembled and calibrated before catheter insertion. This procedure, the equipment used, and the basic principles of hemodynamic monitoring will be described in this chapter. In addition, specific information regarding indications; techniques of insertion, measurement, and interpretation; and nursing responsibilities for each method of hemodynamic monitoring will be discussed.

PRINCIPLES OF HEMODYNAMIC MONITORING

Hemodynamics deals with the interrelationship of pressure, flow, and resistance within the cardiovascular system. Mechanical energy in the circulatory system is produced by the contraction of the heart and the movement of blood. This energy is transmitted throughout the blood vessels in a series of pulses or waves, which can be displayed on a pressure monitor. The configuration of the pressure waveform varies in each part of the vascular system. The nurse must be familiar with the normal configurations and pressures of the waveforms commonly monitored in the critical care unit (ICU).

Equipment

To monitor cardiac and intravascular pressures at the bedside, a catheter is placed in a vessel and connected to a pressure transducer system, which allows the mechanical energy in the vascular system to be converted into an interpretable electrical signal. The four components of a pressure monitoring system are (1) a catheter placed in the appropriate artery or vein and connected to fluid-filled pressure tubing, (2) a transducer, (3) a monitor with an oscilloscope, and (4) a continuous flush system (Figure 6.1). Each component of the pressure transducer system has specific criteria to ensure accurate measurements. The catheter used should have a large internal diameter that allows the mechanical energy to pass out of the vessel without obstruction. The catheter is then connected to pressure tubing that has rigid walls and resists expansion and contraction. This rigidity minimizes the amount of energy lost in transmission of the pulse. The pressure tubing is connected to a transducer, which

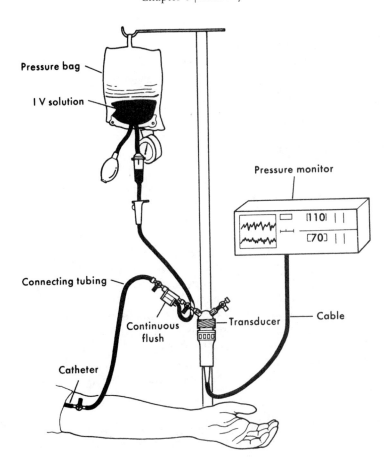

Pressure bag

I V solution

Pressure monitor

[110]

[70]

Connecting tubing

Continuous flush

Transducer — Cable

Catheter

FIGURE 6.1
Four components of the pressure monitoring system: catheter, transducer, monitor, and continuous flush. (From Daily, E. K., and Schroeder, J. S. Techniques in Bedside Hemodynamic Monitoring, 2nd ed. St. Louis: Mosby, 1981. Used with permission.)

actually converts the mechanical energy into an electrical signal. The mechanical energy is transmitted through the pressure tubing onto the diaphragm of the transducer. The diaphragm vibrates and produces an electrical signal that is amplified by the monitor. The waveform of the pulse is then displayed on the oscilloscope.

Waveforms vary in amplitude depending on the pressure within the system. Each monitor has various pressure scales — for example, 0 to 60, 0 to 100, and 0 to 200 mm Hg — that can be used appropriately so that all waveforms will be clearly visible. Low-pressure systems, such as pulmonary artery and left atrial pressure, would be monitored on the 0 to 60 mm Hg scale, whereas high-pressure systems, such as blood pressure, would be monitored on the 0 to 200 mm Hg scale. Pressure monitors are designed to measure the different points on each waveform and to record these values in a digital display. This system allows for continuous observation and assessment of both the pressure waveforms and the exact numerical value of the variable being monitored. Systolic, diastolic, or mean values can be recorded. Low-amplitude pressures such as the CVP, left atrial pressure (LAP), and pulmonary capillary wedge pressure (PCWP) are measured using the mean mode. High-amplitude pressures are measured using both the systolic and diastolic modes; mean pressures are also obtained, however (Figure 6.2).

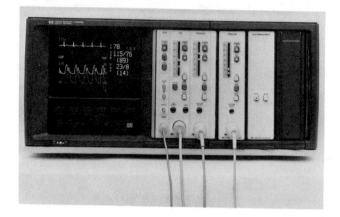

FIGURE 6.2
Waveforms displayed on a monitor, with pressure readings shown at right. (Used with permission from Hewlett Packard Co.)

The last essential component of the pressure transducer system is the continuous flush system. Heparin, in a concentration of 1 to 5 units per milliliter, is added to a bag of normal saline solution, placed under 300 mm Hg pressure by means of a pressure bag, and connected to a flush device (see Figure 6.1). Heparin is added to prevent clots from forming in and around the catheter tip. Counterpressure, from the pressure bag, is required to prevent backflow of blood from the vascular system. The flush device provides for an infusion at a constant 3 ml per hour into the catheter to maintain patency. It may also be operated manually to flush the system whenever necessary.

Obtaining Measurements

Before pressure measurements are obtained, several interventions must be performed to ensure accurate readings: the transducer must be leveled, and the monitor must be calibrated. To ensure accurate readings, the transducer must be leveled to the position of the right atrium. The standard level of reference is called the phlebostatic axis, or the external reference point. This point is found by imagining a line drawn from the fourth intercostal space at the sternum to the side of the chest, and a second line drawn at the midchest position. The point of intersection is marked on the patient's chest and should be used thereafter to obtain readings (Figure 6.3). If the transducer is lower than the patient's external reference point, the pressure will be falsely elevated; if it is higher, the pressure will be lower.

When hemodynamic monitoring was first instituted, it was assumed that the patient had to be in a supine, flat position for measurements to be accurate. It was soon recognized that this constant readjustment of the position of the head of the bed was detrimental to the patient's well-being. Subsequently, one large study conducted by nurse researchers found that reliable pressures can be obtained at backrest angles of 20 degrees or less [42]. Another study found no significant differences when pulmonary artery pressure measurements were taken in the supine and 20-, 45-, and 60-degree positions [27]. It is now recognized that reliable measurements can be obtained at various backrest positions so long as the transducer is releveled to a consistent reference point.

The transducer can be leveled to the position of the external reference point by several methods [32]: use of a carpenter's level, sighting or "eyeball-

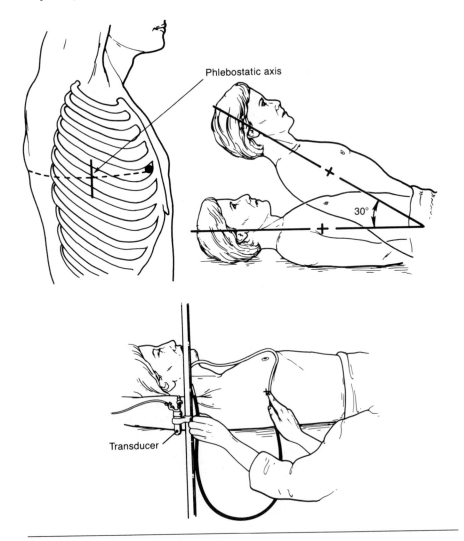

FIGURE 6.3
The phlebostatic axis, with the transducer leveled to that point using the closed-loop method. Measurements are not altered when the head of the bed is elevated so long as the transducer is releveled to the phlebostatic axis.

ing," or use of a closed-loop water leveler (see Figure 6.3). To ensure accuracy, either the carpenter's level or the closed-loop method is recommended. Releveling is generally done on every shift, whenever the position of the bed has been changed, or if measurements obtained are in question.

After positioning the patient, marking the external reference point, and leveling the transducer, the nurse must zero and calibrate the monitor. Pressure transducers are very sensitive, so the calibration must be checked frequently. To zero the transducer, one stopcock is opened to the atmosphere and that pressure is read as zero. If the pressure recorded is not zero, minor adjustments can be made on the monitor to obtain a reading of zero; if major adjustments

TABLE 6.1
Hemodynamic Troubleshooting Guide

Problem	Possible Causes	Interventions
Damped waveform: waveform contours are not sharp; amplitude is reduced	Air or blood in tubing; blood in the transducer; occlusion of the catheter tip	Check tubing and transducer for air bubbles; flush line with small amount of heparinized saline solution
	Loose connections	Check and tighten all connections
Catheter fling: waveform tall with many spikey distortions	Too much tubing between transducer and line	Remove excess tubing; there should be no more than 4 ft of tubing from catheter tip to transducer
	PA line coiled in ventricle	Check CXR; catheter may need to be repositioned
Tracing has disappeared from scope or is present at much lower values	Zero button pushed without the transducer open to air	Open transducer to air and rezero
PA tracing does not go into wedge when balloon is inflated	Balloon ruptured, if no resistance to injection is met	Do not inject more air
	Catheter no longer in good position; may have slipped further back in the pulmonary artery or into the right ventricle	Assess tracing for right ventricular waveform Check CXR for catheter position
Balloon inflation causes tracing to flatten out and escalate toward the top of the screen	Balloon overinflated or occluding the tip of the catheter	Deflate balloon and inflate with less air
Transducer cannot be zeroed	Disposable dome positioned incorrectly on the transducer membrane	Reposition the dome and rezero

PA = pulmonary artery; CXR = chest roentgenogram.

(greater than 10 mm Hg) are required, however, the monitor channel is probably faulty and should be replaced.

Calibrating the monitor ensures that the baseline used to display the various waveforms is exactly on the highest and lowest point of the pressure scale selected. The procedure used for calibration will vary depending on the equipment used and is easily learned in the clinical setting by demonstration. If there is any question about the accuracy of equipment, the transducer can be checked manually with a mercury sphygmomanometer. The transducer and monitor should be leveled, zeroed, and calibrated at least every 8 hours, whenever a major change in the readings occurs, or whenever inaccurate readings are suspected. A problem commonly associated with inaccurate readings is damping of the waveform. *Damping* is the term used to describe a loss of the sharp contours of the waveform. This and other problems associated with hemodynamic monitoring are outlined in Table 6.1, along with the appropriate nursing interventions.

Complications and Related Nursing Care

Invasive hemodynamic monitoring is associated with some risk; the majority of complications, however, can be prevented or minimized with proper maintenance of equipment and quality nursing care. Certain potential complications are common to various types of indwelling vascular catheters.

Infection

The widespread use of invasive hemodynamic monitoring devices in the ICU has resulted in an increased incidence of nosocomial infections. Kaye [23] reports that 45% of all nosocomial infections are device related, and approximately one-quarter of these are due to infusion fluids, intravascular catheters, or monitoring devices. It is essential that critical care staff be aware of this problem and adhere closely to policies and practices that prevent the development of infections in their patients. Infections related to hemodynamic monitoring devices can result from poor aseptic technique during insertion, or from contamination of the equipment during manufacture, set-up, or maintenance.

Several nursing interventions are recommended to prevent the development of infections. The insertion site must be examined for signs of redness, swelling, and drainage, which may indicate a developing infection. All dressings should be dated and initialed when changed. Dressing techniques vary from institution to institution. Generally, the site is cleansed and defatted using alcohol, acetone, or hydrogen peroxide. An iodine preparation is then used for its bacteriocidal and fungicidal properties. Povidone-iodine ointment is then applied to the insertion site, and the area is covered with a dry sterile dressing, which may be either air occlusive or nonocclusive. Air-occlusive dressings are changed every 48 hours, dry sterile dressings are changed daily, and transparent dressings are changed as necessary. In addition, the date of insertion of the catheter should be recorded in a visible place. All invasive lines should be removed as soon as possible or at the first sign of infection. If an infection is suspected, the catheter tip should be sent to the laboratory for culture and sensitivity testing.

Strict aseptic technique must be employed when setting up and manipulating any portion of the pressure transducer system. Any opening into the system must have some type of sterile covering. Use of any extra pieces of equipment, tubing, or stopcocks, and unnecessary manipulation of the equipment, should be avoided, because each increases the risk of contamination. The entire transducer system, including transducer dome, tubing, and intravenous solution, should be changed every 48 hours. Normal saline solution is recommended because 5% dextrose in water has been shown to support growth of various organisms [23]. Residual blood in or around the stopcocks or transducer also may result in increased infection. All stopcocks used for blood drawing must be kept covered and cleansed of blood after a sample has been obtained.

Blood Loss

Bleeding around the catheter insertion site can occur because of movement of the catheter; it can be resolved by suturing the catheter in place. If any connections within the pressure transducer system are loose or broken, bleeding may result. Such bleeding is especially dangerous with arterial catheters because of the high pressure within the artery. If any part of the system becomes completely disconnected, the patient can lose large quantities of blood very quickly. For this reason, all hemodynamic monitoring devices should be connected to systems with alarms that will respond to a fall in pressure. It is also important that all insertion sites and equipment be closely observed for blood loss.

Emboli

Air or blood emboli can also occur with hemodynamic monitoring. Air emboli can result when syringes and tubing are not properly inspected during infusions and when connections are loose. Whenever a foreign body is introduced into a vessel, microemboli may result because of irritation of the vessel. As a preventive measure, catheters should be manipulated as little as possible. The addition of heparin to the flush system and the use of a continuous flush system also help to prevent the formation of microemboli.

Diminished Circulation

The size of the catheter itself may cause diminished blood flow to the tissues beyond the insertion site. The cannulated extremity must be checked routinely for changes in skin color, sensation, temperature, pulses, and capillary filling. Any abnormal findings should be reported immediately to the physician.

ARTERIAL PRESSURE MONITORING

Intra-arterial pressure monitoring is frequently used in the ICU because it provides direct, continuous observation of the systolic, diastolic, and mean arterial pressures. Arterial cannulation can be performed easily by percutaneous puncture of the artery and, in more difficult situations, via surgical cutdown. The most common sites for arterial cannulation are the radial, brachial, and femoral arteries.

Indications

Arterial monitoring is especially valuable in the following patients: (1) those who are hypotensive, hypertensive, or hemodynamically unstable, (2) those receiving potent vasoactive substances, (3) those who need frequent arterial blood sampling, and (4) those who require intra-aortic balloon counterpulsation [16].

In the hypotensive patient it is often difficult for the nurse to auscultate an accurate blood pressure. In this instance an arterial catheter can provide continuous, accurate measurement of the patient's blood pressure. Continuous measurement is especially important when the patient's condition is unstable and the nurse must continually reassess the effects of the interventions used. The patient who is receiving potent vasoconstrictive or vasodilating agents must be monitored constantly for rapid changes in blood pressure that would necessitate either an adjustment in the dose of the medication or additional interventions.

An arterial catheter also provides easy access to arterial blood, permitting frequent blood gas samples and blood for electrolyte evaluation to be obtained with minimal discomfort to the patient. An arterial catheter is essential for the patient with an intra-aortic balloon pump to ensure accurate timing. If the timing is off, the patient will not receive full therapeutic effects from the balloon.

Waveforms

The arterial waveform represents the ejection of blood into the aorta and its movement through the periphery. The waveform begins with the opening of the aortic valve. The initial upslope is rapid and sharp and represents the rapid ejection of blood into the aorta. The peak of the waveform denotes the systolic pressure. The peak is generally slightly rounded, and the downslope is more gradual than the upslope. The dicrotic notch appears in the downslope as a slight hump; it represents the closure of the aortic valve and the end of systole. The diastolic pressure is the lowest point in the waveform and is a product of the resistance in the vessel walls (Figure 6.4A).

Examination of the arterial waveform can yield valuable information regarding both blood pressure and cardiac function. A delay in the rapid rising of the upstroke suggests a decrease in myocardial contractility or aortic stenosis (Figure 6.4B). Occurrence of the dicrotic notch on the lowest third of the downslope indicates a reduced cardiac output (Figure 6.4C). The waveform can also indicate the physiological effects of such abnormalities as tachypnea, irregular cardiac rates, perfusion with premature or ectopic beats, and hypotension.

Nursing Responsibilities

Nursing care of the patient with an intra-arterial catheter includes preparing the patient and the equipment for the procedure; leveling, zeroing, and calibrating the equipment; observing, assessing, and recording pressures; and preventing complications. Many of these techniques and interventions have been described in the section discussing the principles of hemodynamic monitoring. Additional nursing interventions specific to the patient with an arterial line will be mentioned here.

The nurse should ensure against catheter displacement by taping the catheter securely to the skin and immobilizing the extremity on an armboard.

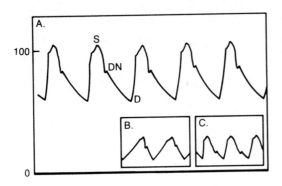

FIGURE 6.4

(A) Normal arterial waveform. (*S* = systole; *D* = diastole; *DN* = dicrotic notch.) (B) Arterial waveform with delayed upstroke. (C) Arterial waveform with low dicrotic notch.

This will also decrease internal catheter movement, which will lessen the incidence of thrombosis and arterial spasm. The cannulated extremity should always be in clear view of the nurse to permit detection of any signs of bleeding.

Arterial catheterization should be discontinued as soon as possible. Some institutions recommend that after catheter removal, the catheter tip be sent to the laboratory for culture and sensitivity testing. After the catheter is removed, direct pressure must be applied over the site for 5 to 10 minutes. This will prevent hemorrhage, hematoma formation, and the development of an aneurysm at the insertion site.

CENTRAL VENOUS PRESSURE MONITORING

Indications

Central venous catheters are commonly used in the clinical area to administer hyperalimentation and potent medications, and to withdraw blood for laboratory studies. In the ICU they are used most often to measure CVP. CVP represents the pressure in the right atrium, which reflects right-ventricular end-diastolic pressure (RVEDP), or preload. This pressure is regulated primarily by blood volume and venous tone. (Chapter 3 provides a review of cardiac physiology.) CVP monitoring is very valuable in assessing the condition of patients with disorders in fluid or blood volume. Serial measurements guide the clinician in fluid and blood replacement and the administration of vasopressors, vasodilators, and diuretics.

Measurements of CVP can be obtained with a thermodilution PA catheter or by insertion of a catheter in a central vein. The thermodilution technique will be discussed in the section describing PA pressure monitoring. The following discussion will focus on obtaining measurements using a CVP catheter and H_2O manometer.

Central venous catheter insertion can be performed at the bedside and involves percutaneous puncture of a vein. Although numerous veins can be used, the most commonly used are the internal or external jugular vein, the basilic or cephalic vein, and the subclavian veins [22]. Once inserted, the catheter is advanced into the superior vena cava or right atrium and connected to a three-way stopcock, manometer, and intravenous solution (Figure 6.5). Proper placement of the catheter tip must be confirmed by chest roentgenogram before measurements are obtained.

Obtaining and Interpreting Measurements

A consistent technique must be used to obtain CVP measurements if the results are to be considered a reliable indication of the patient's hemodynamic state. To obtain a CVP reading, the nurse positions the zero mark on the H_2O manometer at the patient's external reference point (see Figure 6.5). The three-way stopcock is turned off to the patient, thus allowing the manometer to fill with intravenous solution. The stopcock is then opened to the patient. The fluid level will fall until the pressure in the water column equilibrates with the patient's own pressure. When the fluid level stops falling, the numerical value is read and recorded.

With a manometer, CVP is measured in centimeters of water. If a transducer system is used, it is measured in millimeters of mercury. Conversions

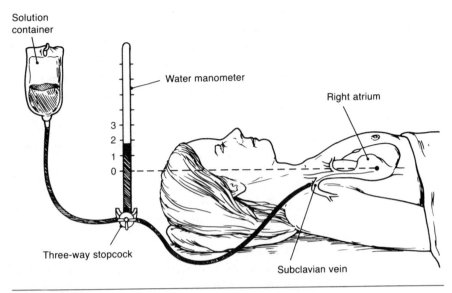

FIGURE 6.5
Central venous pressure monitoring. The zero mark on the manometer is leveled to the phlebostatic axis.

from one form of measurement to the other can be made readily based on the equivalence of 1 mm Hg and 1.36 cm H_2O. Therefore, centimeters of water can be converted to millimeters of mercury by dividing the former by 1.36. One converts millimeters of mercury to centimeters of water by multiplying by 1.36.

The normal CVP ranges from 4 to 10 cm H_2O, or from 2 to 6 mm Hg. A low CVP reading may indicate hypovolemia, dehydration, or vasodilatation. An elevated CVP occurs because of volume overload, right ventricular failure (which may or may not be secondary to left ventricular failure), pulmonary hypertension, tricuspid stenosis or regurgitation, constrictive pericarditis, and cardiac tamponade.

Serial measurements or the identification of trends in the readings is much more reliable than one isolated reading. The interpretation of CVP measurements should always be made in conjunction with evaluation of the patient's appearance and additional laboratory data.

Nursing Responsibilities

Once the CVP catheter has been inserted and baseline readings recorded, the primary goals in caring for the patient are to maintain patency of the system, monitor pressures, and prevent complications.

To maintain patency, the CVP catheter is connected to intravenous solution at a rate specified by the physician. A continuous flow of solution must be maintained to prevent clots from forming in or around the catheter tip. This continuous flow is interrupted while measurements are obtained; therefore, to ensure continued patency, CVP measurements should be obtained quickly. On occasion heparin may be added to the solution or used to flush the tubing. The infusion may be slowed if the tubing is kinked, if blood appears in the tubing, or if the height of the bottle is not sufficient. The CVP system is susceptible to clot formation if the drip rate is too slow or if the line is used frequently to draw blood or administer blood or colloids.

Insufficient or absent fluctuation of fluid in the H_2O manometer can be due to kinked or defective equipment, partial clotting at the catheter tip, or the resting of the catheter tip against the wall of the vein or right atrium. Aspiration with a syringe followed by gentle irrigation may clear the line. Force should never be used during irrigation. If these efforts are unsuccessful, the catheter should be removed.

Monitoring, recording, and interpreting CVP readings are a major responsibility of the nurse. Measurements must be consistent and accurate. Written guidelines for identifying the reference points and for leveling will facilitate consistency among staff members.

Despite the relative ease of insertion and maintenance of CVP catheters, complications can occur. The major complications are dysrhythmias, blood loss, infection, air emboli, and thromboemboli. Most of these complications, and the nursing interventions used in their prevention, have been discussed in the previous section.

Dysrhythmias, specifically ventricular, may occur during insertion, or later if the catheter slips into the right ventricle. Such dysrhythmias result from mechanical irritation of the right ventricular wall by the tip of the catheter. Dysrhythmias can be detected by observing the cardiac monitor or by feeling an irregular pulse. The problem can be resolved if the physician withdraws the catheter several inches.

Air emboli can occur during tubing changes because of pressure differences between the venous system and the atmosphere. The nurse can prevent this complication by placing the patient in a slight Trendelenburg position, instructing the patient to perform a Valsalva maneuver, and changing the tubing rapidly.

Thromboemboli are another potential complication of CVP monitoring. They can be avoided by maintaining a continuous flow of fluid through the system, adding low-dose heparin to the solution, flushing adequately after blood withdrawal, and avoiding the administration of blood or blood products through the line.

PULMONARY ARTERY PRESSURE MONITORING

The development of the flow-directed, balloon-tipped catheter has significantly altered the care of the critically ill patient. In 1970 H. J. C. Swan and W. Ganz designed the first double-lumen catheter. Since that time several types of PA catheters have been manufactured; the one most commonly used today, however, is the thermodilution catheter (Figure 6.6). The thermodilution catheter is designed to measure several variables that provide valuable information about left ventricular function. These include PA pressures (systolic [PAS], diastolic [PAD], and mean [PAM or MPAP]), PCWP, and cardiac output (CO) (see Figure 6.6). Assessment of these variables facilitates early diagnosis and

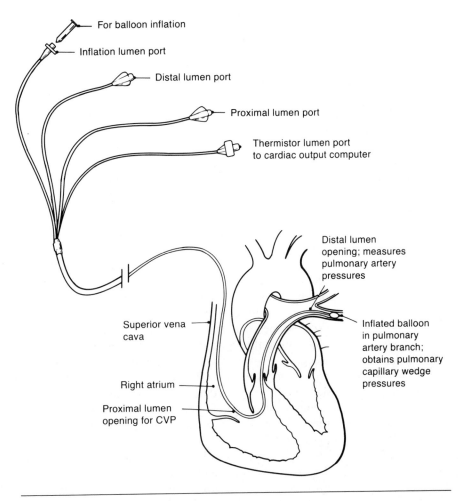

For balloon inflation

Inflation lumen port

Distal lumen port

Proximal lumen port

Thermistor lumen port
to cardiac output computer

Distal lumen
opening; measures
pulmonary artery
pressures

Inflated balloon
in pulmonary
artery branch;
obtains pulmonary
capillary wedge
pressures

Superior vena
cava

Right atrium

Proximal lumen
opening for CVP

FIGURE 6.6
Thermodilution pulmonary artery catheter in position in the heart.

more precise management of critically ill patients such as those with heart failure or cardiogenic shock.

The adequacy of CO is determined mainly by the efficiency of the left ventricle. The volume of blood in the left ventricle just before contraction is called left ventricular end-diastolic volume (LVEDV). This volume of blood creates a pressure called left ventricular end-diastolic pressure (LVEDP), which is a major determinant of left ventricular performance. With a thermodilution catheter, two measurements, PAD and PCWP, can be obtained that are approximately equal to LVEDP. The PCWP is obtained by inflating the balloon, which occludes a smaller pulmonary vessel. At the end of diastole, the mitral valve is open, permitting an unobstructed, and therefore equilibrated, flow of blood from the pulmonary arteries and capillaries to the left atrium and ventricle. An elevated PCWP indicates pulmonary congestion, because the level of

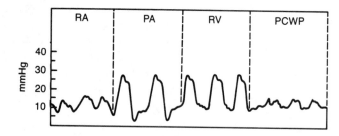

FIGURE 6.7
Waveforms produced during insertion of the
pulmonary artery catheter. (*RA* = right atrium;
RV = right ventricle; *PA* = pulmonary artery;
PCWP = pulmonary capillary wedge pressure.)

this pressure is a critical factor affecting the shift of fluid from the pulmonary capillaries into the interstitial and alveolar space. The PCWP is also important because it reflects LAP, which is an index of left ventricular filling pressure.

Insertion

The catheter can be inserted at the bedside either percutaneously, using the antecubital, jugular, or subclavian vein, or by means of a cutdown. The catheter is flushed with heparinized solution and attached to a pressure transducer, monitor, and oscilloscope. The position of the catheter tip can be estimated by observing the pressure waveform on the oscilloscope (Figure 6.7). The catheter is threaded through the vein until a right atrial wave pattern appears on the oscilloscope. The balloon is inflated at this point and carried by the flow of blood from the right atrium to the right ventricle and on into the PA until it wedges itself in one of the smaller branches. When the catheter is wedged, the pulmonary vessel is occluded, preventing blood flow distal to this point. Care must be taken to deflate the balloon quickly after obtaining wedge measurements to prevent pulmonary infarction. Once in position, the catheter is sutured in place and a chest roentgenogram is ordered to confirm proper placement.

Nursing responsibilities related to this procedure begin prior to insertion. The patient and family should be prepared and informed of the benefit of this invasive procedure. All equipment must be assembled, calibrated, and zeroed as previously described. In addition, it is generally the nurse's responsibility to observe the cardiac monitor for premature ventricular contractions (PVCs). PVCs result from mechanical irritation of the right ventricle by the catheter tip as the catheter is advanced. A prefilled syringe of lidocaine hydrochloride, a cardiac antiarrhythmic, should be at the bedside ready for use.

Measurement and Waveform Interpretation

Pulmonary Artery Pressures
Normal PA pressures and other hemodynamic values are listed in Table 6.2. Changes in intrathoracic pressure caused by labored breathing, mechanical ventilation, or positive end-expiratory breathing (PEEP) will alter PAP measurements. Elevated PAP can occur with disorders causing increased pulmonary vascular resistance, such as pulmonary hypertension and embolization; with increased pulmonary blood flow, as occurs in atrial septal defect (ASD) or ventricular septal defect (VSD); and in instances of increased pulmonary venous pressure, as in mitral stenosis or left ventricular failure [8].

The normal PCWP ranges from 4 to 12 mm Hg. Pulmonary congestion may be indicated early by a rising PCWP. Elevations in pressure will occur before the patient exhibits overt signs and symptoms of failure or fluid over-

TABLE 6.2
Normal Hemodynamic Values

Variable	Range
Pressures (mm Hg)	
Right atrial	2–6 *CVP*
Right ventricular	
Systolic	15–28
Diastolic	0–5
Pulmonary artery	
Systolic	15–30 *PAS*
Diastolic	5–15 *PAD*
Mean	10–20
Wedge	4–12 *Wedge*
Left atrial	4–12
Left ventricular	
Systolic	90–140
Diastolic	4–12
Calculations	
Cardiac output (L/min)	4–6 *CO*
Cardiac index (L/min/m²)	2.5–4.0
Stroke volume (ml/beat)	60–100
Stroke volume index (ml/beat/m²)	35–70
Left ventricular stroke work index (gm/m²)	45–60
Right ventricular stroke work index (gm/m²)	5–10
Pulmonary vascular resistance (dynes/sec/cm⁵)	45–150
Systemic vascular resistance (dynes/sec/cm⁵)	900–1500
Ejection fraction (%)	>60

load. A PCWP of greater than 18 mm Hg may be associated with heart failure, and pulmonary edema may occur if the pressure exceeds 30 mm Hg [7]. Other conditions that elevate the PCWP are mitral stenosis and insufficiency, pericarditis, and cardiac tamponade. A decreased PCWP usually indicates hypovolemia.

Cardiac Output

CO can be measured by several techniques. The most common methods are the Fick method, the indicator dilution method, and the thermodilution method. The thermodilution method is frequently used in the critical care area because it is accurate, it is easy to perform, and it can be done at the bedside using a thermodilution PA catheter.

To obtain a CO value, fluid of known volume and temperature is injected into the right atrium through the proximal lumen of the catheter. This fluid mixes with the blood, and the resulting temperature change is detected by the thermistor in the catheter tip, located in the PA. A temperature–time curve is recorded by the computer, and the CO is calculated and displayed (Figure 6.8).

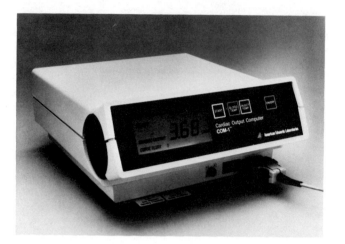

FIGURE 6.8
Thermodilution cardiac output computer, showing digital display. (Used with permission from American Edwards Laboratories.)

The exact procedure for obtaining a CO value will vary from unit to unit depending on the equipment available and individual practices. Certain techniques, however, are commonly used. Most often the injectate is 10 ml of 5% dextrose in water, which is either at room temperature or iced to 0°C. Generally, two or three measurements are obtained and the average computed and recorded. The CO value obtained is then evaluated in conjunction with other hemodynamic measurements and clinical signs and symptoms. The nursing staff must take great care to avoid errors in technique that could result in inaccurate measurements. The most common sources of error are inaccurate volume and temperature of injectate, variations in injection techniques, and altered location of the catheter tip. Errors should be suspected when successive measurements vary by more than 20% [8].

The normal CO ranges from 4 to 6 L per minute. This range reflects variation in individual body size. The average CO for an adult is approximately 5 L per minute, and in general the value for females is about 10% less than that for a male of the same size [17]. There are numerous causes of low CO. The most common are (1) decreased myocardial contractility secondary to myocardial infarction, shock, heart failure, surgery, or the effect of drugs; (2) decreased left ventricular filling pressure secondary to hypovolemia, cardiac rhythm disturbance, pericarditis, or cardiac tamponade; (3) increased systemic vascular resistance or hypertension; and (4) valvular disorders. An increased CO may occur in athletes during exercise and in various conditions that cause or result in decreased total peripheral resistance, such as septic shock, hypoxia, pulmonary disease, and pregnancy [17].

Cardiac Index
The cardiac index (CI) is a more specific indicator of cardiac function than is the CO. This measurement is more accurate because it is based on the person's body surface area (BSA), which is determined by height and weight and obtained from the Dubois Body Surface Chart (Figure 6.9). The CI is computed by dividing the CO by the BSA. The normal resting CI is 2.5 to 4.0 L/min/m^2, with a mean value of 3.2.

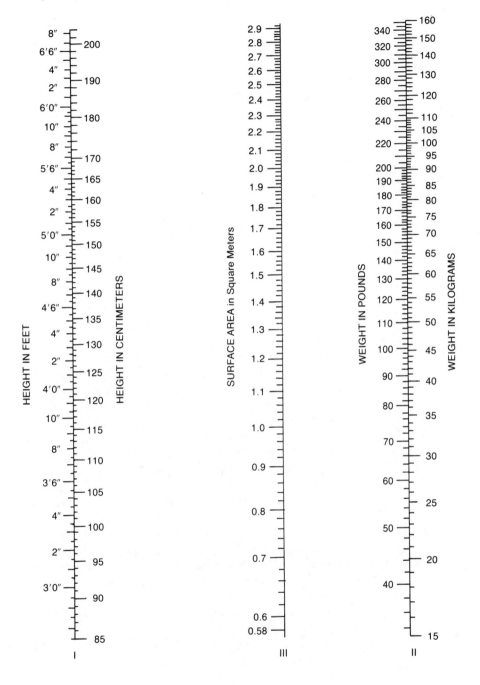

FIGURE 6.9
Dubois Body Surface Chart. To find the body surface area of a patient, locate the height in inches (or centimeters) on scale I and the weight in pounds (or kilograms) on scale II and place a straight edge (ruler) between these two points, which will intersect scale III at the patient's surface area. (From Dubois, E. F. *Basal Metabolism in Health and Disease*. Philadelphia: Lea & Febiger, 1936. Used with permission.)

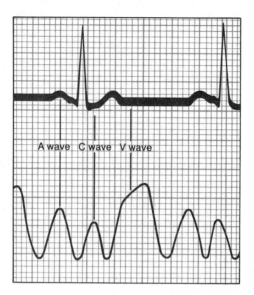

FIGURE 6.10
Atrial waveform with A, C, and V waves correlated with the ECG waveform.

Waveforms

Monitoring both pressures and waveforms is vital to patient care. Each component of the waveform represents various mechanical events of the heart. Events in the cardiac cycle can be evaluated by examining the atrial pressure waveform, as reflected in the CVP, LAP, and PCWP. The atrial waveform has several components (Figure 6.10). Only two, the A and V waves, are clinically significant. The A wave is produced by atrial contraction and corresponds to the P–R interval of the electrocardiogram (ECG). The A wave is absent in atrial fibrillation and pronounced when atrial pressure is elevated, as in pulmonary hypertension or mitral or tricuspid stenosis. The V wave represents ventricular systole and corresponds in time to the T–P interval on the ECG. Elevation of the V wave indicates valvular incompetence, which may develop suddenly as a complication of acute myocardial infarction.

Close observation of the pressure waveform is also essential to assessing the location of the catheter in the PA. If the catheter is inadvertently pulled out slightly, it may move into the right ventricle. This change would be indicated by the presence of a right ventricular waveform on the oscilloscope (see Figure 6.7). Between measurements the catheter can float forward into a wedge position, which can also be detected by observation of the waveform. In such an event, the catheter must be repositioned immediately by the physician to prevent pulmonary infarction.

Complications and Nursing Responsibilities

PA catheterizations are performed routinely in many ICUs. Although the procedure is associated with some risk, most problems can be minimized or prevented with proper maintenance of equipment and quality nursing care. Unless the nursing staff is familiar with the equipment and can use the data obtained to make quick assessments and to intervene when necessary, hemodynamic monitoring is of no benefit to the patient. The nurse must also be aware of the potential complications and the nursing interventions to be used to prevent them.

The potential complications associated with PA catheterization are infection, dysrhythmias, thromboembolism, pulmonary infarction, PA rupture, and air embolism. Most of these complications have been discussed in previous sections.

Although rare, PA rupture can occur. For this reason it is recommended that PCWP measurements be obtained as infrequently as possible. Some institutions are no longer routinely obtaining PCWP measurements and are using the PAD as a reflection of LVEDP.

Air embolism can occur during insertion because of loose connections in the pressure transducer system, air in the tubing, or rupture of the balloon. The balloon should be inflated slowly and only with the recommended volume of air (usually 1 cc). Balloon rupture can be suspected if no resistance is felt during balloon inflation, if the waveform indicates that the catheter is not in wedge position, and if blood can be aspirated from the balloon port. If balloon rupture occurs, the physician should be notified, the balloon port covered to prevent further inflations, and the catheter removed.

Advanced Hemodynamic Assessment

The experienced critical care nurse may want more detailed information regarding a patient's physiological state. With the aid of a calculator or a computer, the nurse can calculate additional hemodynamic variables using the data obtained with a thermodilution catheter. Obtaining measurements of such variables as stroke volume index, CI, and pulmonary and systemic vascular resistance will allow the clinician to assess the patient's condition more closely and to intervene when necessary. The definitions and formulas for these and other hemodynamic measurements are given in Exhibit 6.1.

LEFT ATRIAL PRESSURE MONITORING

LAP can be monitored directly or indirectly. Indirect measurements can be obtained with a PA catheter. Studies have shown a strong correlation between LAP and PCWP [22]. If the PCWP is not obtainable, then the PAD pressure is a reliable index of LAP in the absence of increased pulmonary vascular resistance.

Direct measurements of LAP are frequently instituted during cardiac surgery. Two techniques are used: the surgeon can thread a catheter through a central pulmonary vein into the left atrium, or insert the catheter directly into the left atrium. This method of monitoring LAP is particularly useful for the rare patient with an artificial tricuspid valve, in whom a PA catheter cannot be used.

Once inserted, the LA catheter is connected to a flush system and monitoring equipment that provides a continuous display of the waveform and measurement reading. The amplitude of the LAP waveform is low, and therefore measurements are recorded as the mean value rather than as systolic and diastolic pressures. The normal LAP ranges from 4 to 12 mm Hg. An increased LAP is seen in patients with mitral valve disease, fluid overload, or congestive failure. A decreased LAP indicates hypovolemia. As measurements are

EXHIBIT 6.1
Hemodynamic Terms and Formulas

Cardiac index (CI):
cardiac output adjusted for body surface area (BSA)

$$CI = \frac{CO}{BSA}$$

Cardiac output (CO):
amount of blood ejected from the heart into systemic circulation each minute

$$CO = HR \times SV$$

Ejection fraction (EF):
index of ventricular contractility; the percentage of total ventricular volume that is ejected during each contraction

$$EF = \frac{SV}{EDV} \times 100$$

Left ventricular stroke work index (LVSWI):
index of contractility of the left ventricle

$$LVSWI = \frac{1.36(MAP - PCWP)}{100} \times SVI$$

Right ventricular stroke work index (RVSWI):
index of contractility of the right ventricle

$$RVSWI = \frac{1.36(PAM - PCWP)}{100} \times SVI$$

Stroke volume (SV):
amount of blood ejected from the ventricle with each contraction

$$SV = \frac{CO}{HR}$$

Stroke volume index (SVI):
stroke volume adjusted for body surface area

$$SVI = \frac{SV}{BSA}$$

Systemic vascular resistance (SVR):
measure of the resistance in the systemic vascular system

$$SVR = \frac{MAP - CVP}{CO} \times 80$$

Pulmonary vascular resistance (PVR):
measure of the resistance in the pulmonary vascular system

$$PVR = \frac{PAM - PCWP}{CO} \times 80$$

HR = heart rate; MAP = mean arterial pressure; PCWP = pulmonary capillary wedge pressure; PAP = pulmonary artery pressure; PAM = mean pulmonary artery pressure.

obtained, they should be assessed in conjunction with other hemodynamic values before a final evaluation is made.

Nursing Care

The management of the patient with an LA catheter requires extreme caution on the part of the nursing staff. The potentially fatal complications include air or blood emboli, infection, and bleeding.

To prevent emboli, the nurse should always aspirate until blood is seen before flushing. If a blood return cannot be obtained, no attempt should be made to flush the line, and the catheter should be removed as soon as possible. Medications, blood products, and other intravenous fluids should not be infused into the LA catheter. Infection can be prevented by using the techniques previously described. To prevent potential complications, the catheter is generally removed on the first postoperative day if the patient is hemodynamically stable. Bleeding may occur upon removal; for this reason, mediastinal chest tubes should remain in place for several hours after the catheter is removed [22]. A dry sterile dressing is applied over the insertion site, and the area is assessed, along with chest tube drainage, for bleeding.

SUMMARY

Monitoring arterial, central venous, pulmonary artery, and left atrial pressures has become an invaluable aid in the management of critically ill patients, but consistency and accuracy are essential if the data obtained are to be accepted as a true indication of the patient's condition. Abnormal measurements must be evaluated in conjunction with other clinical signs and symptoms. Close observation, accurate measurement, and skilled care by the nurse will ensure early recognition of abnormalities and prompt treatment. It is essential that the nurse not become so involved in the equipment and measurements that the person in the bed is forgotten. Hemodynamic monitoring is an adjunct to the care of the critically ill patient, not an end in itself.

STUDY QUESTIONS

1. Hemodynamics deals with the interrelationships among _____ , _____ , and _____ .
2. List the four components of a pressure monitoring system.
3. List the indications for continuous arterial pressure monitoring.
4. True or false: The dicrotic notch represents closure of the mitral valve.
5. CVP reflects the pressure in the _____ _____ .
6. Proper placement of the CVP and PAP catheter is determined by _____ .
7. Describe the reference point used to level CVP and PAP using both an H_2O manometer and a transducer. Explain how to locate this point.
8. List two conditions indicated by low CVP readings.
9. List three conditions indicated by elevated CVP readings.
10. Name three primary goals in caring for the patient with a CVP or PAP catheter.

11. List three nursing interventions used to prevent infection.

12. Indicate the normal values or normal range of values for the following variables.
    a. CVP _____ cm H_2O
    b. CVP _____ mm Hg
    c. PAP _____ mm Hg
    d. MPAP _____ mm Hg
    e. PCWP _____ mm Hg
    f. CO _____ L/min

13. PCWP is approximately equal to _____ in the absence of pulmonary disease.

14. Filling pressures of the heart are reflected on the right side by _____ and on the left side by _____ .

15. List four potential complications of both CVP and PAP catheters.

CASE STUDIES

CASE 1

A 48-year-old woman is admitted to the coronary care unit with a diagnosis of acute myocardial infarction complicated by hypotension and ventricular tachycardia. For three days prior to admission, she has complained of nausea, vomiting, and diarrhea. Upon admission, an arterial catheter and PA catheter are inserted, with the following resultant pressure readings: blood pressure, 90/50 mm Hg; PCWP, 4 mm Hg; PAP, 20/6 mm Hg; and CVP, 4 mm Hg.

1. Discuss the patient's fluid status and the possible causes of her hypotension.

2. During the day, the patient's arterial waveform appears to be damped. What are some possible causes of this? What can the nurse do to correct the damping?

3. The nurse notices that the PA tracing appears to be wedged. What actions should she or he take? Explain your rationale.

4. The patient begins to have increasing amounts of ventricular ectopy in spite of continuous antiarrhythmic therapy. Other than myocardial ischemia, what is a possible cause of this increased ectopy?

CASE 2

An 82-year-old woman is admitted to the coronary care unit with a diagnosis of acute pulmonary edema. On admission she is pale, restless, diaphoretic, and dyspneic. Temperature is 98°F, pulse is 130 beats per minute, respirations are 32 per minute, and blood pressure is 140/70 mm Hg. A pulmonary artery catheter is inserted to monitor the patient's fluid balance. Baseline measurements are obtained: PAP, 50/28 mm Hg, CVP, 20 mm Hg; and PCWP, 26 mm Hg.

1. Assess the patient's vital signs and PA pressures. Are they normal or abnormal?

2. Do this patient's vital signs indicate left-sided heart failure, right-sided heart failure, or biventricular failure?

Treatment is instituted immediately. The patient is given 40 mg of Lasix IV bolus, 4 L of O_2 nasally, and 6 mg of MSO4 IV; and 2 inches of nitroglycerine paste.

3. Discuss the rationale for each of these treatments.

4. The treatments are effective. The patient excretes approximately 1,000 cc of urine. Which of the following patterns of vital signs would you expect the patient to exhibit? Why?

Variable	A	B	C
Temperature (°F)	98	98	98
Pulse (beats/min)	120	60	90
Respirations (/min)	26	18	24
Blood pressure (mm Hg)	90/60	84/60	120/70
PAP (mm Hg)	50/30	40/25	35/15
PCWP (mm Hg)	5	25	16
CVP (mm Hg)	15	18	10

5. List three primary goals in caring for a patient with a PA catheter.

REFERENCES

1. Abels, L. F. Hemodynamic monitoring. In L. F. Abels (ed.), *Manual of Critical Care.* St. Louis: Mosby, 1979.

2. Adams, N. R. Reducing the perils of intracardiac monitoring. *Nurs. '76* 6:66, 1976.

3. Armstrong, P. W., and Baigrie, R. S. Hemodynamic monitoring in critically ill patients. *Heart Lung* 9:1060, 1980.

4. Aubin, B. A. Arterial lines: a review. *Crit. Care Q.* 2:57, 1979.

5. Berne, R. M., and Levy, M. N. *Cardiac Physiology.* St. Louis: Mosby, 1981.

6. Brantigan, C. O. Hemodynamic monitoring: interpreting values. *Am. J. Nurs.* 82:86, 1982.

7. Buchbinder, N., and Ganz, W. Hemodynamic monitoring: invasive techniques. *Anesthesiology* 45:146, 1976.

8. Daily, E. K., and Schroeder, J. S. *Techniques in Bedside Hemodynamic Monitoring* (2nd ed.). St. Louis: Mosby, 1981.

9. Daily, P. O. Positions of patients for central venous pressure measurements. *J.A.M.A.* 219:1223, 1972.

10. Dalen, J. E. Bedside hemodynamic monitoring. *N. Engl. J. Med.* 301:1176, 1979.

11. Eckstein, J. W. Position of patient for central venous pressure measurements. *J.A.M.A.* 219:1223, 1972.

12. Fisher, R. E. Measuring central venous pressure: how to do it accurately. . . and safely. *Nurs. '79* 9:74, 1979.

13. Forrester, J. S., et al. Filling pressures in the right and left sides of the heart in acute myocardial infarction. *N. Engl. J. Med.* 285:190, 1971.

14. Forrester, J. S., et al. Medical therapy of acute myocardial infarction by application of hemodynamic subsets. *N. Engl. J. Med.* 295:1356, 1976.

15. Gernert, C. F., and Schwartz, S. Pulmonary artery catheterization. *Am. J. Nurs.* 73:1182, 1973.

16. *Guide to Physiologic Pressure Monitoring.* Waltham, Mass.: Hewlett Packard Co., 1977.

17. Guyton, A. C., and Jones, C. E. Central venous pressure: physiological significance and clinical implications. *Am. Heart J.* 86:431, 1973.

18. Haag, G. Central venous catheters and monitoring. *Crit. Care Q.* 2:51, 1979.

19. Hathaway, R. The Swan-Ganz catheter: a review. *Nurs. Clin. North Am.* 13:389, 1978.

20. Haughey, B. CVP lines: monitoring and maintaining. *Am. J. Nurs.* 78:635, 1978.

21. Jackle, M., and Halligan, M. *Cardiovascular Problems: A Critical Care Nursing Focus.* Bowie, Md.: Brady, 1980.

22. Kaplan, J. A. Hemodynamic monitoring. In J. A. Kaplan (ed.), *Cardiac Anesthesia.* New York: Grune & Stratton, 1979.

23. Kaye, W. Catheter- and infusion-related sepsis: the nature of the problem and its prevention. *Heart Lung* 11:221, 1982.

24. Labet, C. G., and Roderick, M. A. Infection control in the use of intravascular devices. *Crit. Care Q.* 3:67, 1981.

25. Lantiegne, K. C., and Civetta, J. M. A system for maintaining invasive pressure monitoring. *Heart Lung* 7:610, 1978.

26. Laulive, J. L. Nursing management of left atrial pressure monitoring. *Crit. Care Q.* 4:75, 1981.

27. Laulive, J. L. Pulmonary artery pressures and position changes in the critically ill adult. *Dimens. Crit. Care Nurs.* 1:28, 1982.

28. Liebson, P. R. Postoperative hemodynamic monitoring. In M. D. Goldin (ed.), *Intensive Care of the Surgical Patient* (2nd ed.). Chicago: Year Book, 1981.

29. Loeb, H. S., and Gunnar, R. M. Hemodynamic monitoring in the coronary care unit. *Heart Lung* 11:302, 1982.

30. Murray, J., and Smallwood, J. CVP monitoring: sidestepping potential perils. *Nurs. '77* 7(1):42, 1977.

31. Nielsen, M. A. Intra-arterial monitoring of blood pressure. *Am. J. Nurs.* 74:48, 1974.

32. Pennington, L. A., and Smith, C. Leveling when monitoring central blood pressures: an alternative method. *Heart Lung* 9:1053, 1980.

33. Pugh, D. A. Thermodilution cardiac output: what, how and why. *Crit. Care Q.* 2:21, 1979.

34. Sears, M. F., and Heise, C. Troubleshooting the Swan-Ganz catheter. *Heart Lung* 9:303, 1980.

35. Smith, R. N. Invasive pressure monitoring. *Am. J. Nurs.* 78:1514, 1978.

36. Spaccavento, L. J., and Hawley, H. B. Infections associated with intra-arterial lines. *Heart Lung* 11:118, 1982.

37. Spence, M. I., and Lemberg, L. Hemodynamic monitoring in the coronary care unit. *Heart Lung* 9:541, 1980.

38. *Using Monitors.* Horsham, Pa: Intermed Communications, 1980.

39. Vij, D., Babcock, R., and Magilligan, D. J. A simplified concept of complete physiological monitoring of the critically ill patient. *Heart Lung* 10:75, 1981.

40. Visalli, F., and Evans, P. The Swan-Ganz catheter: a program for teaching safe, effective use. *Nurs. '81* 11:42, 1981.

41. Walinsky, P. Acute hemodynamic monitoring. *Heart Lung* 6:838, 1977.

42. Woods, S. L., Grose, B. L., and Laurent-Bopp, D. Effect of backrest position on pulmonary artery pressure in critically ill patients. *Cardiovasc. Nurs.* 18:19, 1982.

43. Woods, S. L., and Mansfield, L. W. Effect of body position upon pulmonary artery and pulmonary capillary wedge pressures in non-critically ill patients. *Heart Lung* 5:83, 1976.

CHAPTER 7

Basic Electrophysiology

Susan Lynn Zorb

INTRODUCTION

Dysrhythmia monitoring has been closely associated with the development of critical care units. In fact, coronary care units were formed to detect and treat life-threatening dysrhythmias in the patient who had experienced a myocardial infarction. Initially, nurses were educated to recognize dysrhythmias from a cardiac monitor, but recently emphasis has been placed on interpretation of the full twelve-lead electrocardiogram (ECG). The anatomy and physiology of the conduction system and the myocardial cell were discussed in Chapter 3. This chapter will review electrophysiology and describe the normal ECG, the changes seen in myocardial infarction, interventricular conduction defects, and determination of electrical axis. Chapter 8 will review the dysrhythmias seen in the critical care unit. It is essential that the critical care nurse be able to diagnose dysrhythmias and interpret subtle changes in the ECG.

ELECTROPHYSIOLOGY

The ECG is a graphic representation of the electrical activity of the heart. Each myocardial cell has a pattern of electrical activity, referred to as an action potential. Examination of the myocardial cell reveals that there is a difference in electrical charge across the cell membrane (Figure 7.1). The cell is said to be polarized, with the inside of the cell negative in relation to the outside. This negative charge is due to the large numbers of nondiffusible negative ions (anions), such as sulfates, phosphates, and proteins, found in the cell. In the resting state the electrical difference between the inside and the outside of the cell is -90 mV and is called the resting membrane potential (RMP).

Because the cell membrane is not permeable to major anions, the polarity

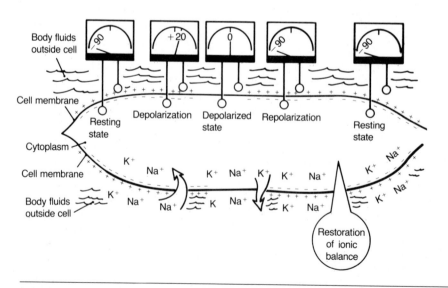

FIGURE 7.1
Polarized cardiac cell. The inside of the cell is negative in relation to the outside of the cell.

of the cell changes because of movement of the more diffusible positive ions (cations) into and out of the cell. Sodium (Na^+) is the predominant extracellular cation, with normal concentration of 140 mg/dl, whereas potassium (K^+) is the predominant intracellular cation. The intracellular concentration of K^+ cannot be accurately measured but is thought to approximate the extracellular Na^+ concentration. The extracellular K^+ concentration is 3.5 to 5.0 mg/dl.

The action potential is the schematic representation of the electrical events occurring in the cell (Figure 7.2). In the resting state the cell membrane is more permeable to K^+ than to Na^+; therefore, K^+ ions are constantly diffusing out of the cell. When the cell is stimulated to the critical threshold level, the permeability of the cell membrane changes, allowing a rapid influx of Na^+ through the fast channels located in the cell membrane. This causes the inside of the cell to become less negative, resulting in a loss of polarity across the cell membrane called depolarization. This is phase 0 of the action potential. In addition to the rapid influx of Na^+ during depolarization, there is a slower inward movement of calcium (Ca^{++}) and magnesium (Mg^{++}). The total movement of cations into the cell produces a slight, transient, positive charge on the inside of the cell.

Repolarization begins with phase 1 of the action potential. During this time the fast channels close and the influx of Na^+ stops. The slow channels in the cell membrane for the movement of Ca^{++} and Mg^{++} remain open throughout this phase and phase 2, referred to as the plateau phase. During phase 2 K^+ begins to leave the cell, which counteracts the continued influx of Ca^{++} and Mg^{++}, resulting in maintenance of the transmembrane potential. At the end of phase 2, the calcium channels close and the movement of K^+ out of the cell increases, leading to phase 3, rapid repolarization. During this

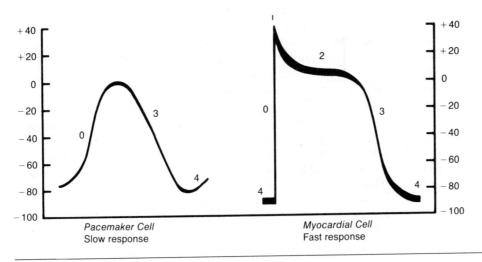

FIGURE 7.2
Fast- and slow-response action potentials. In the slow response, phases 1 and 2 are absent and phase 4 is sloping, which allows for spontaneous depolarization.

phase the membrane potential quickly returns to -90 mV through the movement of K^+ ions out of the cell. At the end of phase 3, the cell is electrically repolarized, but the ionic concentrations across the cell membrane are reversed. Correction occurs during phase 4, often referred to as the resting phase, when the Na^+/K^+ pump expels Na^+ from the cell and returns K^+ to the cell. By the end of phase 4, both the electrical and the ionic concentrations are correct.

An action potential is divided into two phases: depolarization and repolarization. Depolarization is a rapid, one-step (phase 0) process that occurs whenever a myocardial cell is stimulated to a critical membrane potential, usually -70 mV, referred to as the threshold potential. Repolarization, however, is a multistep process that is divided into three parts, reflecting the cell's ability to accept an impulse and depolarize. The first step of repolarization, encompassing phases 1 and 2 of the action potential, is called the absolute refractory phase. During this time the cell cannot be depolarized regardless of the strength of the stimulus. The relative refractory period occurs during phase 3. A strong stimulus received during this time will cause the cell to depolarize again. The action potential produced by this depolarization has a slower upstroke in phase 0 and is less stable than a normal action potential. The supernormal phase of repolarization occurs at the very end of phase 3, when the RMP is reestablished but the ionic concentration is still reversed. During this time the cell can be depolarized by a very weak stimulus. This period is referred to as the vulnerable period of repolarization. The three refractory phases are important in the mechanism of action of the various antiarrhythmic agents.

The action potential just described, termed the fast response, occurs normally in the vast majority of myocardial cells. The slow-response action potential (see Figure 7.2) occurs routinely in the cells of the sinoatrial (SA) and atrioventricular (AV) nodes and accounts for the pacemaker abilities of these cells. There are several differences between the fast- and slow-response action potentials, the most notable of which occurs in phase 4. In the slow-response potential, phase 4 is a gradual upslope that continues until the threshold potential is reached and depolarization (phase 0) begins. This upslope is due to a gradual influx of Na^+ and other cations into the cell, which causes the membrane potential to rise. This process is referred to as diastolic depolarization. In contrast, phase 4 in the fast-response potential is flat. The RMP of the slow response is higher than that of the fast response, and once threshold potential is reached, depolarization (represented by the slope of phase 0) is slowed. The slower rate of depolarization is due to the dependence of the slow-response depolarization on the slower influx of Ca^{++} rather than on the rapid influx of Na^+. Because of these differences in depolarization, phases 1 and 2 are absent from the slow-response action potential. Repolarization begins with phase 3 and is more gradual than in the fast response. These differences in the action potential enable the cells of SA and AV nodes to initiate depolarization without an outside stimulus. These cells are said to be automatic cells. Any myocardial cell can adopt automatic properties under certain conditions, such as ischemia, acidosis, hypoxia, digitalis intoxication, and catecholamine stimulation [14].

PRINCIPLES OF ELECTROCARDIOGRAPHY

The ECG is a graphic recording of the electrical activity of the heart viewed from twelve different perspectives, or leads. The first six leads, I, II, III, aV_R, aV_L, and aV_F, are referred to as the limb leads because the recording sites are on the extremeties. The second six leads, V_1 through V_6, are referred to as the chest leads because the recording sites are on the chest. These leads may be either bipolar or unipolar. In the bipolar leads, I, II, and III, there are positive $(+)$ and negative $(-)$ electrodes that measure the electrical activity between them. The unipolar leads, aV_R, aV_L, aV_F, and V_1 through V_6, measure the electrical activity between the heart, which is considered electrically zero, and the positive electrode. ECG paper is a strip of graph paper in which blocks or small squares are grouped into larger squares by heavy, dark lines. There are five small squares between each pair of heavy lines. The horizontal axis of this graph paper denotes time. In the standard ECG each small square is 0.04 sec in duration. Therefore, each large square is 0.20 sec in duration. The vertical axis denotes voltage; each small square is 1 mM, and each large square is then 5mM (Figure 7.3).

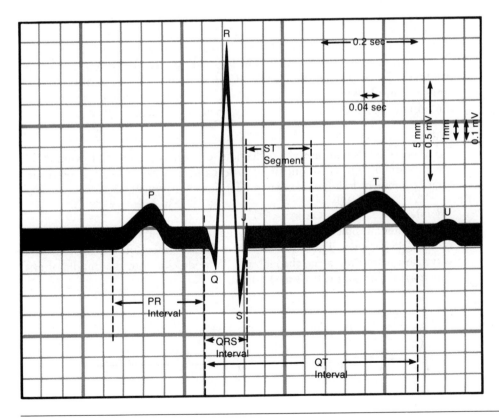

FIGURE 7.3
Normal ECG waveforms and intervals.

The events recorded on the ECG reflect the composite of the transmembrane action potentials that occur in various parts of the heart. Each event displays a characteristic waveform or is reflected in a specific segment or interval of the ECG. It is important to examine each component to interpret the ECG properly (see Figure 7.3).

Waveforms

P Wave

The P wave represents the wave of depolarization spreading throughout the atria. It is generally a small, rounded hump 0.10 sec in duration and less than 2.5 mM in height, reflecting the small muscle mass present in the atria.

QRS Wave

The QRS wave is, collectively, the wave of depolarization spreading throughout the ventricles. The Q wave refers specifically to a negative deflection following the P wave, the R wave to the positive deflection, and the S wave to any negative deflection following the R wave. If there is more than one positive deflection, the second is referred to as R'. Although the letters *QRS* are used to denote ventricular depolarization, all three waves need not be present at all times and various combinations of waves may occur (Figure 7.4). The normal QRS duration is less than 0.10 sec; normal voltage varies widely from person to person, however.

T Wave

The T wave represents ventricular repolarization. It is generally an upright, asymmetrical, rounded wave that coincides with phases 3 and 4 of the action potential. The area from the middle of the upslope to just over the rounded hump is considered to be the vulnerable period, because a weak stimulus here can initiate disordered electrical activity, such as ventricular fibrillation.

U Wave

The U wave is a small, upright deflection sometimes present following the T wave. Normally either absent or of little clinical significance, this wave becomes prominent in hypokalemia and cardiac enlargement.

Intervals and Segments

PR Interval

The PR interval is measured from the beginning of the P wave to the beginning of the QRS complex. This interval reflects the movement of the depolarization wave throughout the atria, through the AV node, and into the bundle of His. The normal duration is 0.12 to 0.20 sec.

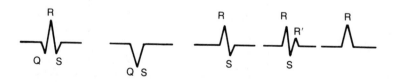

FIGURE 7.4
Potential QRS configurations.

TABLE 7.1
Relationship of Normal QT Interval to Heart Rate

Heart Rate (bpm)	Duration of QT Interval (sec)
60	0.33–0.43
70	0.31–0.41
80	0.29–0.38
90	0.28–0.36
100	0.27–0.35
120	0.25–0.32

QT Interval
The QT interval is measured from the beginning of the QRS complex to the end of the T wave. It reflects the duration of ventricular depolarization and repolarization. The normal interval varies with heart rate, age, and sex (Table 7.1).

ST Segment
The ST segment represents the time between the end of ventricular depolarization and the T wave, or phases 1 and 2 of the action potential. It should normally show no electrical activity, a state represented by an isoelectric or flat line on the ECG paper. Deviations of greater than 1 mM, either positive or negative, are considered abnormal. The ST segment encompasses the J point, which is the junction between the QRS complex and the ST segment.

THE NORMAL ECG

Interpretation of the twelve-lead ECG requires careful attention to the structure of the various waveforms and segments in all twelve leads. The nurse must be familiar with the normal ECG in order to detect subtle changes that may warn of impending complications.

In the standard ECG the heart is viewed from twelve different perspectives. Table 7.2 summarizes these perspectives and the area of the heart monitored by each lead. By changing leads, one changes the viewing perspective only; the direction and magnitude of the depolarization wave remain the same. In learning to understand the normal ECG, it is helpful to remember the position of the positive pole in each lead (see Table 7.2), because this determines the direction of the waveform deflection. If the depolarization wave flows toward the positive pole, the deflection will be upright; if it flows away from the positive pole, the deflection will be negative; if it flows perpendicular to the positive pole, it will generate either a biphasic wave (upright and downward) or an isoelectric line. The magnitude of the deflection depends on the direction of the flow. If the flow is exactly parallel to the lead, the deflection will have a large magnitude. If the flow is less than parallel, it will be of lesser magnitude.

Generally, the direction of depolarization of the heart in the chest is downward and to the left. That direction gives the distinctive waveforms in

TABLE 7.2
The Twelve-Lead Electrocardiogram

Lead	Polarity	Area of Heart Monitored
I	Positive pole: left arm Negative pole: right arm	Lateral wall of LV
II	Positive pole: left leg Negative pole: right arm	Inferior wall of LV
III	Positive pole: left leg Negative pole: left arm	Inferior wall of LV
aV_R	Positive pole: right arm	Superior aspect of LV
aV_L	Positive pole: left arm	Superior aspect of LV
aV_F	Positive pole: left leg	Inferior wall of LV
V_1	Positive pole: 4th intercostal space to the right of the sternum	Anteroseptal LV wall
V_2	Positive pole: 4th intercostal space to the left of the sternum	Anteroseptal LV wall
V_3	Positive pole: midway between V_2 and V_4	Anteroseptal LV wall
V_4	Positive pole: 5th intercostal space, left midclavicular line	Anteroseptal LV wall
V_5	Positive pole: lateral to V_4 at the left anterior axillary line	Anterolateral LV wall
V_6	Positive pole: lateral to V_5 at the left midaxillary line	Anterolateral LV wall

LV = left ventricular.

each of the twelve leads shown in Figure 7.5. Because of the differing positions of the heart in the chest, however, normal variations in the ECG do occur.

Determination of Axis

The term *axis* refers to the mean frontal QRS vector, or the direction of electrical flow. It is determined by examining the first six ECG leads, using the hexaxial reference system (Figure 7.6). This system is created by having the first six ECG leads intersect at the heart. A circle is formed by the poles and is divided into twelve sections of 30 degrees each. Lead I has been assigned the values of 0 degrees at its positive pole and ± 180 degrees at its negative pole. Moving clockwise from 0 degrees, the values are positive; moving counterclockwise from 0 degrees, the values are negative. The normal axis is considered to be from −30 degrees to +110 degrees. Left axis deviation (LAD) runs from −30 degrees to −90 degrees; right axis deviation (RAD) from +100 degrees to +180 degrees. An axis of from ± 180 degrees to −90 degrees is indeterminate and may be either extreme RAD or extreme LAD.

There are many methods for calculation of axis. Several of these have been detailed by Duke [5, 6]. Here we will discuss a method that is easily used at the bedside and that requires no additional equipment. This method places the axis within one of four quadrants. Another technique for further defining the axis, which builds on the quadrant system, will also be described. The following steps facilitate calculation of the electrical axis: (1) Examine leads I and aV_F, which are perpendicular to each other on the hexaxial reference sys-

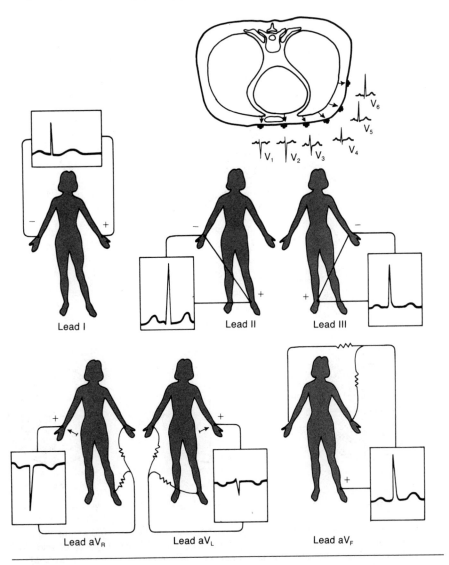

FIGURE 7.5
Normal waveforms in the twelve-lead ECG.

tem. (2) Determine if the QRS complex is positive or negative in each lead. If the complex is positive, then the vector is traveling toward the positive pole of that lead. If it is negative, the vector is traveling away from the positive pole. The axis will be in the quadrant that falls between the direction of lead I and the direction of lead aV_F (Figure 7.7).

We can define the axis further: (1) Find the most equiphasic of the first six leads. (2) Examine the lead that is perpendicular to this lead. (Lead I is perpendicular to aV_F, lead II to aV_L, and lead III to aV_R). The direction of this lead will fall within the previously defined quadrant and will be the electrical axis.

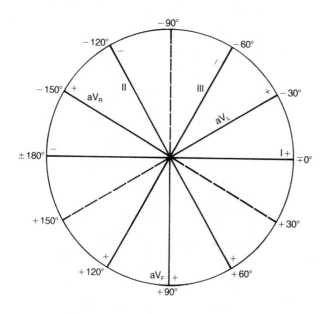

FIGURE 7.6
Hexaxial reference system. The six limb leads
intersect at the heart, forming a circle that is
divided into twelve sections of 30 degrees each.

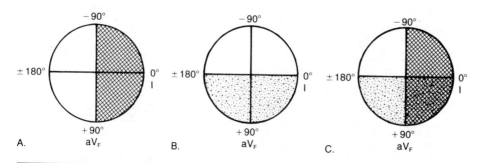

FIGURE 7.7
Determination of axis using leads I and aV_F. (A) The cross-hatched half represents the
positive (+) area of lead I. (B) The dotted half represents the positive (+) area of lead aV_F.
(C) The axis of the ECG lies in the quadrant covering the direction (+ or −) of the QRS
complex in leads I and aV_F.

Changes in electrical axis indicate some alteration in the conduction of
the impulse through the ventricles. The change may be due to ischemia, injury,
fibrosis of the conduction system, or changes in ventricular muscle mass. Determination of axis is especially important in the diagnosis of intraventricular
conduction defects (IVCDs). The normal axis for each person will vary somewhat in relation to the anatomical position of the heart in the chest. A tall
person may have a vertical axis greater than +75 degrees, whereas a heavy-
set, broad-chested person may normally have an axis of between 0 degrees and
−30 degrees.

INTRAVENTRICULAR CONDUCTION DEFECTS

In IVCD, changes in the conduction system cause the impulse to depolarize the ventricles in an abnormal fashion. Because some of the tissue is refractory when the impulse arrives, the impulse must bypass that section of tissue, delaying the impulse and causing the QRS to be wider than normal. The rest of the conduction system may be intact, and depolarization of the tissue will occur normally. The result is a characteristic ECG pattern for each defect, right bundle branch block (RBBB), left bundle branch block (LBBB), left anterior hemiblock (LAH), and left posterior hemiblock (LPH).

Normal Ventricular Activation

The common bundle of His advances from the AV node into the ventricular septum, where it branches into the right bundle branch (RBB) and the left bundle branch (LBB). The RBB continues down the septum and into the right ventricle (RV). The LBB divides almost immediately into the thin anterior fascicle, which travels through the left ventricle (LV) in an anterior-superior direction, and the thick posterior fascicle, which travels through the LV in a posterior-inferior direction.

Ventricular activation occurs in the following sequence. The intraventricular septum is depolarized from left to right. These forces are referred to as the initial forces of depolarization. The ventricles are then depolarized from the endocardium to the epicardium. The time it takes for the impulse to travel from the endocardium to the epicardium is referred to as the ventricular activation time (VAT) and is measured from the beginning of the QRS to the highest peak of the R or R' wave. It is normally 0.02 sec. RV depolarization is completed first, because the RV muscle mass is less than that of the LV. The LV is depolarized from apex to base. The ECG representation of normal ventricular activation in leads V_1 and V_6 is shown in Figure 7.8. The small r wave in V_1 and q wave in V_6 represent the initial forces of septal depolarization. These two leads are the best leads for detecting BBB, because V_1 views the RV and V_6 views the LV.

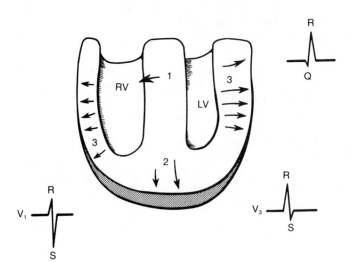

FIGURE 7.8
Normal ventricular activation. The septum is depolarized first from left to right, followed by the apex and ventricles from endocardial to epicardial surfaces. (*RV* = right ventricle; *LV* = left ventricle.)

Right Bundle Branch Block

A block of the RBB may occur in any type of heart disease, as well as in the absence of any cardiac abnormality. It may be evident only with a change in heart rate or may be present continuously.

In RBBB the initial forces of depolarization remain unchanged. The septum is depolarized from left to right, and LV depolarization proceeds normally. RV depolarization is delayed, however, occurring after LV depolarization. In V_1 the ECG will show a normal small r wave followed by a large S wave, depicting LV depolarization. This is followed by a large R' wave, which represents RV depolarization. The QRS duration is prolonged, usually to 0.12 to 0.13 sec. The VAT is lengthened to as much as 0.09 sec, and the T wave is inverted. In V_6, a small q wave is followed by a large R wave, reflecting LV depolarization. A large S wave, representing RV depolarization, completes the complex. The QRS duration is prolonged, but the VAT is normal, because activation of the LV is normal. The T wave is upright. Although V_1 and V_6 are the leads that best reveal RBBB, changes can be discerned in other leads as well. Leads I, aV_L, and V_5 will have patterns similar to those of lead V_6. Lead V_2 patterns will resemble those of V_1 (Figure 7.9).

Incomplete RBBB occurs when only a portion of the RBB is blocked; the ECG features are the same as those in complete RBBB except that the QRS duration is less than 0.12 sec and the VAT in V_1 is less than 0.06 sec. Incomplete RBBB is caused by hypertrophy or strain.

Left Bundle Branch Block

A block of the LBB may occur in persons with myocardial ischemia, left ventricular hypertrophy, hypertension, or virtually any form of heart disease. It is occasionally found in a person with no cardiac abnormality. When the LBB is blocked, the septum must be depolarized from right to left. Then the RV is depolarized, followed by the LV. In V_6 the small q wave is eliminated; instead, there is a tall R wave followed by RV depolarization, which will appear either as an S wave or, more likely, as a notching in the R wave. LV depolarization produces a wide R' wave, and the QRS duration is greater than 0.12 sec. The VAT is more than 0.09 sec, and the T wave is inverted. In V_1, there is a small q wave, reflecting septal depolarization, followed by a small r wave, reflecting RV depolarization. A large S wave indicates LV depolarization. The small r wave is not always present; thus, the QRS complex may evidence a deep, wide Q wave (Figure 7.10).

Incomplete LBBB occurs when the pattern of LBBB is present but the QRS is less than 0.12 sec, and the VAT is less than 0.09 sec. The condition indicates the presence of LV hypertrophy or strain.

Left Anterior Hemiblock

A block of the left anterior fascicle (LAF) is more common than one involving the left posterior fascicle (LPF) because the anterior fascicle is thin and has only a single blood supply. LAH occurs with coronary artery disease, left ventricular hypertrophy, emphysema, and cardiomyopathy. When the anterior fascicle is blocked, LV conduction initially spreads through the posterior fascicle to the inferior posterior wall. The impulse travels through the Purkinje system to activate the anterior lateral wall. This produces a left axis deviation with a mean axis of more than −30 degrees. The QRS complex is of normal duration.

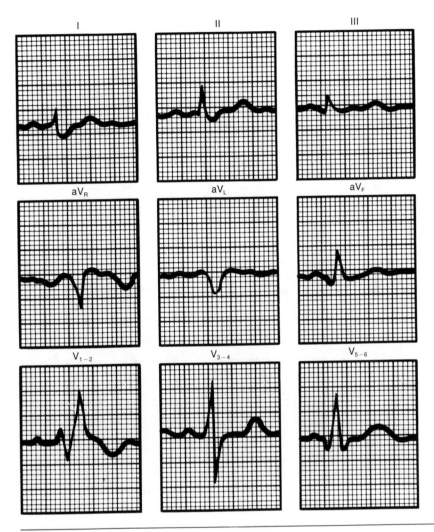

FIGURE 7.9
Right bundle branch block.

There is a small r wave in II, III, and aV$_F$, followed by a large S wave. In leads I and aV$_L$ there is a small q wave followed by a large R wave (Figure 7.11).

Left Posterior Hemiblock

The LPF is less susceptible to block than the LAF because of its greater thickness, its better blood supply, and its position in the outflow tract. Therefore, LPH is relatively rare. It can occur with myocardial ischemia, sclerosis of the conduction tissue, myocarditis, and hyperkalemia. When the LPF is blocked, the LV is initially activated by the anterior fascicle. The impulse then travels through the Purkinje system to the inferior posterior walls. This produces a right axis deviation of more than +120 degrees. In leads I and aV$_L$ there is an rS pattern, and in leads II, III, and aV$_F$ there is a qR pattern. The QRS duration remains normal (Figure 7.12).

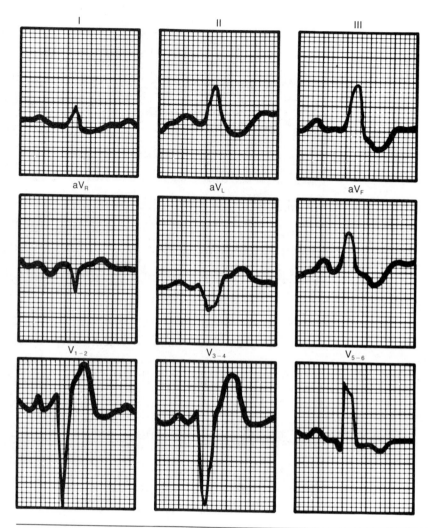

FIGURE 7.10
Left bundle branch block.

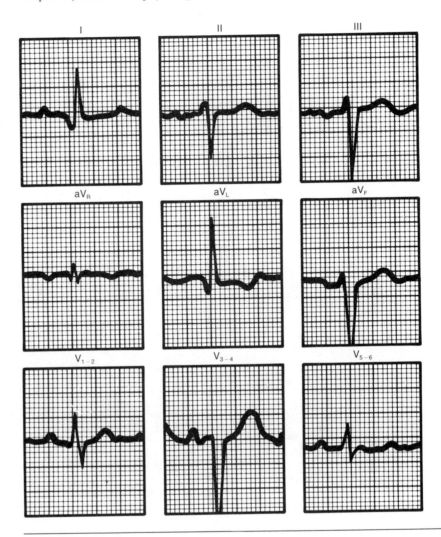

FIGURE 7.11
Left anterior hemiblock.

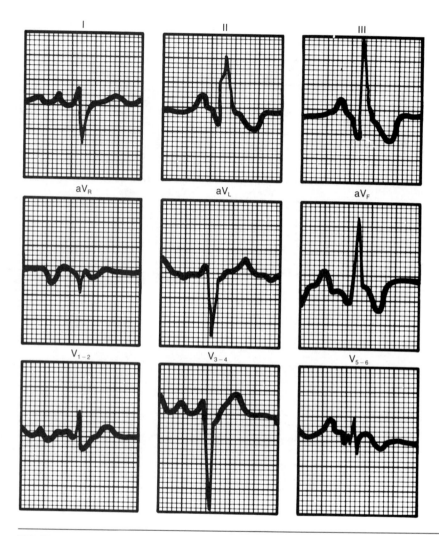

FIGURE 7.12
Left posterior hemiblock.

Bifascicular and Trifascicular Blocks

Concurrent blocks in more than one of the three distal fascicles (RBB, LAF, and LPF) are not rare. When they occur in the setting of an acute myocardial infarction, 40% to 45% of the patients will develop complete heart block [10]. The critical care nurse must be able to recognize this development and understand its implications. Bifascicular blocks commonly occur with anteroseptal myocardial infarctions, because the fascicles receive their blood supply from the left anterior descending artery. There are three possible combinations of bifascicular block: RBBB and LAH, RBBB and LPH, and LBBB. Figure 7.13 shows an example of RBBB with LAH. If the RBBB develops first, the patient should be monitored in lead II to detect any shift in axis that would indicate the advent of LAH.

Trifascicular block may be either complete or incomplete. Complete block of all three fascicles results in complete heart block. Incomplete trifas-

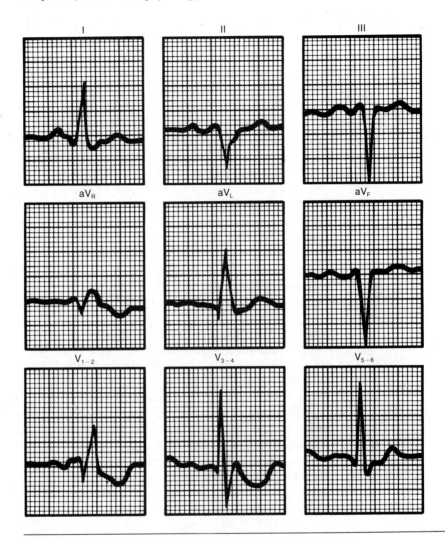

FIGURE 7.13
Right bundle branch block with left anterior hemiblock.

cicular block occurs when a person with bifascicular block begins to show an incomplete block of the third fascicle. Such an incomplete block would result if, in addition to bifascicular block, the person developed a first-degree atrioventricular block or demonstrated alternating complete RBBB and LBBB. This situation is dangerous and requires immediate attention.

ECG CHANGES IN MYOCARDIAL INFARCTION

As described in Chapter 9, a myocardial infarction (MI) is a complex process evolving over time. The process involves ischemic, injured, and infarcted tissue, each of which produces characteristic changes in the ECG. The nurse must be able to recognize and interpret these changes when caring for the cardiac patient.

The tissue affected in an MI may be viewed electrically from more than one perspective. A lead may look directly at the tissue, producing one set of changes, or the tissue may be viewed from the opposite side, producing the reverse, or reciprocal, changes. Analysis of the leads at which the changes occur enables the practitioner to localize the infarct. This allows the skilled nurse to prepare for complications common to specific types of MIs.

Serial ECG Changes in MI

The earliest signs of an MI are peaked T waves or hyperacute T waves, resulting from Na^+ and K^+ shifts in the affected tissue. These changes are brief and may be resolved by the time the person arrives in the emergency room or sees a physician. Elevation of the ST segment over the affected tissue is often the first observed manifestation of the infarction process. The ST elevation is due to the current of injury in myocardial cells that are receiving an inadequate supply of oxygen. Because these cells are poorly activated, there may also be a loss of R wave voltage. During this time, there will be ST depression in the leads that view the opposite wall. The ST elevation will be followed by T wave flattening and inversion, a further manifestation of ischemia. The last sign is the development of abnormal Q waves in the affected leads. An abnormal Q wave is defined as one more than 0.04 sec in duration and more than one-third the total QRS height. Q waves occur because the infarcted tissue is electrically dead; therefore, a lead over this area will view the electrical activity of the opposite wall and a negative deflection will be recorded on the ECG. Q waves may appear immediately or within the first few days. They do not resolve over time and are an indication of previous MIs.

The other ECG changes do resolve over time. Generally, the ST segment returns to baseline level first, and the T waves slowly become upright. In some individuals the T waves remain inverted for years. During this time the T waves may become upright during further episodes of ischemia. This change is referred to as pseudonormalization of the T waves. It emphasizes the importance of comparison of several ECGs; one isolated ECG may appear normal, whereas in fact the myocardium is ischemic.

The ECG pattern just described occurs during the evolution of a transmural MI. A subendocardial MI will produce ST depressions in the affected leads, but Q waves will not develop. There may also be loss of R waves over the affected tissue. These changes will persist for several days. An intramural MI will produce T wave inversions only in the affected leads, and these will persist for several days.

The person experiencing angina generally has a normal resting ECG and demonstrates ST depression and occasional T wave inversion during the anginal episode. These changes return to the baseline when the episode resolves. In variant, or Prinzmetal's, angina, the ECG shows ST elevations consistent with an evolving MI during the anginal episode that completely disappear when the person is pain free.

Localization of Infarct

The importance of localizing the site of the infarction cannot be overstated. The patient's course depends primarily on the location and extent of infarction.

As described in Chapter 9, certain sequelae are common to an anterior MI that are not common to an inferior MI, and vice versa.

Anterior MIs
The anterior wall of the heart is best viewed by means of the precordial leads. Standard leads I and aV$_L$ may also show signs of anterior infarction, although they best demonstrate the lateral wall. Lead III may show reciprocal ST depression early in the infarction process. There are several types of anterior MIs (Figure 7.14):

1. Anteroseptal MI: The changes will occur in leads V$_1$ through V$_3$, because these leads overlie the septum. Changes will usually not be seen in leads I and aV$_L$.

2. Anterolateral MI: The changes will occur in leads V$_4$ through V$_6$ and also in I and aV$_L$.

3. Anteroapical MI: Changes will occur in leads V$_3$ through V$_5$, and not in I or aV$_L$.

Inferior MI
The inferior or diaphragmatic wall of the heart is best seen in leads II, III, and aV$_F$. Reciprocal changes may be seen in leads I and aV$_L$. The precordial leads are usually unchanged in an inferior MI (Figure 7.15).

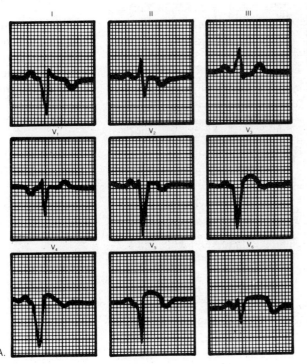

A.

FIGURE 7.14
ECG changes in acute anterior myocardial infarction: (A) anterolateral; (B) anteroapical; (C) anteroseptal.

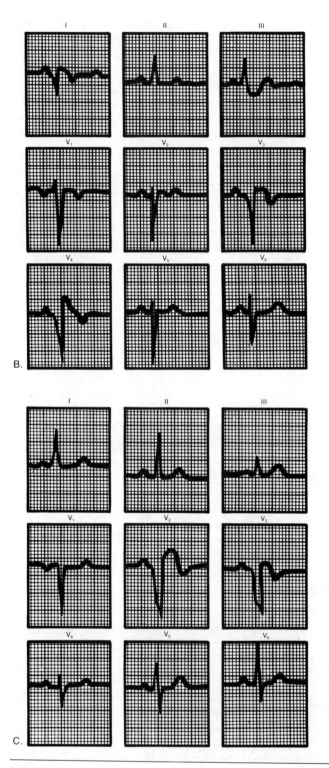

FIGURE 7.14   *(continued)*

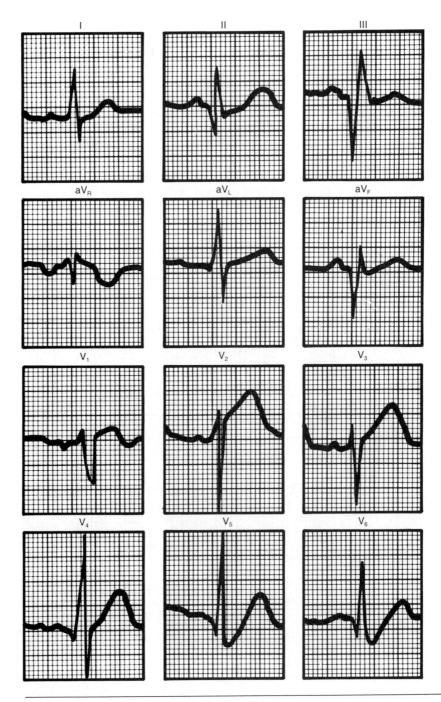

FIGURE 7.15
ECG changes in acute inferior myocardial infarction.

Posterior Wall MI

There are no ECG leads that look directly at the true posterior wall. Therefore, the leads opposite that wall are examined for reciprocal changes. Precordial leads V_1 and V_2 will have large R waves, and V_5 and V_6 will have small R waves. There may be some ST depression in V_3 and V_4 (Figure 7.16). Frequently, posterior infarcts occur with inferior infarcts, a syndrome that produces a picture of tall R waves in V_1 and V_2 and Q waves in II, III, and aV_F.

As previously stated, the ST segment and T wave changes produced by an MI generally resolve in a matter of weeks or months. The Q waves remain, indicating the occurrence of a previous MI. An ECG picture of Q waves in leads II, III, and aV_F, ST elevations, and T wave inversion in leads I, aV_L, and V_5 and V_6 would indicate to the nurse that the person had had a prior inferior

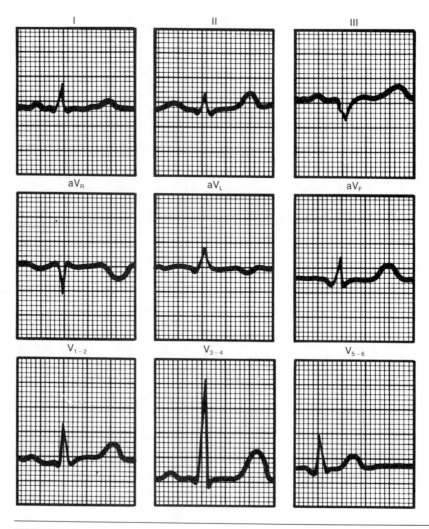

FIGURE 7.16
ECG changes in posterior myocardial infarction.

MI and was evolving an anterolateral MI. In approximately 50% of patients who develop a ventricular aneurysm as a complication of their MIs, ST elevations over the affected area do not return to baseline. Pericarditis may result in diffuse ST elevations of no specific infarction patterns. The diagnosis of MI in the presence of LBBB is difficult, because the presence of the block obscures the development of the Q waves. The presence of an MI is suspected in patients with LBBB if there is marked reduction in QRS voltage or if there is marked ST elevation.

Right Ventricular MI

Right ventricular infarction now appears to be more common than had previously been suspected [9]. It is often associated with infarction of the inferior wall. Although there are no ECG findings that are conclusively diagnostic of a right ventricular MI, some studies have shown that the presence of ST elevations in leads V_{3R} and V_{4R} correlates with the clinical findings of this MI [3] (see Chapter 9).

SUMMARY

The ability to interpret data obtained from the twelve-lead ECG is a crucial skill for the cardiac care nurse. It is not difficult to obtain this skill, but it does require diligence. The nurse who examines the patient's ECGs daily and compares her or his conclusions with those of the other nurses and cardiologists will soon be able to detect the subtle changes that can occur and that can affect the patient's ultimate prognosis. The advanced cardiac nurse is able to detect these changes, validates them against the patient's clinical picture, and seeks the appropriate interventions in a timely manner, thus providing optimal care to the person with cardiac disease.

STUDY QUESTIONS

1. A 56-year-old man is admitted to the cardiac care unit with a 3-hour history of crushing chest pain, nausea, and vomiting. His admission ECG shows Q waves in II, III, and aV_F, with ST elevations in leads I, aV_L, and V_5 and V_6. What area of his myocardium is at risk now? Has he had a myocardial infarction in the past? If so, what type?

2. Define *action potential,* and state the difference between the fast- and slow-response action potential.

3. What is the clinical significance of changes in axis?

4. Changes in polarity across the cell membrane result primarily from the movement of which ions across the membrane?

5. List the normal ECG waveforms and intervals.

6. Define *absolute refractory period.*

7. Define *bifascicular block* and give an example of such a condition.

8. How is the ventricular septum activated normally? How is it activated in LBBB? How is this activity shown on the ECG?

REFERENCES

1. Andreoli, K. G., et al. *Comprehensive Cardiac Care* (5th ed.). St. Louis: Mosby, 1983.

2. Conover, M. *Understanding Electrocardiography* (3rd ed.). St. Louis: Mosby, 1980.

3. Croft, C. H., et al. Detection of acute right ventricular infarction by right precordial electrocardiology. *Am. J. Cardiol.* 50:421, 1982.

4. Dubin, D. *Rapid Interpretation of EKGs* (3rd ed.). Tampa: Cover Publishing Co., 1979.

5. Duke, D. M. Intraventricular conduction blocks. I. *Crit. Care Nurs.* 1(3):30, 1982.

6. Duke, D. M. Intraventricular conduction blocks. II. *Crit. Care Nurs.* 1(4):58, 1982.

7. Goldberger, A. L., and Goldberger, E. *Clinical Electrocardiography* (2nd ed.). St. Louis: Mosby, 1981.

8. Goldman, M. J. *Principles of Clinical Electrocardiography* (11th ed.). Los Altos, Calif.: Lange, 1982.

9. Lorell, B., et al. Right ventricular infarction. *Am. J. Cardiol.* 43:465, 1979.

10. Mandel, W. *Cardiac Arrhythmias.* Philadelphia: Lippincott, 1980.

11. Netter, F. H. *The CIBA Collection of Medical Illustrations. Vol. 5:Heart.* New York: CIBA, 1969.

12. Rice, V. Calcium, the heart, and calcium antagonists. *Crit. Care Nurs.* 1(4):30, 1982.

13. Rice, V. The role of potassium in health and disease. *Crit. Care Nurs.* 1(3):54, 1982.

14. Shepard, N., Vaughan, P., and Rice, V. A guide to arrhythmia interpretation and management. *Crit. Care Nurs.* 1(5):58, 1982.

15. Van Meter, M., and Lavine, P. G. *Reading ECGs Correctly.* Horsham, Pa.: Nursing 81 Books, 1981.

16. Vinsant, M. O., and Spence, M. *Commonsense Approach to Coronary Care.* St. Louis: Mosby, 1981.

17. Winsor, T. *The Electrocardiogram in Myocardial Infarction.* New York: CIBA, 1977.

CHAPTER 8

Alterations in Heart Rate and Rhythm

Susan Lynn Zorb

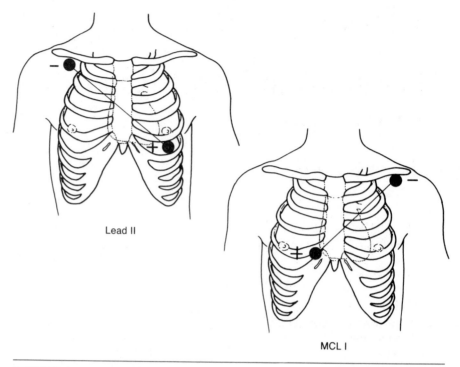

Lead II

MCL I

FIGURE 8.1
Leads most commonly used for continuous ECG monitoring. For lead II the positive pole is at the fifth intercostal space at the left midclavicular line. For modified chest lead (MCL) I the positive pole is at the fourth intercostal space to the right of the sternum.

INTRODUCTION

Recognizing and treating dysrhythmias constitute a major responsibility of the critical care nurse. Dysrhythmias must be promptly and correctly identified by the nurse to prevent the occurrence of serious consequences. In the cardiac critical care area, each patient's electrocardiographic (ECG) tracings are continuously monitored by means of a cable-and-electrode system attached to the patient's chest and connected to a bedside monitor. The electrodes can be placed so that leads similar to the standard ECG leads can be produced. Because they closely parallel the common mean cardiac vector, the most common leads chosen for this purpose are lead II and modified chest lead (MCL) I (Figure 8.1).

The purpose of continuous ECG monitoring is to detect changes in the patient's heart rate and rhythm. Detection of ischemic changes or changes in axis requires analysis of the entire twelve-lead ECG, as discussed in Chapter 7. This chapter will describe the dysrhythmias commonly encountered in the critical care unit (ICU) and their hemodynamic effects on the patient.

MECHANISMS OF DYSRHYTHMIAS

The term *dysrhythmia* refers to a disturbance in rhythm, rate, or conduction of the impulse throughout the myocardium. There are three mechanisms re-

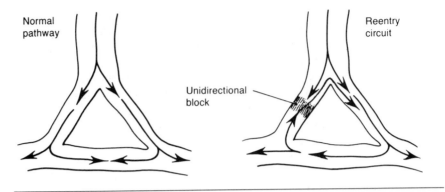

FIGURE 8.2
Mechanism of reentry. In the reentry circuit a unidirectional block permits the impulse to reenter the tissue and set up a circus movement.

sponsible for dysrhythmias: altered automoticity, altered conduction, and reentry. These mechanisms are discussed in terms of action potentials, which are described in Chapter 7. Understanding these mechanisms is crucial to understanding the types of therapy employed in the treatment of specific dysrhythmias.

Altered Automoticity

Enhanced Automoticity
Automoticity — the ability of the cell to generate an impulse — is enhanced if the slope of phase 4 is increased in a slow-response action potential or if a cell with a fast response converts to a slow-response action potential. Several factors enhance automoticity, including catecholamine release, hypokalemia, hypoxia, and hyperthermia. Any agent that blocks the action of the vagus nerve, such as atropine, will also enhance automoticity. Enhanced automoticity predisposes to an increased heart rate and premature beats.

Diminished Automoticity
If the slope of phase 4 is decreased or the threshold potential is increased, the cell will be less able to initiate an impulse. A decreased heart rate will result, as well as firing from sites other than the sinoatrial (SA) node. Factors that diminish automoticity include increased vagal tone, hyperkalemia, and hypothermia. Drugs such as beta blockers, procainamide hydrochloride, and quinidine also work to diminish automoticity.

Altered Conductivity

Dysrhythmias may be caused by changes in the conduction tissue itself. These can be actual physical changes such as fibrosis, or temporary changes resulting from ischemia or tissue injury. Parts of the conduction system may also be altered by surgical procedures, especially replacement of the aortic valve or repair of a ventricular septal defect.

Reentry

In reentry, a single impulse depolarizes the myocardium more than once. Normally, an impulse enters a branching section of the conduction pathway, travels down both branches simultaneously, and is extinguished when it meets itself on the connecting branch (Figure 8.2). In order for reentry to occur, one of the branches must be refractory to the impulse, which then travels down the other branch, across the connecting branch, and back to the refractory branch. This branch has now had a chance to recover and can accept the impulse. The impulse travels back up that branch and reenters the tissue, traveling through the circuit again (see Figure 8.2). If this circus movement is not altered or extinguished it will result in a tachycardia from the reentry point.

Reentry generally occurs in an ischemic or injured heart; such tissue may exhibit a longer refractory time than the surrounding healthy tissue.

DEFINITION OF TERMS

The study of electrocardiography involves a specific vocabulary, and a thorough understanding of these terms is essential for accurate communication of the patient's condition to all members of the health care team. Many of the terms are generic and can be applied to several dysrhythmias. Therefore, the nurse must be specific in applying them — for example, "atrial bigeminy."

Bradycardia. A rate slower then the normal rate for that tissue. Sinus bradycardia is a rate of less than 60 beats per minute (bpm).

Tachycardia. A rate faster than the normal rate for that tissue. Junctional tachycardia is a rate of more than 60 bpm; sinus tachycardia, more than 100 bpm.

Pacemaker. The area in the heart that initiates the depolarization wave; usually the SA node.

Aberrant conduction. Impulse conduction that does not follow the normal pathways.

Ectopic focus. A site of impulse formation other than the SA node.

Capture. To cause depolarization of the entire heart (said of an impulse).

Premature beat. A beat that comes earlier than expected, usually because of altered automoticity or reentry.

Escape beat. A beat that comes later than expected. It is a defense mechanism that operates when higher pacemakers have failed.

Refractory. Unable to accept an impulse and be depolarized (said of tissue).

Interpolation. Occurrence of a rate-related ectopic beat between two normal beats without disruption of rhythm.

Supraventricular. Arising outside of or above the ventricle. The impulse that depolarizes the ventricle is generally supraventricular if the QRS complex is less than 0.11 sec in duration.

Ventricular. Arising within the ventricle. The impulse that depolarizes the ventricle is generally ventricular if the QRS complex is more than 0.11 sec in duration.

Compensatory pause. The interval from the normal beat preceding a

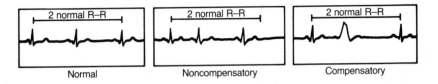

FIGURE 8.3
In a compensatory pause the interval from the normal beat preceding the premature beat to the normal beat following it is exactly equal to two R-to-R intervals. In a noncompensatory pause that interval is less than two normal R-to-R intervals.

single premature beat to the normal beat following the premature beat, if exactly equal to two normal R-to-R intervals (Figure 8.3). Such a pause occurs if the sinus node is not depolarized by the premature beat.

Noncompensatory pause. The interval from the normal beat preceding a single premature beat to the normal beat following it, if equal to less than two normal R-to-R intervals (see Figure 8.3). Such a pause occurs if the sinus node is depolarized by the early beat and resets itself accordingly.

Antegrade conduction. Movement of impulse forward throughout the heart.

Retrograde conduction. Movement of the impulse backward through a part of the heart.

Patterns

Bigeminy. A normal beat followed by a premature beat in a recurring pattern.

Trigeminy. Two normal beats followed by a premature beat in a recurring pattern.

Quadrigeminy. Three normal beats followed by a premature beat in a recurring pattern.

Couplet. Two successive ectopic beats.

Triplet. Three successive ectopic beats.

ANALYSIS OF MONITOR STRIPS

Competent dysrhythmia analysis requires a consistent approach. The specific order of the analysis matters less than the fact that each component is looked at in turn. The components of the ECG that must be analyzed include:

Atrial depolarization

P waves. Presence or absence, configuration, (upright, inverted, biphasic, notched), rate.

PR interval. Duration, constancy.

Ventricular depolarization and repolarization

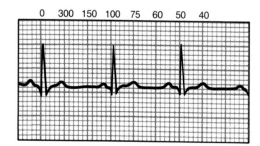

FIGURE 8.4
Method of calculating heart rate. One finds a QRS complex that falls directly on a heavy dark line, labels that line 0, and counts over to the next complex. The heavy line as numbered will indicate the heart rate.

QRS waves.   Presence or absence, one complex for every P wave, duration, configuration, supraventricular or ventricular.

T waves.   Configuration (upright, inverted, flattened).

QT interval.   Normal or prolonged.

Determination of Rate

Rate in both the atria and the ventricles can be an important diagnostic clue. If the person's rhythm is irregular, one can estimate the rate by counting the complexes in a 6-sec (6-inch) rhythm strip and multiplying by 10.

In a rhythm strip with a regular rate, two methods can be employed to calculate the rate. The more accurate is to count the number of small boxes between a point on the waveform being measured to that same point on the next waveform, and then to divide that number into 1,500 (there are 1,500 small boxes in 1 minute). For example, to calculate an atrial rate, one can count the number of small boxes from the beginning of one P wave to the beginning of the next P wave (say, 15) and divide that number into 1,500: 1,500 ÷ 15 = 100 bpm. The ventricular rate can be calculated by measuring from R wave to R wave in the same manner.

Another method of rate calculation involves assigning certain numbers to the heavy black lines on the ECG paper, as indicated in Figure 8.4. One finds a P wave or QRS complex that is directly on a heavy dark line and labels that line 0. If the succeeding heavy lines are then numbered as indicated in Figure 8.4, the label of the line on which the next complex falls will indicate the heart rate. If the next complex falls between lines, one can approximate the rate. This method is intended merely as a quick reference and does not take the place of more accurate rate determination.

DYSRHYTHMIAS

Diagnosis of the dysrhythmia is only the first step in caring for the cardiac patient. The nurse must be able to correlate the dysrhythmia with its effect on the patient's hemodynamic status, and must be familiar with the appropriate interventions for the dysrhythmia. Pharmacological and mechanical intervention is discussed in detail in other chapters of this book. Here we will deal with dysrhythmia recognition (mechanism and ECG criteria), the hemodynamic consequences, and treatment. The dysrhythmias are classified according to the site of impulse formation.

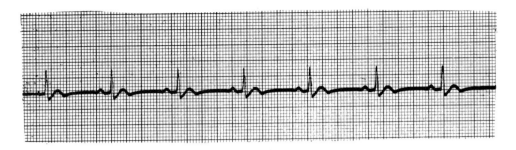

FIGURE 8.5
Normal sinus rhythm.

Sinus Rhythms   *Normal Sinus Rhythm*

Mechanism. The impulse originates in the sinus node and follows the normal conduction system through the heart.

ECG criteria. P, QRS, and T are present with normal configurations. The PR, QRS, and QT intervals are normal. Rate, 60 to 100 bpm, regular (Figure 8.5).

Hemodynamic effects. The hemodynamically ideal rhythm. Atrial and ventricular contraction is synchronized and allows adequate time for atrial emptying and ventricular filling.

Intervention. None.

Sinus Arrhythmia

Mechanism. The impulse arises in the sinus node and is conducted normally through the heart. The heart rate increases on inspiration and decreases on expiration. The acceleration and deceleration with respiration are due to changes in intrathoracic pressures and venous return to the heart.

ECG criteria. P, QRS, and T are present with normal intervals. Rate, usually 60 to 100 bpm, with irregular rhythmic pattern related to respiration (Figure 8.6).

Hemodynamic effects. Generally no adverse effects. Condition may be more pronounced in patients who are hypovolemic or who are receiving positive-pressure ventilation. May make the diagnosis of other dysrhythmias more difficult by disturbing the regular rhythm.

Intervention. Usually none required.

Sinus Bradycardia

Mechanism. The impulse originates in the SA node and is conducted normally throughout the heart; the rate of sinus firing is less than 60 bpm, how-

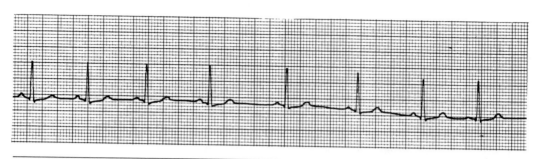

FIGURE 8.6
Sinus arrhythmia.

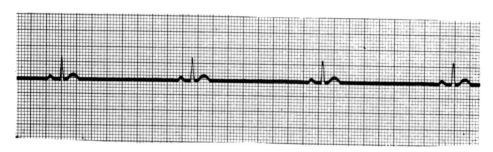

FIGURE 8.7
Sinus bradycardia.

ever, possibly because of increased vagal tone, or beta blockade. This rhythm is normally present in conditioned athletes.

ECG criteria.   P, QRS, and T are present with normal intervals. Rate, less than 60 bpm, regular (Figure 8.7).

Hemodynamic effect.   Cardiac output is usually normal, with heart rates between 40 and 60 bpm; with rates of less than 40 bpm, however, cardiac output may be significantly decreased. Sinus bradycardia is often a desired effect of beta blockade therapy, because it reduces myocardial oxygen consumption.

Intervention.   Atropine sulfate or isoproterenol hydrochloride administration; pacemaker if patient is severely symptomatic.

Sinus Tachycardia

Mechanism.   The impulse arises in the SA node and is conducted normally; the rate of sinus firing is more than 100 bpm, however, and is possibly related to fever, dehydration, increased sympathetic stimulation, exercise, and stress.

ECG criteria.   P, QRS, and T are present with normal intervals. The T and P waves may blend together because of the increased rate, making it difficult or impossible to measure the intervals (Figure 8.8).

Hemodynamic effect.   May either increase or decrease cardiac output, de-

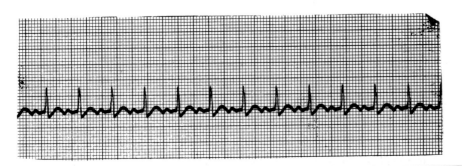

FIGURE 8.8
Sinus tachycardia.

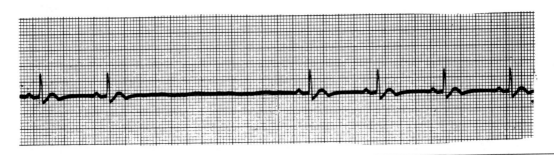

FIGURE 8.9
Sinus arrest.

pending on the state of the ventricles, blood volume, and rate. Tachycardia increases myocardial oxygen consumption.

Intervention. Diagnosis and treatment of the underlying cause.

Sinus Arrest and Sinus Exit Block

Mechanism. In sinus arrest the sinus node does not generate an impulse. In sinus exit block it generates an impulse that is blocked before it can leave the SA node. The block is thought usually to result from increased vagal tone.

ECG criteria. Normal sinus rhythm with pauses. The pause can either be an exact multiple of the normal R-R interval, indicating probable sinus exit block, or bear no relation to the normal R-R interval, indicating sinus arrest (Figure 8.9).

Hemodynamic effect. Depends on the duration of the block. If the pause is short, there is no detrimental hemodynamic effect; if prolonged, however, this rhythm can decrease cardiac output.

Intervention. Atropine or isoproterenol administration, or pacemaker insertion if the patient is severely symptomatic.

Atrial Rhythms   *Premature Atrial Contraction*

Mechanism.   The impulse originates from an atrial focus, not the SA node, and is conducted aberrantly through the atria. Conduction through the atrioventricular (AV) junction depends on the timing. If the premature atrial contraction (PAC) is very early, it may find the AV node refractory, and the impulse will be blocked. If the AV node is partially refractory, it may conduct the impulse more slowly than normal. If it has completely recovered, it will conduct at the normal rate. PACs can result from increased sympathetic stimulation, caffeine or nicotine ingestion, and fatigue.

ECG criteria.   The P wave comes early and may have a configuration different from that of the other P waves. The PR interval may be either short, long, or normal in duration. The QRS complex, if present, is supraventricular in origin. Incomplete or noncompensatory pause generally is present (Figure 8.10).

Hemodynamic effect.   Isolated PACs have little detrimental hemodynamic effect. Frequent PACs reduce cardiac output and may be a precursor of more serious atrial rhythms.

Intervention.   No treatment is required for isolated PACs. Frequent PACs may be treated with one of the following antiarrhythmic agents: quinidine, procainamide, beta blockers, calcium channel blockers, and digitalis.

Atrial Tachycardia

Mechanism.   An atrial focus becomes the dominant pacemaker, through either enhanced automoticity or reentry, with a rate of between 150 and 250 bpm. Conduction through the AV node is either normal, in which case every atrial impulse is conducted, or blocked so that only occasional impulses are conducted. Atrial tachycardia may have a sudden onset and termination, a condition referred to as paroxysmal atrial tachycardia (PAT) or paroxysmal supraventricular tachycardia (PSVT), or may be more sustained. Atrial tachycardia is a common occurrence in young adults, or it can indicate the presence of underlying cardiac disease.

ECG criteria.   P waves are present, but the configuration is often changed from that in a sinus beat; P waves are often buried in the preceding T wave. The PR interval is often hard to measure because of the TP combination. QRS complexes are present and supraventricular. The atrial rate is between 150 and 250 bpm and regular. The ventricular rate is usually the same as, but occasionally less than, the atrial rate (Figure 8.11).

Hemodynamic effect.   Cardiac output is decreased because of the reduced ventricular filling time. Patients may complain of palpitations and lightheadedness.

Intervention.   Maneuvers to increase vagal tone, such as carotid sinus massage and Valsalva maneuver, and drugs such as verapamil hydrochloride, quinidine, procainamide, beta blockers, and digitalis.

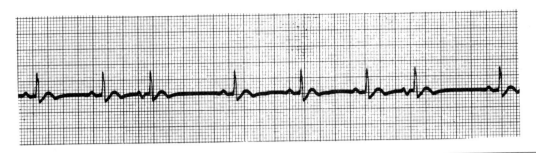

FIGURE 8.10
Premature atrial contraction.

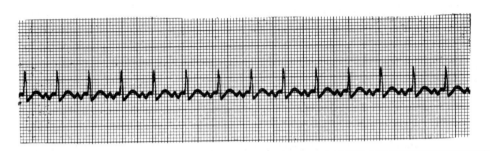

FIGURE 8.11
Paroxysmal atrial tachycardia.

Atrial Flutter

Mechanism. An atrial focus is the dominant pacemaker, with a rate of 250 to 400 bpm. Conduction through the AV node is intermittent because of the rapid atrial rate. Impulses may be conducted in a pattern — for example, every other impulse is conducted (2:1) or every third impulse is conducted (3:1) — or randomly.

ECG criteria. P waves are present; the configuration is generally sawtoothed. The PR interval is impossible to measure accurately. The QRS complex is present and supraventricular. The T wave is present but may be distorted by the P waves. Atrial rate, 250 to 400 bpm, regular. Ventricular rate, usually slower than atrial rate; may be either regular or irregular, depending on AV node conduction (Figure 8.12).

Hemodynamic effect. Cardiac output is decreased because atrial kick is lost and ventricular filling time is decreased.

Interventions. Aimed at controlling the ventricular response via carotid sinus massage and drugs such as verapamil, quinidine, procainamide, digitalis, and beta blockers. Occasionally cardioversion is required if drug therapy is ineffective or the patient is symptomatic.

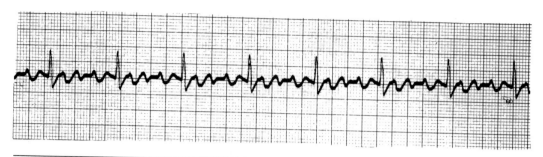

FIGURE 8.12
Atrial flutter.

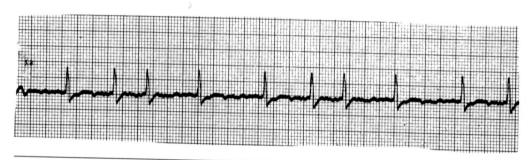

FIGURE 8.13
Atrial fibrillation.

Atrial Fibrillation

Mechanism. The atrial muscle mass fibrillates because each cell depolarizes at its own rate. There is no synchrony in the atrial contraction. Conduction of these rapid, random atrial impulses through the AV node is irregular.

ECG criteria. P waves show no evidence of organized atrial activity; baseline wavers. The QRS complex is present and supraventricular. Ventricular rate may be rapid or slow and is irregular (Figure 8.13).

Hemodynamic effects. Decreased cardiac output because atrial kick is lost and ventricular filling time is reduced. Some patients can tolerate this rhythm well; others begin to decompensate immediately. Generally, the faster the ventricular rate, the greater the decrease in cardiac output.

Intervention. Reduce ventricular rate, as discussed in the section describing atrial flutter.

Junctional Rhythms

Mechanism. The mechanism of all junctional beats is the same regardless of the timing of the beat. An impulse arises in the AV node or junctional tissue, where the inherent rate is 45 to 60 bpm. It is conducted retrograde into the atrium and antegrade through the ventricle. The timing of atrial and ventric-

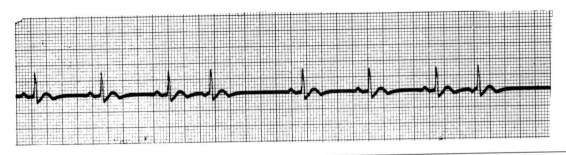

FIGURE 8.14
Premature junctional contraction.

ular depolarization determines the distance of the P wave from the QRS complex. If the depolarization is simultaneous, no P wave will be evident. If the atrium is depolarized before the ventricle, there will be an inverted P wave less than 0.12 sec prior to the QRS complex. If the atrium is depolarized after the ventricle, there will be an inverted P wave after the QRS.

ECG criteria. P waves are inverted prior to the QRS, absent, or inverted after the QRS. The PR interval is less than 0.12 sec in duration. QRS complexes are present and supraventricular.

Premature Junctional Contraction

Mechanism. Possibly enhanced automoticity or reentry.

ECG criteria. P waves are described for junctional rhythms. The QRS complex comes early and is supraventricular. A noncompensatory pause is present (Figure 8.14).

Hemodynamic effects. Minimal effects with isolated beats; decreased cardiac output with frequent premature junctional contractions.

Intervention. This dysrhythmia requires treatment only if the patient is hemodynamically unstable. Procainamide, quinidine, or beta blockers can be used.

Escape Junctional Contraction

Mechanism. Normal response to failure of higher pacemakers (SA node, atria) to function.

ECG criteria. P waves are as described for junctional rhythms. The QRS complex occurs after the normal R-to-R interval and is supraventricular (Figure 8.15).

Hemodynamic effect. Improves cardiac output by providing for ventricular depolarization when higher pacemakers have failed.

Intervention. Treatment of the cause of the higher pacemaker failure.

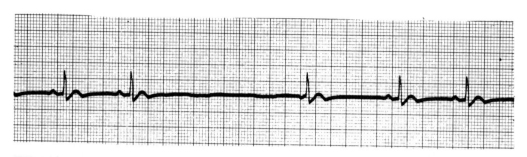

FIGURE 8.15
Escape junctional contraction.

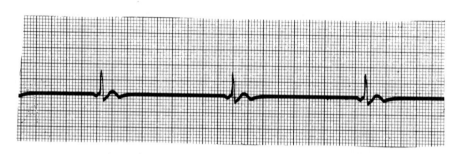

FIGURE 8.16
Junctional rhythm.

Junctional Rhythm

Mechanism. The junctional tissue becomes the dominant pacemaker of the heart by default of the higher pacemakers.

ECG criteria. P waves are as described for junctional rhythms. The QRS complex is supraventricular. Rate, 45 to 60 bpm, regular (Figure 8.16).

Hemodynamic effect. Decreased cardiac output caused by loss of synchrony of atrial and ventricular contraction, as well as the slow rate.

Intervention. Treatment of the cause of higher pacemaker failure.

Junctional Tachycardia

Mechanism. Junctional tissue becomes the dominant pacemaker through either enhanced automoticity or reentry.

ECG criteria. QRS complex is supraventricular. Rate, more than 60 bpm, regular (Figure 8.17).

Hemodynamic effect. Depending on the rate, the cardiac output may be either normal or decreased.

Intervention. If there is evidence of an adequate cardiac output, no interven-

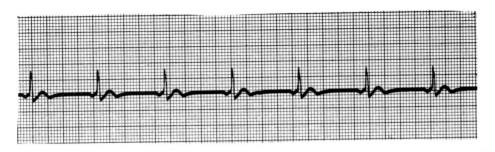

FIGURE 8.17
Junctional tachycardia.

tion is necessary. If cardiac output is decreased, antiarrhythmic agents such as procainamide, quinidine, propranolol, and digitalis are used.

Ventricular Rhythms

Premature Ventricular Contraction

Mechanism. The impulse arises in the ventricles and is conducted abnormally through the ventricles, resulting in a wide (more than 0.11 sec), bizarre QRS configuration. Repolarization is also abnormal, and ST and T waves are usually opposite in deflection from the initial deflection of the QRS. There is no associated atrial activity unless the impulse is conducted retrograde into the atria. If the premature ventricular contraction (PVC) occurs after normal atrial depolarization has begun, a fusion of the normal P wave with the PVC may occur. PVCs can result from either enhanced automoticity or reentry. If they arise from one focus (are unifocal), each PVC will have the same configuration. If they arise from more than one focus (are multifocal), each PVC will have a different configuration. PVCs can occur in the patterns listed on page 177.

ECG criteria. P waves are usually absent. QRS complexes are more than 0.11 sec in duration, are bizarre looking, and occur early. The ST-T wave occurs in a direction opposite from that of the initial QRS complex. Usually a full compensatory pause is evident (Figure 8.18).

Hemodynamic effect. Depends on the frequency. Cardiac output is decreased with frequent PVCs because of decreased diastolic filling time. PVCs that occur in the vulnerable period of the T wave can initiate more serious ventricular dysrhythmias.

Intervention. Treatment depends largely on the frequency and timing of the PVCs. The goal of therapy is to suppress the ectopic focus or to interrupt the reentry pathway. Antiarrhythmic agents such as lidocaine hydrochloride, procainamide, bretylium tosylate, mexilitine, and phenytoin may be used. Most cardiac care units have established treatment protocols for PVCs that are instituted in the following situations: couplets, triplets, multifocal PVCs, occurrence of more than 6 to 8 PVCs per minute, and bigeminy.

The next two dysrhythmias to be discussed — ventricular tachycardia and ventricular fibrillation — are considered life-threatening dysrhythmias.

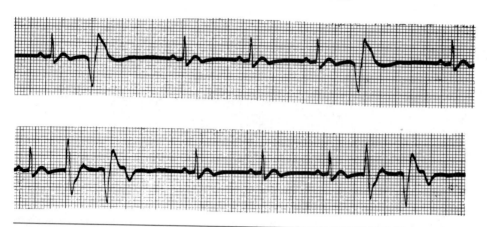

FIGURE 8.18
Premature ventricular contractions, multifocal couplet.

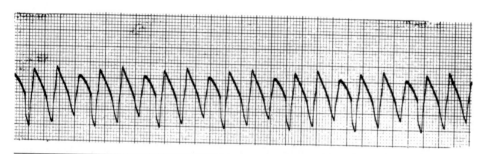

FIGURE 8.19
Ventricular tachycardia.

Development of either of these rhythms is a medical emergency requiring immediate intervention.

Ventricular Tachycardia

Mechanism. Impulse arises in the ventricle and is conducted abnormally throughout the ventricles. Defined as more than three PVCs in a row at a rate of more than 100 bpm.

ECG criteria. QRS complex is wide and bizarre. Rate, more than 100 bpm, usually regular. P waves are usually absent (Figure 8.19).

Hemodynamic effect. Decreased cardiac output because atrial–ventricular synchrony is lost and diastolic filling time is decreased.

Intervention. Lidocaine, bretylium, procainamide, or mexilitine administration, or defibrillation.

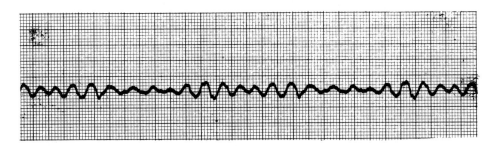

FIGURE 8.20
Ventricular fibrillation.

Ventricular Fibrillation

Mechanism. Multiple ectopic foci firing at random, producing chaotic depolarization of the ventricles with no organized contraction. May be either coarse, in which case the ECG shows wide variations, or fine, in which case the ECG is nearly a straight line.

ECG criteria. Disordered, chaotic electrical activity; no discernible complexes (Figure 8.20).

Hemodynamic effect. Causes cessation of cardiac output, a situation incompatible with life.

Intervention. Defibrillation; bretylium administration. Cardiopulmonary resuscitation must be performed until the patient returns to a stable rhythm.

Escape Ventricular Contraction

Mechanism. A ventricular focus is activated in response to a failure of higher pacemakers. The configuration of the escape beat is the same as that of a PVC, but the former occurs after the normal R-to-R interval.

ECG criteria. Ectopic beat occurs after a normal R-to-R interval. QRS complexes are more than 0.11 sec in duration and of bizarre configuration (Figure 8.21).

Hemodynamic effect. Escape beats act as a compensatory mechanism to maintain cardiac output in the event of higher pacemaker failure.

Intervention. Therapy is aimed at restoring a higher pacemaker site. Drugs such as atropine or isoproterenol may be used alone or in combination with a pacemaker.

Idioventricular Rhythm

Mechanism. An escape rhythm in which a ventricular focus becomes the dominant pacemaker through default of the higher pacemakers.

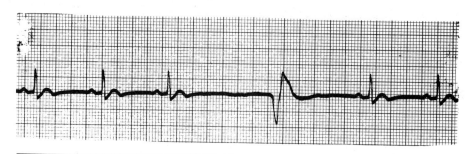

FIGURE 8.21
Escape ventricular contraction.

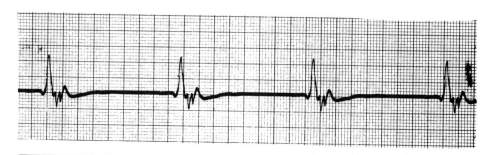

FIGURE 8.22
Idioventricular rhythm.

ECG criteria.   P waves are absent; QRS complexes are wide and bizarre. Rate, less than 40 bpm, regular (Figure 8.22).

Hemodynamic effect.   Cardiac output is reduced because of the decreased rate.

Intervention.   Atropine or isoproterenol administration; pacing.

Accelerated Idioventricular Rhythm

Mechanism.   A ventricular rhythm with a rate of from 40 to 100 bpm. Type I occurs in response to failure of an idioventricular rhythm to maintain an adequate cardiac output in the face of higher pacemaker failure. Type II occurs when an ectopic focus becomes the dominant pacemaker at this rate and follows a PVC. The causative mechanism affects the treatment selected.

ECG criteria.   P waves are absent. The QRS complex is more than 0.11 sec in duration, bizarre, and regular. Rate, 40 to 100 bpm (Figure 8.23).

Hemodynamic effect.   An adequate cardiac output is usually maintained.

Intervention.   Type I: restore the higher pacemakers, as discussed for idioventricular rhythm. Type II: suppress the ectopic focus with lidocaine, procainamide, or mexilitine.

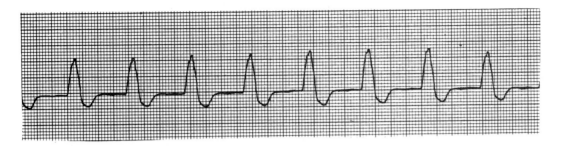

FIGURE 8.23
Accelerated idioventricular rhythm.

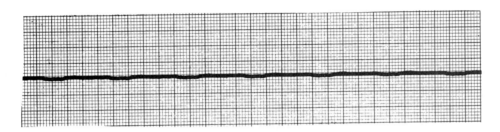

FIGURE 8.24
Asystole.

Asystole

Mechanism.   Complete electrical standstill.

ECG criteria.   Flat baseline; no electrical activity (Figure 8.24).

Hemodynamic effect.   No cardiac output.

Intervention.   Cardiopulmonary resuscitation; epinephrine or calcium chloride administration.

Electromechanical Dissociation
A phenomenon in which there is electrical activity of the heart but no resulting cardiac output. Clinically, this produces an ECG pattern with no palpable pulses. The condition occurs most frequently in the dying heart and in rupture of the heart.

Aberrancy versus Ventricular Ectopy
Atrial impulses may be conducted throughout the ventricles aberrantly — that is, along pathways other than those through normal conduction tissue. Distinguishing between aberrancy and ventricular ectopy will determine the appropriate intervention. An aberrant QRS complex will be wide and bizarre and will appear ventricular in origin. Certain factors favor the occurrence of aberrancy.

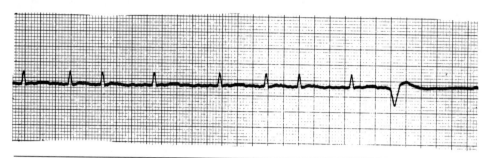

FIGURE 8.25
Ashman's phenomenon.

1. If the rate is increased from the individual's norm, parts of the conduction tissue may be refractory when the next impulse arrives.

2. RSR′ picture in V_1 is frequently evident in aberration, because the right bundle branch has the longer refractory time and is the more likely to be refractory when the next impulse arrives, giving a picture of right bundle branch block (see Chapter 7).

3. Ashman's phenomenon: In atrial fibrillation one frequently encounters a "long–short" pattern in which the short cycle ends with an aberrantly conducted impulse. In the mechanism involved, the long cycle resets the refractory period of the conduction tissue. When the next impulse occurs after a shorter period, it finds some of the tissue refractory and is conducted aberrantly through the ventricles (Figure 8.25).

AV Blocks

First-Degree AV Block

Mechanism. The impulse arises in the SA node and is conducted normally throughout the heart. It does encounter an increased delay in conduction through the AV node. This delay may indicate disease of the conduction system or may be produced by drugs such as digitalis and quinidine.

ECG criteria. P, QRS, and T waves appear normal; each P wave is followed by a QRS complex. The PR interval is more than 0.20 sec in duration (Figure 8.26).

Hemodynamic effect. There are no detrimental hemodynamic effects.

Intervention. If the first-degree AV block (1° AVB) is drug related, the drug may be held. Usually no intervention is needed for 1° AVB.

Second-Degree AV Block

In second-degree AV block (2° AVB), some of the atrial impulses are blocked completely at the AV junction. There are two major types of 2° AVB, with a third group for those that cannot be classified as either type I or type II.

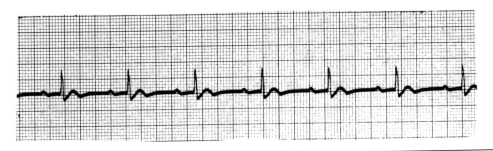

FIGURE 8.26
First-degree AV block.

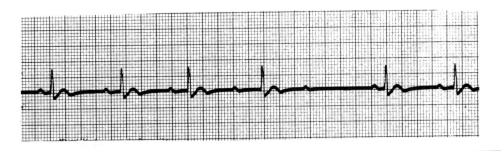

FIGURE 8.27
Second-degree AV block, Mobitz type I.

Mobitz Type I (Wenckebach)

Mechanism.   Impulses originate in the sinus node and are conducted at increasing intervals through the AV node until an impulse is blocked completely. The impulse following the blocked impulse is conducted through the AV node with the shortest delay, and the interval increases progressively until another impulse is blocked. Type I 2° AVB generally occurs in the presence of myocardial ischemia and is usually transitory. It is the most common type of 2° AVB, constituting about 90% of all cases.

ECG criteria.   P waves are present and of normal configuration. Atrial rate is regular. The PR interval progressively lengthens until a QRS complex is dropped, shortens with the next conducted impulse, and lengthens again until a QRS complex again is dropped. Generally, the PR intervals after the dropped QRS complexes are constant, reflecting the best conduction through the AV node. The R-to-R interval is irregular; the QRS complexes appear in groups set off by the pause created by the dropped beat (Figure 8.27).

Hemodynamic effect.   If the dropped beats occur with sufficient frequency, the heart rate may be slow enough to cause a decreased cardiac output.

Intervention.   Unless there are signs of a decreased cardiac output, type I 2° AVB is usually not treated.

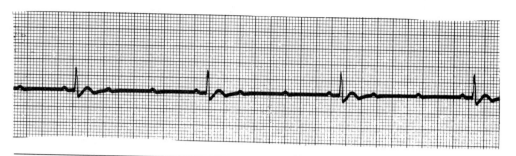

FIGURE 8.28
Second-degree AV block, Mobitz type II.

Mobitz Type II

Mechanism. The impulse arises in the sinus node and is conducted normally throughout the atria and ventricles. Intermittently, an impulse is blocked completely at the AV node. Otherwise, conduction through the AV node is normal. The cause of this intermittent block is not understood, although the block is thought to indicate disease of the conduction system rather than ischemia. Mobitz type II is a high-grade form of AV block. It is often found in conjunction with intraventricular conduction defects, described in Chapter 7.

ECG criteria. P waves are of normal configuration and regular rate. The PR interval is constant. QRS complexes may be normal or aberrant; the rate is irregular because of occasional blocked beats (not every P wave is followed by a QRS complex) (Figure 8.28).

Hemodynamic effect. If impulses are blocked with sufficient frequency, cardiac output may be diminished.

Intervention. If the cardiac output is decreased, the patient may be treated temporarily with atropine or isoproterenol. A permanent pacemaker may be inserted in those at high risk for development of complete heart block, such as those with an intraventricular conduction defect or an anteroseptal myocardial infarction. Otherwise, the patient is closely observed for evidence of a decrease in cardiac output.

2:1 Second-Degree AV Block

This is not a separate category of 2° AVB; rather, it is a descriptive label that is used when the differentiation between Mobitz types I and II cannot be made. When every second QRS complex is dropped, the PR intervals are constant and it is impossible to know whether the rhythm is Wenckebach or Mobitz type II. In order to avoid misdiagnosing the rhythm, it is simply labeled 2:1 AVB.

Third-Degree (Complete) Heart Block

Mechanism. Impulses arise in the sinus node but are completely blocked at the AV node. Therefore, the ventricles must initiate their own rhythm to main-

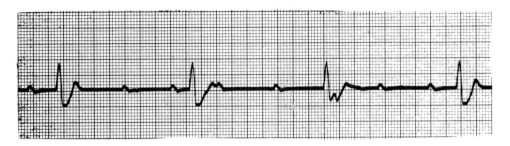

FIGURE 8.29
Third-degree AV block.

tain cardiac output. This ventricular rate is slower than the atrial rate. Complete heart block (CHB) is a result of disease in the conduction system and can be sustained or intermittent (Stokes-Adams attacks).

ECG criteria.   P waves are present, of normal configuration and regular rate. PR intervals are inconsistent. QRS complexes are present, ventricular in origin, and of regular rhythm. Ventricular rate is usually less than 40 bpm (Figure 8.29).

Hemodynamic effect.   Cardiac output can be markedly decreased because of the slow heart rate and the loss of synchrony between atrial and ventricular contraction.

Intervention.   Short-term treatment with drugs such as atropine and isoproterenol. A permanent pacemaker may be required.

AV Dissociation

Mechanism.   Two pacemakers are present, one in the SA node or atria and one in the AV node or junctional tissue. The AV pacemaker is usually more rapid and is the dominant pacemaker. AV dissociation may be complete, in which case the atrial focus never activates the ventricles, or incomplete (interference dissociation), in which case the atrial focus occasionally activates the ventricles. AV dissociation differs from CHB in that atrial impulses are able to activate the ventricles, whereas in CHB, the atrial impulses are blocked entirely at the AV node.

ECG criteria.   The dominant rhythm is usually junctional, with an independent, slower atrial rhythm that occasionally captures the ventricle and thereby disrupts the regularity of the junctional rhythm (Figure 8.30).

Hemodynamic effect.   No major detrimental hemodynamic effects.

Intervention.   Usually none required.

Preexcitation Syndromes

Mechanisms
Preexcitation syndromes are said to exist when part or all of the ventricular myocardium is activated by an atrial impulse earlier than would be expected

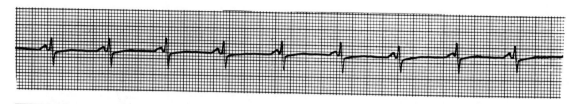

FIGURE 8.30
AV dissociation.

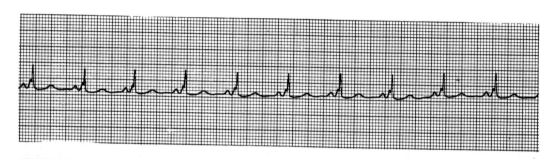

FIGURE 8.31
Preexcitation.

if the impulse were conducted through the normal pathway [5]. The most common preexcitation syndrome is Wolff-Parkinson-White (WPW) syndrome, in which one or more accessory pathways connect the atrial to the ventricular myocardium. Additional types of preexcitation occur in two other instances: (1) when Manheim fibers connect the distal AV node or bundle of His with part of the ventricular myocardium, and (2) when accessory pathways connect the atrial myocardium to the bundle of His, bypassing the AV node but depolarizing the ventricles in the normal manner. The latter pattern occurs in Lown-Ganong-Levine syndrome (LGL).

ECG Findings

WPW syndrome.   Conduction of the impulse through the accessory pathway causes early depolarization of part of the ventricle. The results are a shortened PR interval, a slurring of the initial portion of the QRS complex (referred to as a delta wave), and, often, ST and T wave changes in a direction opposite to that of the deflection of the QRS. (Figure 8.31).

Manheim pathways.   In this instance, because the AV node itself is not bypassed, the PR interval is normal. The QRS complex exhibits a delta wave.

LGL syndrome. The AV node is completely bypassed but ventricular depolarization is normal, producing a shortened PR interval with a normal QRS complex.

Clinical Significance

In and of themselves, preexcitation syndromes have no clinical significance. However, persons with these syndromes are prone to developing atrial tachycardias that are often unresponsive to drug therapy. These tachycardias are due to the reentry phenomenon discussed earlier. If not successfully treated, these rhythms can degenerate quickly into ventricular fibrillation. In patients who develop frequent atrial tachycardias, surgical treatment is often advised to sever the accessory pathways and thereby eliminate the problem.

SUMMARY

Accurate dysrhythmia recognition is an essential skill for the critical care nurse to acquire, and one that develops only through diligent practice. The inexperienced critical care nurse should take every opportunity to analyze rhythm strips with assistance from more experienced nurses and cardiologists. The nurse must be careful to analyze the monitor strip in a systematic fashion so that important information is not overlooked, and to correlate the ECG findings with the patient's clinical picture. A change in a cardiac rhythm can have a profound effect on the patient's hemodynamic status. Therefore, the critical care nurse must be alert to these changes and be able to interpret them correctly so that appropriate intervention can be instituted.

STUDY QUESTIONS

1. Define *supraventricular complexes* and *ventricular complexes,* and state the defining characteristic of each.
2. An impulse that arises from ischemic tissue is an example of which mechanism of ectopy?
3. List the intrinsic rate for the following areas of the conduction tissue: SA node; AV node; Bundle of His; ventricles.
4. What two conditions are necessary in order for reentry to occur?
5. What effect does tachycardia have on myocardial blood supply and cardiac output?
6. Define *preexcitation syndromes.* What clinical significance do they have?
7. What are the ECG criteria for atrial fibrillation?
8. Why are ventricular tachycardia and ventricular fibrillation considered life-threatening rhythms?
9. What hemodynamic effects would one expect to see in a patient who suddenly develops complete heart block?
10. What is the mechanism responsible for Wenckebach?

REFERENCES

1. Andreoli, K. G., et al. *Comprehensive Cardiac Care* (5th ed.). St. Louis: Mosby, 1983.

2. Arbert, S. R., Rubin, I. L., and Gross, H. *Differential Diagnosis of the Electrocardiogram* (2nd ed.). Philadelphia: Davis, 1975.

3. Conover, M. *Understanding Electrocardiography* (3rd ed.). St. Louis: Mosby, 1980.

4. Dubin, D. *Rapid Interpretation of EKG's* (3rd ed.). Tampa: Cover Publishing Co., 1979.

5. Gallagher, J. J., et al. The preexcitation syndromes. *Prog. Cardiovasc. Dis.* 20:285, 1978.

6. Goldberger, A. L., and Goldberger, E. *Clinical Electrocardiography* (2nd ed.). St. Louis: Mosby, 1981.

7. Goldman, M. J. *Principles of Clinical Electrocardiography* (11th ed.). Los Altos: Lange Medical Publishers, 1982.

8. McCarthy, E. Hemodynamic effects and clinical assessment of dysrhythmias. *Crit. Care Q.* 4(2):9, 1981.

9. Rice, V. Calcium, the heart, and calcium antagonists. *Crit. Care Nurs.* 1(4):30, 1982.

10. Rice, V. The role of potassium in health and disease. *Crit. Care Nurs.* 1(3):54, 1982.

11. Shepard, N., Vaughan, P., and Rice, V. A guide to arrhythmia interpretation and management. *Crit. Care Nurs.* 1(5):58, 1982.

12. Van Meter, M., and Lavine, P. G. *Reading EKGs Correctly.* Horsham, Pa.: Nursing '81 Books, 1981.

13. Vinsant, M. O., and Spence, M. *Commonsense Approach to Coronary Care.* St. Louis: Mosby, 1981.

PART III

Alterations in Cardiac Function

In Major Cardiac Disorders

CHAPTER 9

Coronary Artery Disease: Clinical Sequelae

Barbara Homer Yee

INTRODUCTION

Coronary artery disease (CAD) progressing to myocardial infarction (MI) is the leading cause of death in the United States and other Western countries. It is estimated that as many as 1.5 million Americans suffered an MI in 1982, and about 555,000 of these infarctions were fatal [2]. Atherosclerosis, an accumulation of lipids on the intima of arteries, is the major underlying cause of CAD. Although the atherosclerotic process actually begins at a very young age, symptoms may not appear until the fifth or sixth decade of life, when the coronary arteries are approximately 75% occluded. The initial clinical manifestations of the disease vary widely and include angina, MI, and sudden death. Because of the early development of this disease and the late presentation of symptoms, it is clear that prevention, through risk factor reduction, is the key to management of CAD.

RISK FACTORS

Several factors have been identified as contributing to an increased risk of developing CAD. A number of classification systems for risk factors exist; the American Heart Association uses the following three categories: (1) nonmodifiable factors, (2) modifiable factors, and (3) contributing factors [2]. The probability of a specific individual's developing CAD is determined by the number of risk factors present and the level of each factor.

Nonmodifiable Risk Factors

Age and Sex

Atherosclerosis becomes more prevalent with increasing age. It is a major cause of death in men aged 35 to 45 years, however, and causes 40% of deaths in men between the ages of 55 and 64 [3]. For women, the incidence of CAD increases sharply after menopause, approaching that among men of the same age. Before the age of 60, women have a 10% chance of having a cardiovascular event, compared with a 27% probability for men [22].

Race and Family History

Nonwhite individuals have a greater risk of developing CAD than do whites. Individuals with a family history of CAD are at greater risk for CAD and tend to develop it at a younger age.

Modifiable Risk Factors

Cigarette Smoking

The evidence linking cigarette smoking to increased risk is overwhelming and distinguishes the habit as one of the three major coronary risk factors. The incidence and mortality of CAD associated with smoking are influenced by several factors: the number of cigarettes smoked, the duration of smoking, the age at initiation of smoking, and the pattern of inhaling. Male smokers have a 70% higher mortality from CAD than male nonsmokers. Young women who smoke increase their risk of MI 20-fold. Individuals who smoke pipes or cigars are at slightly greater risk than nonsmokers; their risk is less than that of cigarette smokers, however. Once an individual quits smoking, the risk begins to decline and within ten years approaches that of a nonsmoker [48].

Cigarettes contain three compounds considered detrimental to health: tar, nicotine, and carbon monoxide. The chief physiological effects of these substances are peripheral vasoconstriction; cardiac stimulation, which increases heart rate, stroke volume, cardiac output, and contractility; increased oxygen consumption and incidence of dysrhythmias; and reduced O_2-carrying capacity of the blood.

Hypertension

Hypertension has long been associated with increased coronary risk and is also considered one of the three major risk factors. The degree of risk is directly related to the severity of hypertension. Individuals with mild hypertension (diastolic blood pressure of 90 to 104 mm Hg) are now being treated, however, with the impetus for early treatment being the increased cardiovascular risk associated with the condition. Hypertension is known to accelerate atherogenesis of the coronary and other arteries. The elevated arterial pressure also causes increased systemic vascular resistance, ventricular hypertrophy, and eventual cardiac failure.

Increased Cholesterol Levels

An increased serum cholesterol level is the third major risk factor. Studies have repeatedly demonstrated a distinct relationship between cholesterol levels and coronary risk. Here, also, the degree of risk is related to the amount of elevation. The Framingham Heart Study demonstrated that a man with a serum cholesterol level of more than 259 mg/dl is three times more likely to develop CAD than a man whose level is less than 200 mg/dl [21]. The optimal cholesterol level is less than 200 mg/dl.

Cholesterol is transported in the blood by two categories of lipoproteins: high density (HDLs) and low density (LDLs). An elevated concentration of HDLs seems to have a protective effect against the development of atherosclerosis. The level of HDLs is related to (1) gender — women have higher HDL levels than men; (2) physical activity — HDL increases with increased activity; and (3) body weight — the higher the weight, the lower the HDL level [48]. High levels of LDLs, in contrast, appear to promote the development of atherosclerotic lesions and therefore increase coronary risk.

Diabetes

The precise mechanism by which diabetes predisposes an individual to coronary disease is unclear. Individuals with diabetes have a 50% greater risk of developing CAD. In addition, diabetic patients seem to develop CAD at an earlier age, regardless of sex.

Contributing Factors

Obesity

The true effect of obesity on coronary risk is presently controversial. Obesity is so frequently associated with diabetes, hypertension, hyperlipidemia, inactivity, and other risk factors that it is difficult to study in isolation. Reports to date have yielded conflicting evidence.

Physical Inactivity

There is no conclusive evidence demonstrating an increased risk of CAD with physical inactivity, but studies supporting such a relationship seem to outnumber those refuting it. Therefore, most practitioners feel that exercise is beneficial in preventing or minimizing CAD. Physical activity is known to raise the level of HDLs, increase cardiovascular functional capacity, and decrease myocardial O_2 demand.

Personality and Stress

Researchers have long associated a particular personality type with an increased risk of developing CAD. In addition, the role of psychological stress as a risk factor and as a possible initiating factor of acute MI is currently receiving increased attention [27]. The coronary-prone type A personality is a behavioral syndrome or style of living characterized by an unusual sense of time urgency and competitiveness, excessive job involvement, aggressiveness, haste, impatience, and restlessness [13]. Type B individuals are more relaxed and easygoing. These two personality types have been compared on a number of variables, including morbidity and mortality, response to acute myocardial infarction, and length of hospital stay. Type A individuals are more prone toward recurrent and fatal acute MI, more likely to use denial as a psychological defense mechanism in coping with life-threatening situations, and more likely to remain anxious and depressed during recovery from acute MI [13]. Patients with a type A personality have a significantly shorter average hospital stay (12 days) than do type B individuals (17 days). This finding is attributed to the more active involvement in their own care demonstrated by type A individuals [13].

PATHOLOGY

The pathogenesis of atherosclerosis remains unknown. The lesions of atherosclerosis develop in three stages, fatty streak, fibrous plaque, and complicated or advanced lesion.

Fatty Streak

Fatty streaks appear as yellowish, lipid-rich lesions that protrude slightly into the arterial lumen. The lesions consist of an increased number of smooth muscle cells and macrophages, both of which contain deposits of cholesterol and cholesterol oleate. The lesions cause little or no arterial obstruction and are not associated with any clinical symptoms. Although evident shortly after birth, the lesions appear in increasing numbers in childhood. Whether a fatty streak always progresses to the next stage of atherosclerosis, a fibrous plaque, remains controversial [19].

Fibrous Plaque

A fibrous plaque is elevated and protrudes into the lumen of the artery to varying degrees, possibly resulting in complete occlusion. The lesions are white and consist of a proliferation of smooth muscle cells, which form a fibrous cap and cover deeper deposits of extracellular lipids and cell debris [19].

Advanced Lesion

The advanced lesion of atherosclerosis represents a fibrous plaque that has become calcified. Hemorrhage, ulceration, and thrombus formation may also occur, causing arterial occlusion, which may result in ischemia or infarction.

The severity of atherosclerotic lesions varies considerably in different arteries. CAD occurs most frequently in the left anterior descending artery, less

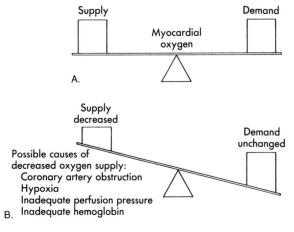

A.

Supply

Myocardial
oxygen

Demand

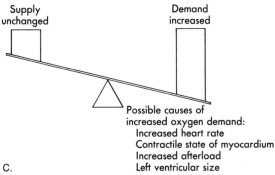

Supply
decreased

Possible causes of
decreased oxygen supply:
  Coronary artery obstruction
  Hypoxia
  Inadequate perfusion pressure
B. Inadequate hemoglobin

Demand
unchanged

Supply
unchanged

Demand
increased

Possible causes of
increased oxygen demand:
  Increased heart rate
  Contractile state of myocardium
  Increased afterload
  Left ventricular size

C.

FIGURE 9.1
Balance between myocardial oxygen
supply and myocardial oxygen demand.
(A) Normal balance. (B) Imbalance:
supply is decreased but demand remains
unchanged. (C) Imbalance: supply is
unchanged but demand is increased.
Atherosclerotic coronary vessels are
limited in their ability to increase the
oxygen supply. (From Phipps, W. J., Long,
B. C., and Woods, N. F. *Medical-Surgical
Nursing: Concepts and Clinical Practice*,
2nd ed. St. Louis: Mosby, 1983. Used with
permission.)

often in the right coronary artery, and even less frequently in the circumflex
[3]. As previously mentioned, symptoms occur late in the disease process, usually when the artery is more than 75% occluded.

The pathophysiological effect of CAD on the myocardium ranges from
potentially reversible injury of muscle cells to irreversible destruction of tissue
[48]. Symptoms result because of an imbalance between myocardial O_2 supply
and demand. Numerous factors affect the supply/demand ratio (Figure 9.1).
Most commonly, however, myocardial ischemia or infarction occurs because
the coronary arteries are obstructed as a result of atherosclerosis, thrombi, or
spasm, and the demand for O_2 therefore cannot be met. Initial clinical manifestations of this imbalance in supply and demand include angina, myocardial
infarction, and sudden death.

ANGINA

Angina pectoris, or chest pain, is the cardinal symptom of myocardial ischemia
and is most often caused by obstructive coronary atherosclerosis. Classic angina has a characteristic pattern. It is usually precipitated by physical exertion
and relieved within 2 to 5 minutes by rest, nitroglycerin administration, or
both. Most often the discomfort is located in the retrosternal region, although
it often radiates to the neck, jaw, shoulders, and arms, particularly the left arm.

Occasionally, patients will complain of discomfort only in the area of radiation. Because angina is a subjective symptom, it should be referred to as chest discomfort, rather than chest pain, when attempting to elicit information from the patient. Patients often describe the feeling as a tightness, aching, squeezing, burning, heaviness, or smothering feeling rather than as pain. All too often the patient attributes the discomfort to indigestion. The duration is usually two to five minutes, or occasionally as long as 5 to 15 minutes. The onset is frequently precipitated by physical activity but can also be brought on by cold, heavy meals, smoking, emotional stress, or excitement.

Angina can be described as stable, unstable, Prinzmetal's (variant), or nocturnal, or as angina decubitus. Stable angina is angina that is predictable and that has not changed in frequency, duration, or precipitating factors in the previous 60 days. Unstable angina is chest pain that is unprecedented, that has been present for less than 60 days, that is increasing in frequency or duration, or that is precipitated by less than the usual stimuli [19]. Prinzmetal's, or variant, angina produces some symptoms similar to those of classic angina. Variant angina, however, is usually of longer duration, occurs at rest, and is thought to result from coronary artery spasm. Nocturnal angina usually awakens the patient; angina decubitus occurs at rest when the patient is supine.

Diagnosis, Physical Findings, and Electrocardiographic Changes

The diagnosis of angina is usually based on a characteristic history, because findings on the physical examination are usually normal and the electrocardiogram (ECG) is usually normal at rest. During acute periods of angina, signs and symptoms of ischemia are evident but transient. The patient may appear anxious or pale, and blood pressure as well as pulse may be elevated. Pulmonary congestion may develop, and an S4, transient paradoxical splitting of S2, or an S3 may be heard on auscultation. An ECG obtained during angina, will often show transient ST segment depression (Figure 9.2). Patients with Prinzmetal's angina will demonstrate ST segment elevation on ECG. The changes evident on ECG provide valuable clues as to which coronary arteries are involved and, to some degree, of the amount of myocardium that is in jeopardy from ischemia [20] (Table 9.1).

Management

Angina resulting from CAD is conventionally managed medically, with various medications, control of risk factors and lifestyle changes, or surgically, with coronary artery bypass grafting. Other treatments, such as percutaneous transluminal coronary angioplasty, are also being used. Considerable debate remains regarding the benefits of medical management of CAD versus surgical intervention. This controversy is addressed briefly in Chapter 12, which also discusses surgical management. Our discussion here will focus on the medical management of angina.

Such management has two major goals: (1) relief of acute attacks of angina, and (2) optimal prevention of subsequent episodes.

Relief of Acute Angina
During an acute attack of angina, nursing interventions are aimed toward minimizing or eliminating the myocardial demands producing ischemia, which could potentially progress to infarction [48]. Any physical activity that the

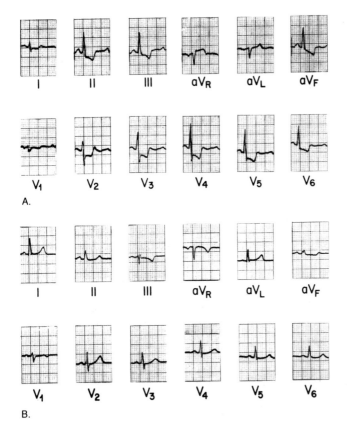

A.

B.

FIGURE 9.2

Twelve-lead ECG (A) during and (B) after an episode of severe ischemic pain in a 58-year-old man. During pain, marked downsloping depression of the ST segments is present in leads II, III, aV_F, and V_2 through V_6, reading 4 mm in lead V_4. There is a shift in the frontal plane QRS axis to +90 during pain, and a return to +20 when the pain resolves; this axis shift suggests transient left posterior hemiblock. Minor ST segment changes remain after the pain has subsided (B). Global ischemia is suggested by the widespread nature of the changes and the severity of the ST segment depressions. Coronary arteriography disclosed a 70% narrowing in the left main coronary artery and an 80% narrowing in the proximal right coronary artery. (From Johnson, R. A., Haber, E., and Austen, W. G. *The Practice of Cardiology.* Boston: Little, Brown, 1980. Used with permission.)

TABLE 9.1
Correlation Between ECG Location of Ischemic Changes and Area of Myocardium and Coronary Artery Involved

ECG Leads Reflecting Ischemic Changes	Area of Myocardium Involved	Coronary Artery Involved
II, III, aV_F	Inferior	RCA
V_1 to V_2 (reciprocal changes)	Posterior	RCA
V_2 to V_4	Anteroseptal	LAD branch of LCA
V_3 to V_5	Anterior	LAD branch of LCA
I, aV_L	High lateral	Circumflex marginal or diagonal branch of LCA
V_5 to V_6	Apical	Usually LAD branch of LCA; can be posterior descending branch of RCA

RCA = right coronary artery; LCA = left coronary artery; LAD = left anterior descending.

Adapted from Johnson, R. A., Haber, E., and Austen, W. G. *The Practice of Cardiology.* Boston: Little, Brown, 1980. Used with permission.

patient may be engaged in at the onset of angina must be stopped. Physical activity increases myocardial O_2 demands, and demand is already greater than supply during an anginal episode. Complete rest and relaxation are therefore recommended for the duration of the episode.

The characteristics of the chest discomfort, including location, radiation, quality, and quantity, are quickly assessed. It is helpful to ask the patient to quantify the severity of the discomfort by rating it on a scale of 1 through 10. Although pain is a purely subjective experience, this technique allows the nurse to evaluate the efficacy of treatment and compare the severity of subsequent attacks. Heart rate and rhythm, and blood pressure, are rapidly measured as nitroglycerin is administered sublingually. A twelve-lead ECG is obtained during the chest discomfort and evaluated for ST segment and T wave changes. If relief is not obtained after 3 to 5 minutes, subsequent doses of nitroglycerin are given, or an analgesic such as morphine sulfate may be added.

When the acute episode has subsided, the patient may slowly resume activities. The nurse must carefully document all information about the attack. Data recorded should include characteristics of the chest discomfort (including any possible precipitating factors, duration, and frequency), vital signs, ECG changes, and treatment. This information provides a baseline from which the disease process can be monitored and treatment regimens evaluated.

Prevention

Long-term management of angina is aimed at preventing ischemic episodes, primarily by administering medications and by modifying the patient's lifestyle to delay the progression of atherosclerosis and conserve energy. The medication regimen may include long-acting nitrates, beta-adrenergic blocking agents, and calcium channel blockers. The precise actions, clinical uses, dosages, administration, and side effects of these drugs are discussed in detail in Chapter 14. Patients with angina may also be prescribed sedatives, tranquilizers, and antiarrhythmic agents. The effectiveness of anticoagulants, antilipid drugs, and agents that alter platelet function, such as aspirin, remains controversial.

Patients with angina may find it necessary to modify their lifestyles. Initially, habits, activities, occupations, and cardiac risk factors are thoroughly assessed. Based on this assessment, an individualized treatment plan is instituted to eliminate or reduce risk factors such as smoking, obesity, and hypertension. Any coexisting medical problems are evaluated and treated. Physical activity is reduced to just below that amount that produces chest discomfort, and in some cases a supervised exercise program is prescribed. Cardiac rehabilitation programs may be contraindicated for some patients with unstable angina. If closely monitored, patients with stable angina can progressively increase their exercise capacity. Over time, with conditioning, heart rate and, therefore, myocardial O_2 consumption become only minimally affected by an increase in activity. Consequently, patients can do more with less energy expenditure.

Patient and family education is another important aspect of the long-term control of angina. Chapter 15 provides additional information on patient teaching in relation to CAD.

Percutaneous Transluminal Coronary Angioplasty

Although angina can be a debilitating condition, it does not result in permanent damage to the myocardium. The patient is, however, always at risk for a myocardial infarction. One technique that may reduce that risk by reducing coronary artery stenosis is the percutaneous transluminal coronary angioplasty (PTCA), an invasive procedure that involves dilatation of the lumen of a stenotic coronary artery. Originally performed in 1977 by Dr. Andreas Gruentzig, this technique has gained widespread popularity because of the impressive results and ease of performance. A select group of patients with CAD who might otherwise require coronary artery bypass grafting (CABG) can now be offered this mode of therapy.

The criteria used for selecting patients for PTCA vary among institutions and physicians. The factors taken into consideration are the anginal history, the coronary artery anatomy and degree of stenosis (determined by cardiac catheterization), the number of vessels obstructed, and the patient's overall physical condition. The ideal patient has single-vessel disease of a dominant artery with a proximal lesion. Patients with a recent history (less than one year) of angina most often have soft, compressible atheromas that are easily dilated. The structural characteristics of the artery and the stenosis must allow for passage of the catheter [15]. Patients undergoing PTCA must also be candidates for CABG, because certain complications can occur during the procedure that warrant emergency open heart surgery.

Preparation of the patient for the procedure involves diagnostic tests such as chest roentgenograms; ECG; blood studies including a complete blood count, coagulation survey, electrolyte studies, and typing and cross matching; and myocardial radionuclide imaging [30] (see Chapter 4). The patient is informed by the physician of the benefits and risks of the procedure. The nurse can minimize the patient's anxiety by providing information about the procedure itself and post-PTCA care, as well as answering any questions that may arise.

The angioplasty is done in the cardiac catheterization laboratory under fluoroscopy. A balloon-tipped catheter is introduced through the femoral artery and advanced to the site of the lesion, where it is inflated and deflated several times. The atheroma is compressed, thereby enlarging the lumen of the artery. Successful dilatation occurs in 85% to 90% of all cases and is defined by Gruentzig as (1) significant reduction of the pressure gradient across the stenotic lesion and angiographic evidence of increased luminal diameter, and (2) improvement in the patient's ability to perform exercise without precipitating angina or evidence of perfusion defects [31]. Complications that may occur during or after the procedure include MI, thrombosis, bleeding, coronary spasm or laceration, angina, dysrhythmias, and fluid and electrolyte imbalances.

The patient may be transferred to a medical unit or to a coronary care unit for continuous observation. Nursing care is directed toward prevention and early detection of complications. Upon admission, a thorough cardiovascular assessment is made. Vital signs, peripheral pulses, and cardiac rhythm are assessed every 15 to 60 minutes; the ECG is also assessed frequently. Bed rest and leg immobilization are maintained for 18 to 24 hours. The groin insertion site is checked frequently for bleeding, hematoma formation, and swelling. In addition, intake and output, coagulation studies, and electrolyte levels are closely monitored. Unless complications arise, the usual hospital stay is 36 to 48 hours.

Statistics are currently being compiled to determine the long-term patency rate of the dilated arteries. In the future, considerable controversy is likely regarding the relative risks and benefits of this mode of therapy and CABG for the patient with coronary artery stenosis.

MYOCARDIAL INFARCTION

When myocardial ischemia is severe or prolonged, irreversible injury or infarction of tissue results.

Diagnosis

The diagnosis of an MI is made when at least two of the following three clinical features are present: (1) chest discomfort that is characteristic of myocardial ischemia, (2) abnormal Q waves or ST-T wave changes that are typical of myocardial ischemia or infarction, and (3) abnormal elevations in the serum level of cardiac enzymes [19]. Approximately 10% to 15% of patients who have an MI do not exhibit one of these three criteria; that is, a small percentage of patients with MI either do not describe typical chest discomfort, fail to demonstrate typical ECG changes, or show no enzyme level elevation.

A large number of patients have had an unrecognized MI. The Framingham Heart Study has reported that more than 25% of MIs are unrecognized (silent) [23]. Within this group, half of the patients had no symptoms at the time of the event and the other half had symptoms that were so atypical that neither the patient nor the doctor suspected an MI. The diagnosis of MI was made during routine biennial ECG examination.

Chest Discomfort

Typically, patients present in the emergency room with severe, crushing substernal chest pain. Patients may describe the chest discomfort as "someone standing on my chest" or "a truck running over my chest." Occasionally patients complain only of mild discomfort, and others have no pain at all (silent MI). The pain may radiate to the arms, shoulders, neck, jaw, or back. The onset is usually sudden, and the pain persists for more than 15 to 30 minutes. Unlike angina, the discomfort of an MI is not relieved by rest or nitroglycerin and often requires potent analgesics. In addition to chest discomfort, patients may evidence nausea, vomiting, diaphoresis, syncope, palpitations, weakness, anxiety, and fear.

ECG Changes

The ECG changes that occur with an MI are caused by alterations in ventricular depolarization and repolarization that result from ischemic, injured, and necrotic tissue. Microscopic or pathological examination of myocardial tissue after MI reveals three distinct zones, demonstrating different levels of myocardial damage. Each zone creates different alterations on the ECG (Figure 9.3). The inner core, described as the necrotic zone, produces abnormal Q or QS waves. Beyond the necrotic core is the zone of injury, which produces ST seg-

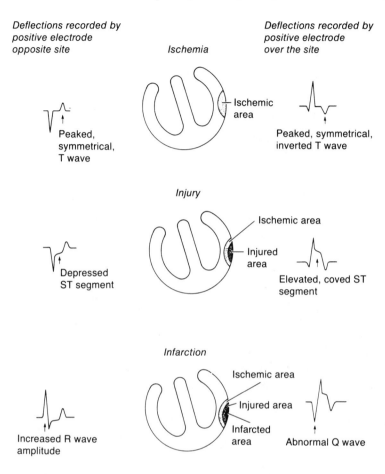

Deflections recorded by positive electrode opposite site

Peaked, symmetrical, T wave

Depressed ST segment

Increased R wave amplitude

Ischemia

Ischemic area

Peaked, symmetrical, inverted T wave

Injury

Ischemic area

Injured area

Elevated, coved ST segment

Infarction

Ischemic area

Injured area

Infarcted area

Abnormal Q wave

Deflections recorded by positive electrode over the site

FIGURE 9.3
ECG patterns of myocardial ischemia, injury, and infarction. As damage progresses, signs are superimposed on earlier changes. For example, the pattern of infarction includes the abnormal Q wave (produced by the infarcted area), an elevated ST segment (from the surrounding injured area), and an inverted T wave (from the surrounding ischemic area). (Adapted from Holloway, N. M. *Nursing the Critically Ill Adult,* 2nd ed. Menlo Park: Addison-Wesley, 1984. Used with permission.)

ment displacement on ECG, and the ischemic zone, which causes symmetrical T wave inversion. These ECG changes will occur in those leads that overlie or view the affected region of the myocardium. The ECG changes that occur with each type of MI are summarized in Figure 9.4 and discussed in detail in Chapter 7.

Enzyme Level Elevation
With necrosis of myocardial tissue, enzymes that are normally confined within the cells leak out into the serum. Measurements of creatine phosphokinase (CPK), lactic dehydrogenase (LDH), and serum glutamic oxaloacetic transaminase (SGOT) levels are used to confirm the diagnosis of MI, estimate the size of the infarct, and assess the patient's prognosis. Each of these enzymes can be found in several other tissues in the body; thus, an elevation is not specific for myocardial damage. LDH and CPK, however, can be broken down further into distinct forms called isoenzymes, which are organ specific. Cardiac enzymes are assayed upon admission and every 6 to 24 hours thereafter for three days, depending on hospital protocol and physician preferences. Each cardiac enzyme level rises, peaks, and declines at various times within the first

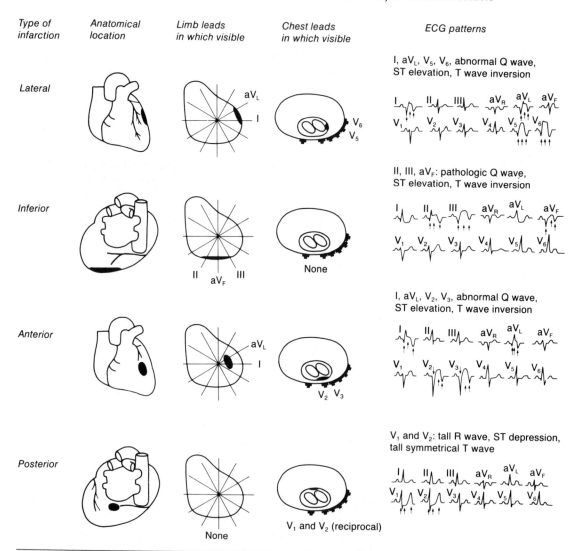

Type of infarction	Anatomical location	Limb leads in which visible	Chest leads in which visible	ECG patterns

FIGURE 9.4

Localization of infarcts. Lateral infarction usually results from occlusion of the left coronary artery, circumflex branch. Inferior infarction usually is due to occlusion of the right coronary artery, posterior descending branch. Anterior infarction usually is caused by occlusion of left coronary artery, anterior descending branch. Posterior infarction usually is due to occlusion of right coronary artery. (Adapted from Holloway, N. M. *Nursing the Critically Ill Adult.* 2nd ed. Menlo Park: Addison-Wesley, 1984. Used with permission.)

week after MI; thus, the pattern developed and the peak values are examined and correlated.

Total CPK level begins to rise within 3 to 6 hours of an MI, peaks in 12 to 24 hours, and returns to normal in three to five days. This enzyme is found predominantly in skeletal muscle, heart, bowel, lung, bladder, and brain. Three isoenzymes have been identified and are labeled as CPK-BB (in brain), CPK-

MM (in muscle), and CPK-MB (in heart). Elevations in CPK-MB level are highly specific for myocardial necrosis and begin 4 to 8 hours after infarction, peak in 24 hours, and last for 72 hours.

LDH is distributed widely throughout the body, but the highest concentrations are found in the liver, skeletal muscle, kidney, heart, and red blood cells. Total LDH level increases within 12 hours of an MI, peaks at 36 to 72 hours, and returns to normal within approximately ten days. Five isoenzymes of LDH have been identified and are numbered 1 through 5. LDH1 is the predominant form in the heart. The ratio of LDH1 to LDH2 is less than 1 (25% LDH1 and 35% LDH2) [40]. After an acute MI, the ratio is reversed, and the patient exhibits a "flipped" pattern; that is, there is more LDH1 than LDH2. This profile usually develops within 12 to 24 hours. Although LDH isoenzymes are relatively specific for an acute MI, CPK isoenzymes are more specific. Clinically, the most diagnostic enzyme pattern for an acute MI is an elevated CPK-MB level and a "flipped" LDH concentration.

SGOT level rises sharply within the first 12 hours, peaks in 24 to 48 hours, and returns to normal in approximately five days after an MI. This enzyme is also found in high concentrations in such tissues as skeletal muscle, brain, liver, and kidney.

In addition to their diagnostic value, cardiac enzyme levels have been found to correlate with infarct size and prognosis. Serial CPK blood levels measured during the first few hours after infarction can be used to determine infarct size, whereas peak CPK values have been used to quantify the extent of the myocardial damage [48]. Because the extent of myocardial damage is a powerful determinant of outcome, peak enzyme levels are one of the many factors used in estimating prognosis [19]. Another important factor is the location or type of the infarction.

Types of Infarctions

A myocardial infarction is classified in two ways: by (1) the layers of the myocardial tissue involved and (2) the location of the myocardial damage. The pathogenesis, clinical cause, prognosis, and mortality rate differ depending on the type of MI. The amount of myocardial damage certainly influences outcome. A study by Thanavaro and colleagues [45] concluded, however, that the location of the MI may independently affect the patient's prognosis.

Classification by Layer
Subendocardial MI. In a subendocardial infarct, the area of necrosis is confined to the subendocardial layer (Figure 9.5). This area of the myocardium is most at risk for ischemia or infarction because of several anatomical and physiological factors. Recall that the coronary arteries lie on the epicardial surface of the myocardium; thus, the epicardium is better oxygenated than the endocardium. Furthermore, during systole, the high pressure in the subendocardium and the wringing effect of contraction diminish perfusion to this area. Consequently, although the endocardium needs more O_2 because of its long myofibrils, the supply is decreased as a result of its location and physiological functions [18].

A subendocardial infarction is caused by a relatively insufficient coronary blood flow that lasts long enough for necrosis to develop. The tissue damage

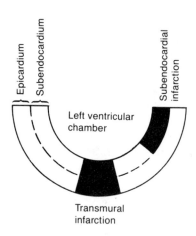

FIGURE 9.5
Cross section of left ventricle, differentiating subendocardial infarction, which involves inner half of ventricular wall, and transmural infarction, which involves full thickness of wall. (From Goldberger, A. L., and Goldberger, E. *Clinical Electrocardiography,* 2nd ed. St. Louis: Mosby, 1981. Used with permission.)

may be localized, occurring in the area supplied by one coronary vessel, or diffuse. Although the initial hospital course of patients with a discrete subendocardial infarction is generally benign, there is a risk of extension of the infarction and a resultant transmural infarction [20].

Transmural MI.   A transmural infarction involves the entire thickness of the myocardium (see Figure 9.5). Unlike a subendocardial infarct, a transmural infarct results from a process involving either complete occlusion of an artery or a very severe reduction in the lumen of the coronary vessel. Postmortem examination shows a very high incidence of thrombotic occlusion at the site of severe atherosclerotic narrowing [20].

Classification by Location
Myocardial infarctions are further described according to their locations of the left ventricular wall: anterior, inferior, posterior, and lateral. Recently, however, right ventricular infarctions are being recognized as more common than previously suspected [8].

Anterior MI.   An acute anterior MI (AMI) usually involves occlusion of the left anterior descending (LAD) coronary artery. Although such an MI may be present exclusively, other areas of the myocardium are frequently involved, resulting in anteroseptal or anterolateral infarctions. Acute AMIs constitute 26% of all MIs, with an associated mortality of 25.6% [48]. Compared with patients with inferior or posterior MIs, those with anterior or lateral MIs have more myocardial damage, significantly higher mortality, and a significantly greater prevalence of congestive heart failure and cardiogenic shock. In addition, the prevalence of sinus tachycardia, paroxysmal atrial tachycardia, right bundle branch block, left anterior hemiblock, and intraventricular conduction defects is significantly higher [45]. Patients with AMIs also seem to develop left ventricular (LV) aneurysm, LV thrombus, and myocardial rupture more often.

   Another problem associated with AMIs is sympathetic overactivity. Shortly after the onset of infarction, there is increased activity of both the parasympathetic and sympathetic nervous systems; usually, however, one component predominates. Patients with AMI show evidence of increased sympathetic activity and high levels of circulating catecholamines. These factors reduce the threshold for ventricular fibrillation and may increase the extent of the infarct [20]. The response of the autonomic nervous system to acute MI will be explained further in the section on local and systemic response to MI.

Inferior MI.   An inferior MI (IMI) typically occurs with occlusion of the right coronary artery (RCA). IMIs are also referred to as diaphragmatic infarctions. Approximately 17% of infarctions are IMIs, and the associated mortality is 10%. Patients with IMIs frequently develop conduction disturbances in the atrioventricular node, which also receives its blood supply from the RCA. Compared with patients with AMIs, those with IMIs demonstrate less myocardial damage, a significantly lower in-hospital death rate, and significantly fewer complications [45]. The response of the autonomic nervous system to an IMI is usually increased parasympathetic activity, evident in bradyarrhythmias, a normal or low cardiac output, and low peripheral vascular resistance [20, 48].

Posterior MI.   A posterior MI (PMI) results from occlusion of the RCA or the circumflex branch of the left coronary artery. Most posterior infarcts also involve the lateral or inferior wall of the left ventricle. True posterior infarcts are relatively rare; the incidence is approximately 2% [48].

Lateral MI.   A myocardial infarction confined to the lateral wall is also relatively rare, with an incidence of approximately 3%. If the lateral wall is infarcted, it is often in combination with the anterior wall.

Right ventricular infarction.   A right ventricular infarction (RVI) usually results from occlusion of the RCA. The incidence is higher than previously realized: 3% to 8% of all patients with acute MI [8]. Right ventricular infarcts most often occur in patients with IMIs. The clinical features of an RVI represent dysfunction of the right ventricle and include neck vein distention, elevated central venous pressure, and right ventricular end-diastolic pressure. Commonly, patients also have hypotension, bradycardia, and vasodilatation. These clinical features are quite different from those accompanying all other types of infarcts, which demonstrate left ventricular dysfunction. The clinical features of this and other types of MIs are due to both local (myocardial) and systemic responses to acute infarction.

Local and Systemic Response to Acute MI

Soon after an acute MI, the myocardium undergoes numerous electrical and mechanical changes that affect its ability to function. The hemodynamic changes vary and depend on the size and location of the MI. The core of the infarct or necrotic zone is electrically and functionally silent. Ventricular contractility and compliance diminish or may be absent. During systole the affected myocardium bulges out, and asynchronous movement results. Stroke volume and ejection fraction are decreased, and left ventricular end-systolic as well as end-diastolic volume increases. Signs of pulmonary congestion will be evident if left atrial or pulmonary capillary wedge pressure exceeds approximately 25 mm Hg [19]. Signs of cardiogenic shock are evident when 40% of the left ventricle has been damaged. Acidosis results from anaerobic glycolosis, which is also thought to decrease contractility.

Dysrhythmias are very common during the immediate postinfarction period, because ischemia alters cell membrane permeability. During this period there are disturbances in refractoriness, depolarization, and conductivity, as well as increased excitability. The most common dysrhythmias are ventricular ectopic activity and ventricular fibrillation [20].

Many of the signs and symptoms evident in the immediate postinfarction period are due to the normal response of the sympathetic nervous system to stress. The adrenal medulla releases catecholamines, including epinephrine, which acts as a cardioaccelerator. Epinephrine exerts its effect on the heart, blood vessels, lungs, and liver. Consequently, heart rate, contractility, cardiac output, blood pressure, and systemic vascular resistance all increase. These effects are detrimental to the already ischemic myocardium, because afterload, myocardial work, and, therefore, myocardial O_2 consumption rise. Additional effects of catecholamine release include dysrhythmias and hyperglycemia.

Some patients with acute MI, particularly those with inferior or posterior infarcts, demonstrate an increased parasympathetic response. These patients have bradycardia, low systemic vascular resistance, and a normal or low cardiac output [48].

The complications resulting from the local tissue and systemic response to an acute MI vary in severity. A small group of patients experience no complications at all. Some patients, however, die immediately because of ventricular fibrillation. If MI is suspected, patients are admitted as soon as possible to the coronary care unit (CCU), where they are closely and constantly monitored for acute cardiovascular complications that might warrant emergency interventions.

Psychological Response to Acute MI

The patient being admitted to the CCU after an episode of acute chest pain is most often extremely anxious, fearful, or shocked. Fears of death or disability may be overwhelming for both the patient and the family. The response to the event may be influenced by the patient's age, perception of the illness, and health history, and by the condition of family members or friends who have suffered heart attacks in the past. The diagnosis of heart attack is especially difficult to accept for young individuals with no history of heart disease. Patients with a history of angina may have adapted somewhat to their diagnosis and altered lifestyle.

The overwhelming anxiety and fear that occur in response to acute MI may escalate if chest pain persists, other complications arise, or the patient perceives a threat to life, self-image, or job. The responses used to cope with anxiety include denial, anger, and depression. After one or two days in the CCU, the threat of death decreases and the patient may begin to deal with the realities of the situation. By this time, serial isoenzyme values have been obtained and the physician usually has explained the extent of the attack to the patient and family. Some patients and families react to the news with anger and depression, which may persist. Others can comprehend the meaning of the illness and after discharge begin to deal with the consequences.

Patient Management

After the development of CCUs in the early 1960s, traditional management of the patient with acute MI centered on prevention and prompt treatment of life-threatening dysrhythmias as well as provision of an environment that promoted rest and recovery. Today, however, the primary goal in the management of an acute MI is to preserve the ischemic myocardium and limit the size of the infarct. Numerous techniques are being researched today, many of which are directed toward reducing the discrepancy between myocardial O_2 supply and demand. The major determinants of myocardial O_2 demand include heart rate, contractility, preload, and afterload; the major determinants of myocardial O_2 supply are coronary arterial and collateral blood flow.

Recent therapeutic approaches directed toward increasing flow and thereby preserving the myocardium are PTCA (discussed earlier) and intra-coronary streptokinase infusion. Streptokinase, a fibrinolytic agent, has been shown to lyse coronary artery thrombi. When patients are treated within the first few hours after the onset of chest pain suggestive of an MI, successful reperfusion of the myocardium can be achieved in most cases. Thus, streptokinase may prevent myocardial necrosis.

Medical interventions used to decrease myocardial O_2 demand are aimed at manipulating the determinants of myocardial work, namely, preload, afterload, contractility, and heart rate [32]. These goals are achieved mainly by administering various pharmacological agents and controlling the environment. The goals of therapy for the patient with acute MI are (1) reduction in myocardial workload, (2) prevention and early detection of complications, and (3) early participation in a rehabilitation program. Because myocardial workload is related to the patient's psychological as well as physiological state, quality nursing care must be directed toward both aspects.

Reduction in Myocardial Workload
Because heart rate is one of the major determinants of myocardial O_2 demand, any and all factors that would increase the patient's heart rate should be controlled. Upon admission the patient must be assessed quickly, and priorities established. After quick assessment of the patient's cardiovascular status through blood pressure, pulse, and ECG evaluation, the priority of care is to relieve chest discomfort. Hypotension and life-threatening dysrhythmias, if present, must be treated immediately.

Chest discomfort. Chest discomfort is treated immediately, because it increases the patient's heart rate and anxiety level and consequently increases myocardial O_2 consumption during an acute ischemic episode. Morphine sulfate (MSO_4) administered by direct intravenous (IV) push is the drug of choice; it is a potent analgesic and anxiolytic agent and also has the ability to decrease preload by peripheral vasodilatation. Meperidine hydrochloride is usually given to patients who are allergic to morphine or who have an undesirable reaction. The IV route is preferred, because intramuscular (IM) injections will result in elevations of the serum CPK level. Thus, the CPK concentration cannot be used to evaluate cardiac muscle necrosis accurately in patients who have had IM injections. Because of the potential side effects of MSO_4, particularly hypotension, it is advisable to select the minimal dose that relieves pain. Therefore, the drug is administered in small doses, usually 2 to 4 mg, every 5 to 15 minutes until relief is obtained. The patient's blood pressure, pulse, respiratory rate, and cardiac rhythm are monitored closely during, and for several hours after, drug administration. The total dose of MSO_4 needed and the time required to relieve pain are quite variable. If chest discomfort persists or recurs, additional medications may be administered, such as a continuous IV drip of nitroglycerin or propranolol.

Patients with severe, persistent, or recurrent chest pain may require intra-aortic balloon pumping until angiography can be scheduled or other modes of treatment explored. Percutaneous insertion of a balloon can be performed in the CCU if fluoroscopy is available. This mode of therapy usually results in prompt relief of pain; balloon pumping is continued for approximately two to three days, however, until the patient is in stable condition or is treated surgically.

Dyspnea and hypoxia.   Dyspnea may be evident during the acute episode of chest pain and may increase the patient's anxiety level. Oxygen is administered, via nasal prongs, upon admission in an attempt to relieve dyspnea and hypoxia. Oxygen therapy may also optimize the delivery of O_2 to the ischemic myocardium. Additional nursing interventions that may relieve dyspnea and hypoxia include elevating the head of the bed, decreasing all physical activity, and approaching the patient in a calm, reassuring manner. The necessity for continued O_2 use for several days after the MI can be determined on the basis of the patient's clinical appearance or arterial blood gas values. Even after O_2 therapy is discontinued, however, it is recommended that the equipment be readily available at all times. If the patient complains of subsequent episodes of chest pain or dyspnea, O_2 therapy can be reinstituted immediately.

Activity restrictions.   All physical activities, including getting out of bed, washing, eating, shaving, and walking, are closely monitored during the entire recovery period. Because any physical activity increases myocardial O_2 demand, bed rest is instituted upon admission. Usually the patient is allowed to use a bedside commode, because this requires less physical exertion than using a bedpan. All activities are then gradually increased from day to day once the patient's condition is stable. If the patient develops any complications, such as chest pain or dysrhythmias, activity progression is halted temporarily. The physiological effects of exercise and the usual activity protocol in the CCU are discussed in detail in Chapter 15.

Activity restrictions may be very difficult for the patient to accept, particularly the patient who has no further symptoms. A thorough explanation of the rationale for and necessity of activity restrictions may promote compliance. In addition, the patient should be allowed as much independence and control as possible and permitted to make decisions concerning his care when appropriate.

Stress reduction. One of the major goals of care in the CCU is to decrease stress and promote rest. As we have described, the normal physiological response to stress involves sympathic overactivity, resulting in elevated blood pressure and tachycardia. Consequently, myocardial O_2 consumption is increased.

Numerous interventions can be used in the CCU to ensure a calm environment in which anxiety can be allayed. Once the immediate physiological problems, such as chest pain, are effectively managed, the patient should be oriented to the CCU. Explanations of nursing routines, the cardiac monitor, and the nurse's call light, and descriptions of symptoms to report to the nurse, should be included. The patient and family need to be informed about the events of the next few days, including checking of vital signs, laboratory work, activity progression, and visiting hours. Brief explanations using general terms, rather than specific details, are best when attempting to decrease anxiety. Consistency in care is important, so that the patient can develop trust in the health care system and feel secure. Specific concerns and questions from the family or patient should be solicited throughout the hospital stay.

During the day, the nurse plans and coordinates rest periods with other members of the interdisciplinary team. At night, all nursing activities should be organized so as to allow the patient at least 6 hours, if possible, of uninterrupted sleep. If the patient's personality or psychological status inhibits his or her ability to relax, sedatives or tranquilizers may be ordered.

Diet. Dietary recommendations in the period immediately following the MI are variable and depend on the patient's condition. In the first few hours after admission, patients may be unstable, with nausea or vomiting; therefore, food and fluids are generally withheld. After approximately 6 to 12 hours, small, frequent meals are given. Large meals are avoided because of the associated potential increase in splanchnic blood flow, which may increase cardiac work [48]. Myocardial stimulants, particularly caffeine, should be avoided. In some CCUs hot and cold fluids are restricted. Caplin [5], however, based on a review of the literature related to ingestion of cold fluids, has concluded that there is insufficient evidence to support this practice. Based on her review, three guidelines are recommended for nursing practice: (1) the patient may ingest 240 cc of cold water, (2) the patient must not drink more than one cup of cold water in a 30-minute period, and (3) the patient must be in an upright position during ingestion [5].

During the recovery period, a balanced diet that is low in cholesterol, saturated fat, and salt is usually ordered. Overweight patients are also put on a reducing diet. Electrolyte levels are carefully monitored; if hypokalemia, which usually occurs secondary to diuretic therapy, is detected, foods rich in potassium are offered in addition to potassium supplements.

The potential for constipation is great in the CCU because of the sudden decrease in activity and the administration of MSO_4, which decreases peristalsis. Straining with elimination is avoided because it results in a Valsalva maneuver, which can cause bradycardia and hypotension. The patient's dietary intake should therefore contain an adequate amount of bulk and fluids. Stool softeners are usually ordered during the entire hospitalization period or until the patient's normal evacuation pattern has returned.

Prevention and Early Detection of Complications

The rationale for admitting patients to the CCU after MI is to prevent potentially life-threatening complications. Some complications are evident at the onset of chest pain, whereas others appear several months later, such as a ventricular aneurysm or Dressler's disease. The severity and incidence of complications are determined by the extent of injury and infarction of the heart muscle and the total degree of coronary artery disease [6]. The most common physiological complications evident in the CCU unit during the first few days after MI are dysrhythmias and cardiac failure. Less common, but no less devastating, are complications that involve heart structures, such as papillary muscle rupture, ventricular septal defect, pericarditis, cardiac tamponade, and thromboembolic complications.

Many of the complications described here are discussed in more detail in other chapters. Dysrhythmias and conduction disturbances are discussed in Chapters 7 and 8. Heart failure, including pulmonary edema and cardiogenic shock, is covered in detail in Chapter 10. Mechanical complications involving heart structures are explained in depth in Chapter 11. Here we present an overview of complications as they relate specifically to the patient with acute MI.

Dysrhythmias. The incidence of dysrhythmias in the early hours after acute MI is nearly 90%. Consequently, cardiac monitoring is instituted immediately upon admission and evaluated continuously. Abnormalities in rate, rhythm, and conduction can be detected from a monitor strip. A full twelve-lead ECG, however, is required to detect changes related to ischemia, myocardial infarction, axis deviation, and hemiblocks. Various modes of therapy are used in the management of dysrhythmias, depending on the patient, the cardiac rate, and the rhythm. Defibrillation, cardioversion, cardiac pacing, and administration of antiarrhythmic agents are the most common interventions. Because many dysrhythmias are treated with medications administered by IV push, it is essential that the patient have an IV line inserted on admission and an IV or heparin lock maintained for approximately one week. These interventions are discussed in detail in Chapters 13 and 14.

Life-threatening dysrhythmias include complex premature ventricular contractions, ventricular tachycardia (VT), ventricular fibrillation (VF), and conduction disturbances that result in severe bradyarrhythmias. Less severe dysrhythmias include sinus tachycardia and bradycardia, heart blocks, and supraventricular dysrhythmias. The cause is related to electrophysiological disturbances created by myocardial ischemia and injury. The mechanisms responsible for the dysrhythmias include enhanced automaticity and reentrant activity (see Chapter 8). Treatment protocols for each dysrhythmia are also discussed in Chapter 8.

Ventricular dysrhythmias. Ventricular dysrhythmias are the most frequent dysrhythmias accompanying acute MI. Premature ventricular contractions

(PVCs) occur in approximately 80% of patients. Malignant PVCs are defined as those that (1) occur in pairs (couplets or triplets), (2) are frequent (more than six to eight per minute), (3) are multifocal, or (4) occur close to the T wave, in the vulnerable period. The characteristics and frequency of PVCs should be monitored closely, because malignant PVCs frequently degenerate into VT and VF, severe, life-threatening dysrhythmias that require immediate treatment. Although VT and VF are often preceded by ventricular ectopic activity, they may occur spontaneously.

Sinus dysrhythmias.   Sinus tachycardia (ST) is common, occurring in approximately 35% to 45% of patients with MIs. Although ST is often viewed as a benign dysrhythmia, the mortality is high, especially if the cause is congestive heart failure [48]. Other causes of ST include fever, stress, anxiety, and sympathetic stimulation. Because ST increases myocardial O_2 demands, the cause of this dysrhythmia should always be investigated and treated immediately.

Sinus bradycardia may also develop early after MI and occurs most often with inferior infarctions. The cause may be either ischemic damage to the sinoatrial node or increased stimulation of the vagus nerve. The dysrhythmia may be transient or permanent. Sinus arrest and sinoatrial block are also associated with acute MI. The significance of sinus dysrhythmias is related to the ventricular rate and the hemodynamic effect on the patient. A normal cardiac output is usually maintained if the pulse is approximately 45 to 160 beats per minute.

Atrial dysrhythmias.   Atrial flutter or fibrillation occurs in approximately 3% to 10% of patients with acute MI, whereas premature atrial contractions (PACs) occur in approximately 37% to 52% [48]. PACs frequently degenerate to atrial fibrillation or flutter, however. Although many patients with chronic atrial fibrillation or flutter remain in stable condition with these rhythms, new-onset atrial fibrillation or flutter is often associated with rapid ventricular rates and subsequent symptoms of cardiac failure. These changes are due to a loss of atrial kick and a shortened period of diastolic filling. Prompt treatment to control the ventricular rate is essential.

Conduction disturbances.   The patient with an acute MI may develop a variety of conduction disturbances originating anywhere along the normal conduction pathway. The incidence of first-, second- and third-degree block (complete heart block [CHB]) are, respectively, 4% to 13%, 6% to 10%, and 6% to 8%. Wenckebach (Mobitz type I) second-degree atrioventricular block is much more common than type II and is usually seen with IMIs. Mobitz type II is more often seen with AMIs and is more dangerous because it often degenerates to CHB. Although the incidence of CHB is relatively low, the death rate, depending on the extent of the MI, can be between 25% and 75% [48]. Bundle branch blocks are also common after acute MI. The treatment of choice for certain conduction disturbances is emergency insertion of a temporary transvenous pacemaker. Early recognition and prompt intervention by the nurse–physician team in the CCU can influence the outcome and thus the mortality related to dysrhythmias.

Thromboemboli.   Thromboembolic disorders, such as deep vein thrombosis (DVT) and pulmonary emboli, can complicate the clinical course for the patient who has experienced an MI. The incidence of DVT after MI is reported to be 22% to 37% [11]. Cardiac patients most at risk for developing emboli, besides the patient with MI, include (1) the severely ill, (2) those with valvular heart disease — mitral disease in particular, (3) those over the age of 60, (4) those with varicose veins, infections, obesity, leg trauma, or previous thromboembolism, (5) those undergoing prolonged immobility, and (6) those with atrial fibrillation or flutter [48]. Because of the increased risk of emboli, patients are usually given small doses of heparin (5,000 units every 12 hours). In addition, transferring from bed to chair, and ambulation, are started as soon as the patient's condition warrants. Ankle and leg exercises are encouraged while bed rest is maintained.

Cardiac failure.   Although many of the complications of acute MI can be successfully managed in the CCU, the treatment of congestive heart failure remains a challenge. Acute heart failure results when the metabolic demands of the body cannot be met because of inadequate LV pumping. Normal mechanical functioning of the LV, and thus hemodynamics, is altered in response to an acute MI. The severity of the symptoms is directly related to the amount of LV muscle mass damaged. Heart failure is manifested when 20% to 25% of the LV is damaged, and cardiogenic shock develops if more than 40% is lost. Clinical signs and symptoms of failure include fatigue, weakness, shortness of breath, dyspnea, crackles, ventricular gallop (S3), tachycardia, hypotension, and peripheral vasoconstriction. Patients are best managed by close hemodynamic monitoring of intracardiac pressures, such as pulmonary capillary wedge pressures, cardiac output, and index. A thermodilution catheter, inserted at the bedside, can aid the physician in the evaluation of the patient's hemodynamic status. Left-sided as well as right-sided pressure measurements can be obtained, in addition to cardiac output values. With this information, decisions regarding fluid and drug administration can be made in an attempt to optimize cardiac performance. Management of acute LV failure is discussed in greater detail in Chapter 10.

Congestive failure can occur as a direct result of myocardial tissue damage or secondary to damage to such heart structures as the papillary muscle or ventricular septum.

Papillary muscle dysfunction.   Because of their high level of O_2 consumption and their location distal to the origination of the coronary artery, the LV papillary muscles are highly susceptible to ischemia and thus rupture or dysfunction. Although the incidence of this complication is low, 0.5% to 2%, the associated mortality is reported to be as high as 50% to 80% [48]. When the papillary muscle is damaged, the mitral valve does not close properly and blood regurgitates back into the left atrium during systole. A murmur of mitral insufficiency is then evident. The first indication of papillary muscle dysfunction, however, may be a prominent V wave evident on a pulmonary artery wedge pressure tracing. If papillary muscle rupture occurs, acute symptoms of congestive heart failure will ensue.

Ventricular septal rupture.   This complication occurs in a small percentage of patients, 1% to 2%, usually three to four days after MI. Ventricular septal rupture is associated most often with anteroseptal or inferior infarctions. When the septum ruptures, blood is shunted from the higher-pressured LV into the lower-pressured RV. Patients often complain of severe chest pain and abruptly display signs and symptoms of right-sided congestive heart failure. Ventricular septal rupture is discussed in more detail in Chapter 11.

Additional complications.   Additional complications that may occur in the early post-MI period include pericarditis, cardiac rupture, and cardiac tamponade. Transmural infarctions, which extend through the entire myocardial wall, may produce a localized pericarditis. Signs and symptoms of pericarditis are usually evident on the second to fourth day after the MI. Characteristically, patients complain of chest pain that is aggravated by deep inspiration or changes in position. A pericardial friction rub can be auscultated over the inflamed area, and the patient may be febrile. The goal of treatment for pericarditis is to relieve the symptoms with analgesics, anti-inflammatory agents, steroids, or a combination of these. Anticoagulants are contraindicated because of the increased risk of bleeding into the pericardial space [19].

Rupture of the myocardium is a rare complication of acute MI. Factors that appear correlated with a greater incidence of rupture include (1) a transmural infarct with poor collateral circulation, (2) systemic arterial hypertension, and (3) dilatation and thinning of the infarct [19]. This complication occurs most often in patients in their sixth or seventh decade of life. When the rupture occurs, most patients die suddenly. Others may initially show signs and symptoms of cardiac tamponade (see Chapter 11).

Early Participation in Cardiac Rehabilitation
After MI, patients may begin a cardiac rehabilitation program as soon as they are in physiologically stable condition, possibly within 24 hours after admission. The three major parts of the rehabilitation program — education, exercise, and psychological support — can be initiated in the CCU if the patient's physiological and psychological status warrants participation. Cardiac rehabilitation, with emphasis on the acute care period, is covered in depth in Chapter 15.

SUDDEN CARDIAC DEATH

Although sudden death resulting from cardiac disease has been recognized for decades, sudden cardiac death (SCD) as a distinct medical phenomenon has recently been defined and is under intense investigation. It is commonly defined as unexpected cardiac death occurring without symptoms or with symptoms of less than 1 hour's duration.

Characteristically, cardiac arrest occurs out of the hospital, in men of approximately 60 years of age, and during the routine activities of daily life [19]. SCD accounts for more than 400,000 deaths annually. In approximately 75% of these cases the individual has extensive CAD; the remaining 25% of deaths are due to various cardiac problems, such as cardiomyopathy, and to noncardiac causes, such as pulmonary hypertension [48].

In an attempt to decrease deaths from SCD, patients at risk have been identified. Four major characteristics have been associated with enhanced risk of SCD: (1) ventricular electrical instability, particularly complex premature ventricular contractions, which degenerates into VT and VF; (2) extensive coronary arterial narrowing (usually 70% or greater obstruction in two or more vessels); (3) abnormal left ventricular function, such as an aneurysm; and (4) ECG conduction and repolarization abnormalities (prolongation of the QT interval and ST-T changes) [19].

Efforts to decrease deaths resulting from SCD have been directed toward improving cardiac resuscitation efforts in the community and preventing lethal dysrhythmias with antiarrhythmic drugs and implantable defibrillators. With further research on this topic, it is hoped that more deaths will be prevented and effective treatment protocols will be developed.

SUMMARY

The presenting clinical manifestations of CAD vary widely and include angina, myocardial infarction, and SCD. Unfortunately, symptoms do not appear until the coronary arteries are approximately 75% occluded. Many patients die without any history of cardiac disease because of ventricular fibrillation, massive MI, or SCD.

Tremendous achievements have been made over the last several decades, as evidenced by the decreasing death rate. The American Heart Association has spent millions of dollars toward improving patient care, providing public education and community service programs as well as supporting research and educational programs to help Americans cope with cardiovascular disease [1]. Further improvements can be expected as new treatments are developed and rehabilitation programs become more prevalent.

STUDY QUESTIONS

1. List the nonmodifiable and modifiable cardiac risk factors. Which three are the major risk factors?
2. Which coronary arteries are most frequently diseased?
3. What are the physiological effects on the myocardium of coronary artery obstruction?
4. Describe the characteristics of angina, including location, duration, quality, and precipitating and relieving factors.
5. Define *unstable angina* and *variant angina*.
6. Describe a typical treatment protocol for a patient with newly diagnosed angina.

7. Which patients are the best candidates for PTCA, and what is the goal of this mode of therapy?

8. Design a nursing care plan for a patient after PTCA. What complications should you watch for?

9. How is the diagnosis of MI made?

10. Describe the typical signs of symptoms of an acute MI.

11. What are the characteristic ECG changes evident with an acute MI, and why do they occur?

12. What is the typical enzyme level pattern of a patient 24 hours after acute MI?

13. Describe the difference between a subendocardial and a transmural MI.

14. List the different types of MIs, their incidences and mortalities.

15. Describe the hemodynamic changes that result from an MI.

16. List the complications most often seen within the first 48 hours after MI.

17. Define *malignant PVCs*.

18. List the causes of congestive failure in the patient with acute MI.

19. What are the major goals of care for the patient with acute MI?

20. Identify the risk factors for SCD.

CASE STUDIES

CASE 1

A 50-year-old man is admitted to the CCU via ambulance. He is complaining of severe substernal chest pain and is diaphoretic. Vital signs are as follows: blood pressure, 140/80 mm Hg; pulse, 120 beats per minute; respirations, 20 per minute. An ECG reveals an acute anteroseptal MI.

1. List, in order of priority, your next ten nursing interventions. Give your rationale for each.

2. What feelings and concerns may this patient be having?

3. What is the physiological basis for the vital signs given?

4. Describe the local and systemic response to acute MI.

5. After the chest pain is relieved and the patient is physiologically stable, what are the goals of care?

CASE 2

A 60-year-old woman is admitted to the progressive coronary care unit (PCCU) with a diagnosis of unstable angina. She is retired and lives alone. She has a history of smoking (one pack a day) and of hypertension. The patient stopped taking her prescribed medications months ago because she felt she was getting sicker while taking them.

1. What would the treatment protocol consist of if this patient had an acute anginal attack?

2. What are your long-term goals for this patient?

REFERENCES

1. American Heart Association. *1982 National Annual Report*. Dallas: American Heart Association, 1982.

2. American Heart Association. *Heart Facts 1985*. Dallas: American Heart Association, 1985.

3. Andreoli, K. G., et al. *Comprehensive Cardiac Care* (5th ed.). St. Louis: Mosby, 1983.

4. Barden, R. M., Cardin, S., and Urrows, S. T. Right ventricular infarction. *Cardiovasc. Nurs.* 19:7, 1983.

5. Caplin, M. Restriction of cold fluids in myocardial infarction patients: myth or fact? *Focus* 11(1):42, 1984.

6. Chatterjee, I., and Parmley, W. Therapy of acute infarction. In F. Cohn (ed.), *Diagnosis and Therapy of Coronary Artery Disease*. Boston: Little, Brown, 1979.

7. Cimini, D. M., and Goldfarb, J. Standard of care for the patient with percutaneous transluminal coronary angioplasty. *Crit. Care Nurs.* (3):76, 1983.

8. Cohn, J. N. Right ventricular infarction revisited. *Am. J. Cardiol.* 43:666, 1979.

9. Conner, R. P. Coronary artery anatomy: the electrocardiographic and clinical correlations. *Crit. Care Nurs.* 3(3):68, 1983.

10. Dunkel, J., and Eisendrath, S. Families in the intensive care unit: their effect on staff. *Heart Lung* 12:258, 1983.

11. Frishman, W. H., and Ribner, H. S. Anticoagulation in myocardial infarction: modern approach to an old problem. *Am. J. Cardiol.* 43:1207, 1979.

12. Gentry, W. D., and Williams, R. B. *Psychological Aspects of Myocardial Infarction and Coronary Care* (2nd ed.). St. Louis: Mosby, 1979.

13. Gentry, W. D., et al. Type A/B differences in coping with acute myocardial infarction: further considerations. *Heart Lung* 12:212, 1983.

14. Gruentzig, A. Results from coronary angioplasty and implications for the future. *Am. Heart J.* 103:779, 1982.

15. Gruentzig, A. R. Technique of percutaneous transluminal coronary angioplasty. In J. W. Hurst (ed.), *The Heart* (5th ed.). New York: McGraw-Hill, 1982.

16. Hansell, H. N. The behavioral effects of noise on man: the patient with intensive care unit psychosis. *Heart Lung* 13:59, 1984.

17. Harper, R. W., Gold, H. K., and Leinbach, R. C. Acute myocardial infarction. In R. A. Johnson et al. (eds.), *The Practice of Cardiology*. Boston: Little, Brown, 1980.

18. Holloway, N. M. *Nursing the Critically Ill Adult*. Menlo Park: Addison-Wesley, 1979.

19. Hurst, J. W., et al. *The Heart*. New York: McGraw-Hill, 1982.

20. Johnson, R. A., Haber, E., and Austen, W. G. *The Practice of Cardiology*. Boston: Little, Brown, 1980.

21. Kannel, W. B. Recent finding of the Framingham study. *Resident Staff Physician* 24:56, 1978.

22. Kannel, W. B., et al. Menopause and risk of cardiovascular disease: The Framingham Study. *Ann. Intern. Med.* 85:447, 1976.

23. Kannel, W. B., and Abbott, R. D. Incidence and prognosis of unrecognized myocardial infarction. *N. Engl. J. Med.* 311:1144, 1984.

24. Kent, K. M. Percutaneous transluminal coronary angioplasty: report from the registry of the National Heart, Lung and Blood Institute. *Am. J. Cardiol.* 49:2011, 1982.

25. Kouchoukos, N. T. Surgical treatment of acute complications of myocardial infarction. *Crit. Care Cardiol.* Philadelphia: Davis, 1981.

26. Lewis, P. S. Evaluation of the patient sustaining a right ventricular infarction and nursing implications. *Crit. Care Nurs.* 3(1):50, 1983.

27. Madias, J. E. Psychological distress: risk factors for acute MI. *Primary Cardiol.* 9:141, 1983.

28. Maroko, P. R., Deboer, L. W. V., and Davis, R. F. Infarct size reduction: a critical review. *Adv. Cardiol.* 27:127, 1980.

29. Miller, D. H., and Schreiber, T. Early management of acute myocardial infarction: limitation of infarct size. *Clin. Cardiol.* 1:4, 1984.

30. Ng, L. Percutaneous transluminal coronary recanalization with streptokinase: nursing care and implications. *Cardiovasc. Nurs.* 19:25, 1983.

31. Purcell, J. A., and Giffin, P. A. Percutaneous transluminal coronary angioplasty. *Am. J. Nurs.* 81:1620, 1981.

32. Rackley, C. E., et al. Clinical interventions for the preservation of ischemic myocardium. *Crit. Care Cardiol.* Philadelphia: Davis, 1981.

33. Rackley, C. E., et al. Modern approach to myocardial infarction: determination of prognosis and therapy. *Am. Heart J.* 101:75, 1981.

34. Roberts, W. C., and Gardin, J. M. Location of myocardial infarctions: a confusion of terms and definitions. *Am. J. Cardiol.* 42:868, 1978.

35. Rogers, W. J., et al. Clinical methods for assessment of myocardial infarct size. *Crit. Care Cardiol.* Philadelphia: Davis, 1981.

36. Rossi, L. Nursing care for survivors of sudden cardiac death. *Nurs. Clin. North Am.* 19:411, 1984.

37. Rossi, L., and Haines, V. Nursing diagnosis related to acute myocardial infarction. *Cardiovasc. Nurs.* 15:11, 1979.

38. Russel, R. O., et al. Management of unstable angina pectoris. *Crit. Care Cardiol.* Philadelphia: Davis, 1981.

39. Rutsch, W., et al. Percutaneous transluminal coronary recanalization: procedure, results, and acute complications. *Am. Heart J.* 102:1178, 1981.

40. Ryan, A. M. What cardiac enzymes tell you about acute MI. *RN* 47(3):46, 1984.

41. Scheer, E. Enzymatic changes and myocardial infarction: a nursing update. *Cardiovasc. Nurs.* 14:5, 1978.

42. Scheidt, S. Prognosis after myocardial infarction. *Clin. Cardiol.* 1:43, 1984.

43. Scordo, K. A. This procedure called PTCA: your patient's CABG substitute. *Nurs. '82* 12(2):50, 1982.

44. Solack, S. D. Assessment of psychogenic stresses in the coronary patient. *Cardiovasc. Nurs.* 15:16, 1979.

45. Thanavaro, S., et al. Effect of infarct location on the in-hospital prognosis of patients with first transmural myocardial infarction. *Circulation* 66:742, 1982.

46. Trevino, S., and Massey, J. A. Risk factors for arrhythmias after myocardial infarction. *Heart Lung* 12:240, 1983.

47. Tuggle, D. J. Meeting the emotional needs of survivors of sudden cardiac arrest. *Cardiovasc. Nurs.* 18:25, 1982.

48. Underhill, S. L., et al. *Cardiac Nursing.* Philadelphia: Lippincott, 1982.

49. University of Washington Critical Care Unit. Nursing care plan for MI patients. *Crit. Care Nurs.* 2(4):78, 1982.

50. Vaughan, P., and Rice, V. Complications of myocardial infarction. *Crit. Care Nurs.* 2(3):44, 1982.

51. Zullo, M., and Scheidt, S. Treatment of arrhythmias in acute myocardial infarction. *Clin. Cardiol.* 1:12, 1984.

Cardiac Failure

Cynthia Moores

INTRODUCTION

Cardiac failure can be defined as a condition that occurs when the heart fails to meet the metabolic requirements of the body. It is an extremely broad term that should be thought of as a clinical manifestation of other underlying diseases rather than a diagnosis in and of itself.

Cardiac failure appears in varying forms, which are generally determined by the underlying causes. This chapter will discuss the causes, pathophysiology, clinical manifestations, and management of left ventricular failure (LVF), right ventricular failure (RVF), and cardiogenic shock. The specific definitions tend to describe the clinical manifestations associated with the various forms of failure. For example, LVF is manifested in pulmonary congestion, which follows left ventricular dilatation and increases in left-sided pressures [28]. RVF is manifested in peripheral edema, liver enlargement, and an increase in jugular venous pressure. Cardiogenic shock is complete failure of the heart to supply the body with blood and oxygen appropriate for its needs.

LEFT VENTRICULAR FAILURE

Definition and Causation

LVF is manifested in pulmonary congestion secondary to left heart dilatation with accompanying pressure increases. The major symptoms of dyspnea, orthopnea, and fatigue all relate to the presence of pulmonary congestion.

Although there are many causes of LVF, there is one factor common to all: an impaired force of contraction that does not allow the heart to meet the metabolic needs of the body. Any condition that places a continuous strain on the heart by increasing the workload, decreasing the contractility, or hindering blood flow is capable of causing heart failure [22]. The most common underlying causes of LVF are hypertension, coronary artery disease, and valvular disease. Other, less common causes include cardiomyopathies, left-to-right shunts, and congenital heart lesions [28]. Appropriate management or correction of the underlying problem may prevent the development or recurrence of failure.

When LVF does occur, it can generally be traced to some precipitating event that has caused an increased cardiac workload. LVF often occurs suddenly, and the heart's compensatory mechanisms are ineffective. Common precipitating events include dysrhythmias, systemic or cardiac infection, pulmonary embolism, anemia, myocardial infarction, fluid and sodium overload, and environmental or emotional stress [2].

Pathophysiology

When the heart is subjected to a continuous stress over time, heart failure may occur unless sufficient cardiac reserve is present. The extent of the cardiac reserve is determined mainly by the ability of the heart's compensatory mechanisms to handle a stressor. When the cardiac reserve is successful in maintaining adequate blood flow (cardiac output), clinical symptoms are absent and a state of compensation exists. When the compensatory mechanisms of the heart fail, a state of decompensation exists and clinical symptoms are manifested. Decompensation often occurs in response to a precipitating event, such as a dysrhythmia, that suddenly increases the workload of the heart.

The pathophysiology of cardiac failure involves three major compensatory mechanisms that the heart employs when faced with increased workload: (1) myocardial hypertrophy, (2) increased muscle fiber stretch, and (3) a sympathetic response. These three mechanisms are capable of maintaining a relatively normal cardiac output for a time. Each mechanism has a limited potential, however, and eventually will fail. When the compensatory mechanisms actually fail, symptoms of cardiac failure become evident [2].

Myocardial Hypertrophy

Hypertrophy of myocardial muscle occurs when the increased workload stems from an increased resistance to ventricular ejection. Aortic stenosis and systemic hypertension are two common conditions that cause such increased resistance. Hypertrophy is defined as an increase in the muscle mass thickness. The increased thickness causes a decrease in left ventricular compliance, and thus the left ventricular end-diastolic pressure (LVEDP) is elevated while left ventricular volume remains normal [30]. The increased LVEDP is useful in augmenting cardiac output for a period of time.

Any condition resulting in a loss of ventricular compliance is capable of increasing the LVEDP. For example, a stiff and less compliant left ventricle follows an acute myocardial infarction. The elevated LVEDP serves to augment the cardiac output, which tends to fall with loss in muscle compliance. This relationship is based on the Frank-Starling law of the heart.

As the hypertensive or valvular disease progresses, the left ventricular volume does begin to rise. The hypertrophied muscle and the elevated LVEDP are unable to compensate. The rising left ventricular volume causes further increases in the already elevated LVEDP, and eventually the ventricle fails.

Increased Stretch of Muscle Fiber

The capacity of the intact ventricle to vary its force of contraction on a beat-to-beat basis as a function of its initial (end-diastolic) size constitutes one of the major principles of cardiac function. It is referred to as the Starling law of the heart [2]. The greater the stretch of the myocardial muscle fiber, the more forceful the subsequent contraction will be, and hence the greater the cardiac output will be.

This law can be used to demonstrate how the failing heart attempts to maintain its pump requirements through ventricular dilatation [7]. When the muscle fiber stretch in end diastole is increased, a greater stroke volume is ejected and the cardiac output is enhanced. Over time, however, the muscle fiber dilates, and elasticity is lost. The stroke volume and cardiac output fall as fiber stretch is lost. The end-systolic ventricular volume increases, and the clinical manifestations of heart failure begin to appear.

Sympathetic Response

The normal heart is richly supplied with sympathetic nerve endings. Stimulation of the sympathetic nervous system causes the release of norepinephrine, which exerts a strong positive inotropic and chronotropic effect on the myocardial muscle and plays an important role in compensating for acute cardiac failure. When sympathetic stimulation occurs, the heart responds with an increased force of contraction and increased rate. Cardiac output (CO) is augmented by the increased heart rate (HR) and the stroke volume (SV), as demonstrated in the equation $CO = HR \times SV$.

Evidence suggests that the failing heart is accompanied by a depletion of cardiac norepinephrine stores and increased levels of catecholamines in the blood and urine. The failing heart may be supported by the circulating catecholamines and dependent on this extracardiac adrenergic support for maintaining hemodynamic function [2]. Extreme caution should be exercised in the use of any adrenergic blocking agents in the treatment of patients with limited cardiac performance, because of the compensatory role the sympathetic nervous system plays.

Cardiac failure or decompensation occurs when these compensatory mechanisms can no longer maintain a normal hemodynamic state. The elevated LVEDP and left ventricular volume are transmitted back into the left atrial chamber. Consequently, pulmonary congestion occurs as the elevated left atrial pressure is transmitted further backward. The result is interstitial and alveolar edema in the lungs. Clinically, all the symptoms of left ventricular failure become evident.

Clinical Manifestations

Symptoms

The major symptoms of LVF include dyspnea, orthopnea, paroxysmal noctural dyspnea (PND), and pulmonary edema. The principal manifestation of LVF is shortness of breath. This cardinal symptom may range in severity from exertional dyspnea to acute pulmonary edema. Dyspnea occurs as the pulmonary congestion and interstitial edema reduce the lung compliance and the work of the respiratory muscles is increased. It is an insidious symptom. Often the patient complains of difficulty in completing activities that were easily accomplished before without breathlessness. Specific questioning about the patient's usual activities of daily living may be necessary for the identification of this symptom.

Orthopnea is dyspnea that develops in the supine position. When an individual assumes the supine position, less pooling of blood occurs in the lower extremities and venous return to the heart is increased. A failing left ventricle is unable to handle the additional volume effectively, and the patient becomes short of breath when lying flat in bed. Treatment consists of elevating the head of the bed, having the patient sleep on additional pillows, or, in the case of severe orthopnea, having the patient sleep in a chair. The nurse's assessment should specify the number of pillows the patient requires for comfortable sleep and whether this number has recently increased. This is a general indication of the severity of the orthopnea.

PND is an exaggerated form of orthopnea. Bronchospasm may also be present and will produce inspiratory and expiratory wheezing. PND usually occurs suddenly and awakens the patient. It may be relieved by assumption of the upright position, or it may progress to pulmonary edema.

Pulmonary edema is an acute manifestation of LVF that results from the rapid transudation of fluid into the pulmonary alveoli because of a high pulmonary capillary pressure. Clinically, patients present with acute shortness of breath, extreme anxiousness and restlessness, diaphoresis, cool and clammy

EXHIBIT 10.1
Clinical Manifestations of Left Ventricular Failure

Symptoms	Physical Signs
Dyspnea	Pulmonary rales
Orthopnea	Ventricular gallop (S3)
Paroxysmal nocturnal dyspnea	Pulsus alternans
Pulmonary edema	Tachycardia
Fatigue	Left ventricular heave
Weakness	Cheyne-Stokes respirations
Nocturia	
Anxiety	
Restlessness	

skin, frothy sputum, cyanosis, and hemoptysis. Aggressive treatment is required for symptom stabilization in acute pulmonary edema.

Other clinical manifestations that may accompany LVF include fatigue, weakness, nocturia, and insomnia (Exhibit 10.1).

Physical Signs

The major physical findings associated with failure of the left side of the heart are pulmonary rales, a ventricular gallop, tachycardia, pulsus alternans, cardiomegaly, and occasionally Cheyne-Stokes respirations.

Pulmonary rales are due to the transudation of fluid into the pulmonary alveoli because of an elevated pulmonary capillary pressure. Rales are usually bilateral but may predominate on the patient's recumbent side. Pulmonary rales are moist, crackling sounds heard with the diaphragm of the stethoscope on inspiration.

A ventricular gallop, or S3, is commonly heard in early LVF. It is thought to result from vibrations that occur during the rapid ventricular filling phase, when the chamber has limited distensibility. An S3 can be difficult to hear if proper technique is not used. It is a low-pitched sound, heard best with the bell of the stethoscope placed lightly at the apex of the heart with the patient in the left lateral recumbent position. This brings the heart closer to the chest wall. The sound is heard in early diastole, approximately 0.12 to 0.14 sec after the second heart sound. The word *Kentucky* ("Ken-tuc'-ky") can be used to simulate the sound of a ventricular gallop and its relationship to S1 and S2.

Pulsus alternans is characterized by a regular rhythm, with alternation of strong and weak impulses felt at the peripheral pulse site. This pattern occurs most commonly when LVF is secondary to conditions that produce increased resistance to ejection. Aortic stenosis and hypertension are the two best examples. The pulsus alternans is attributed to alterations in the stroke volume ejected by the left ventricle [2].

Cardiomegaly, or enlargement of the heart, is due to the hypertrophy and dilatation that occur as part of the compensatory process in heart failure. The chest roentgenogram, electrocardiogram, and echocardiogram can confirm the presence of this physical sign. During physical examination, a left ventricular heave may be evident on the precordium. This is the clinical sign most indicative of left ventricular hypertrophy. The left ventricular heave is an abnormal, outward motion of the left ventricle during systole. Normally, ventricular contraction may be palpated in the fourth or fifth intercostal space at the mid-clavicular line. This palpable left ventricular contraction is referred to as the point of maximal impulse. In patients with left ventricular failure secondary to myocardial hypertrophy, the abnormal impulse may be felt more laterally and inferiorly than usual.

The major compensatory mechanism for a decreasing stroke volume is tachycardia. As stroke volume decreases, the heart rate increases in an effort to maintain the cardiac output. A rising heart rate may indicate cardiac decompensation and should always be investigated.

Cheyne-Stokes respirations are generally not evident until cardiac failure is advanced. The abnormality is due to the effect on the respiratory center of increased carbon dioxide levels, which occur secondary to the cardiac failure.

RIGHT VENTRICULAR FAILURE

Definition and Causation

RVF is characterized by systemic congestive symptoms, such as peripheral edema, liver enlargement, and engorgement of jugular veins. RVF is commonly caused by failure of the left ventricle. The increases in pressure on the left side of the heart are eventually transmitted to the right side, and systemic congestive symptoms are the result.

Isolated RVF is most commonly secondary to mitral stenosis and acute right ventricular infarctions. Other, less common causes include pulmonic valve disease, pulmonary hypertension, cor pulmonale, tricuspid valve disease, and septal defects.

Pathophysiology

The pathophysiological processes underlying failure of the right ventricle involve the same three compensatory mechanisms discussed in the section on LVF, except that the chamber involved is on the right side instead of the left side of the heart. The three compensatory mechanisms are myocardial hypertrophy, increased stretch in the muscle fiber, and a sympathetic response; they have been described in detail in our discussion of LVF.

Clinical Manifestations

Symptoms
RVF typically involves congestive symptoms that are evident systemically rather than in the pulmonary system. Pulmonary congestion will not be present unless the patient also has LVF. Peripheral edema, fatigue, liver enlargement, and gastrointestinal symptoms are typically evident.

Dependent or peripheral edema is usually not manifested until cardiomegaly, neck vein engorgement, and hepatomegaly are clinically evident. Peripheral edema tends to appear when 5 L or more of extracellular fluid volume has accumulated. Obesity and venous stasis seem to intensify the symptom [7]. The edema typically appears in the feet and ankles; bedridden patients, however, will accumulate fluid in the sacral area. Nursing care must include ad-

EXHIBIT 10.2
Clinical Manifestations of Right Ventricular Failure

Symptoms	Physical Signs
Peripheral edema	Jugular vein distention
Fatigue	Hepatojugular reflux
Liver engorgement	Right ventricular heave
Nausea	Pleural effusion
Anorexia	Auscultatory abnormalities
	Split second heart sound
	Right ventricular gallop
	Tricuspid insufficiency

herence to any sodium and fluid restrictions, measures to preserve skin integrity, and daily monitoring of intake and output as well as obtaining daily weights.

Hepatomegaly occurs because of the elevated central venous pressure. The liver is considered enlarged when the distance between its dull edge and the palpable lower border is greater than 11 cm [7]. The enlarged liver may produce pain in the right upper quadrant or epigastrium.

Gastrointestinal symptoms may be manifested as nausea, a sense of fullness after meals, or anorexia. The symptoms are thought to be due to liver and visceral engorgement.

Physical Signs

The physical manifestations of RVF are typically jugular venous engorgement, a right ventricular heave, hepatojugular reflux, auscultatory abnormalities, and pleural effusion (Exhibit 10.2). Jugular venous engorgement results from increased pressure and volume in the right side of the heart as congestion occurs and right ventricular stroke volume falls. The internal jugular vein can be used to estimate the central venous pressure if more accurate techniques are not available. The upper limit of normal for the jugular venous pressure is a level of 3 cm above the sternal angle [2]. An elevation of greater than 3 to 4 cm is considered abnormal and is taken as evidence of right ventricular congestion. The appropriate technique for estimating central venous pressure at the bedside is described in detail in Chapter 4.

To assess for hepatojugular reflux, apply firm pressure to the right upper quadrant of the abdomen in the region of the liver for 1 minute. This maneuver displaces blood from the liver to the inferior vena cava and increases the venous pressure. A hepatojugular reflux reflects both a congested liver and the ability of the right ventricle to accept and to eject effectively the increased venous return that occurred with compression.

A right ventricular heave may be palpated in patients with right ventricular hypertrophy. The heave may be felt with the palmar surface of the hand applied to the midsternal area of the precordium.

Auscultatory abnormalities of the heart may reveal a widely split second heart sound (S2), an abnormal right ventricular gallop, and a murmur indicating tricuspid insufficiency [13]. The increased volume and pressure that occur in RVF result in a delay in the ejection of blood from the right ventricle in systole. The pulmonary valve is therefore delayed in closure, which causes S2 to be widely split. The aortic valve closes first, before the pulmonary valve. A right ventricular gallop (S3) occurs as a result of rapid ventricular filling. The sound is heard best in early diastole with the bell of the stethoscope placed lightly in the third or fourth intercostal space at the left sternal border. A murmur indicating tricuspid insufficiency may be due to right ventricular dilatation. The dilated ventricle causes alterations in normal tricuspid valve closure, producing a leak during ventricular systole. The murmur is heard best with the diaphragm of the stethoscope placed in the third or fourth intercostal space at the left sternal border.

Pleural effusion may accompany either RVF or LVF. The pleural veins drain into both systemic and pulmonary venous beds. An effusion occurs most commonly with hypertension involving both pulmonary and systemic systems, but it may accompany marked elevation of pressure in either venous bed [2]. The fluid is often reabsorbed as the heart condition improves.

CARDIOGENIC SHOCK

Definition and Causation

Cardiogenic shock is a state of profound LVF. The heart is unable to supply the body with an adequate supply of O_2 and blood. The hemodynamic manifestations include a low cardiac output accompanied by systemic hypotension and elevated LVEDP.

Most commonly, cardiogenic shock occurs as a complication of myocardial infarction. Of patients who develop myocardial infarction and survive to reach the hospital, 10% to 15% develop cardiogenic shock [2]. Most of these patients exhibit three-vessel coronary artery disease with extensive left anterior descending artery involvement. The myocardial infarction involves large portions of the left ventricle. The development of shock is generally associated with impairment of 40% of the left ventricular wall. Despite current therapies, cardiogenic shock continues to carry a high mortality, 75% to 90% [21].

Other potential, although less common, causes of cardiogenic shock are chronic progressive cardiomyopathies, papillary muscle dysfunction or rupture, ventricular septal rupture, end-stage valvular disease, and ventricular aneurysm [2].

Pathophysiology

When cardiogenic shock occurs as a complication of a myocardial infarction, at least 40% of the left ventricle is involved in necrosis and ischemia. The infarcted left ventricle is stiff, with impaired contractility. The primary defect responsible for the development of cardiogenic shock is the impaired myocardial contractility [2]. The degree of impairment is directly related to the amount of muscle mass involved in the infarct.

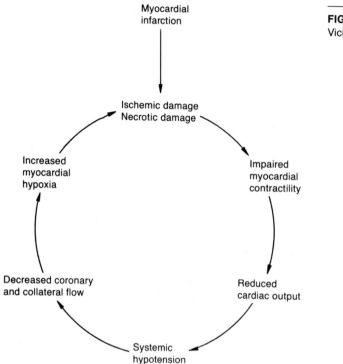

FIGURE 10.1
Vicious cycle of cardiogenic shock.

Impaired contractility is manifested in two major hemodynamic alterations, a decreased cardiac output and an elevated LVEDP. A low cardiac output is associated with a low stroke volume and decreased left ventricular work, resulting from depressed or impaired contractility. (Remember the relationship $CO = SV \times HR$.) The reduced cardiac output generally leads to systemic hypotension and a reflexive compensatory tachycardia [2]. The second major alteration, the rise in the LVEDP, is also associated with a rise in left atrial pressure and in pulmonary venous as well as arterial pressure. The eventual consequence is pulmonary congestion.

The diminished cardiac output, usually associated with systemic hypotension and an elevated LVEDP, sets the vicious shock cycle in motion (Figure 10.1). Ongoing myocardial ischemia and necrosis, which occur secondary to reduced coronary artery blood flow, continue the shock cycle.

The reflexive compensatory tachycardia further reduces the coronary artery blood flow. The coronary arteries fill during diastole. Tachycardia shortens the diastolic period, thereby reducing the time for coronary artery filling [21].

The reduced coronary artery filling time, and arterial pressure that is insufficient to maintain adequate blood flow through the coronary arteries, perpetuate the shock cycle. Myocardial hypoxia increases, resulting in further cell ischemia and necrosis. Table 10.1 compares the typical hemodynamic profile of a normal patient with that of a patient in shock [2].

TABLE 10.1
Hemodynamic Profile

Variable	Normal Individual	Individual in Shock
Arterial pressure (mm Hg)		
Systolic	> 90–< 140	< 80
Mean	> 60–< 100	< 60
Diastolic	> 60–< 90	< 50
Pulmonary artery diastolic pressure (mm Hg)	< 18	> 18
Heart rate (bpm)	60–100	> 95
Cardiac index (L/min/m²)	> 2.2	< 2.2
Systemic vascular resistance (dyne/sec/cm^{-5})	800–1,200	> 2,000

Clinical Manifestations

Symptoms

The clinical features of cardiogenic shock are all manifestations of impaired perfusion to vital organs and the peripheral tissues. The patient is often restless and confused, with cool, moist skin. The pulse pressure is narrowed, and peripheral pulses are rapid and thready. The systemic arterial pressure is usually reduced by 30 mm Hg from the normal level [20]. As kidney perfusion declines, the urine output decreases. A urine output of less than 20 cc per hour is consistent with the shock state [2, 20, 21]. Perpetuation of the shock cycle adds to the persistence or recurrence of ischemic chest pain [2]. Various dysrhythmias occur in patients with cardiogenic shock, particularly sinus tachycardia, ventricular tachydysrhythmias, heart blocks, bradydysrhythmias, and ventricular premature beats.

Pulmonary symptoms vary. Dyspnea, bronchospasm, and pulmonary edema may be evident in varying degrees. A pulmonary capillary wedge pressure (PCWP) of more than 20 mm Hg warns of worsening failure and pulmonary edema. Severe pulmonary congestion ensues when the PCWP exceeds 25 mm Hg. Auscultatory findings of pulmonary congestion will be evident in the lung fields. Respirations may be rapid and shallow. Cheyne-Stokes respirations are common as the shock state becomes increasingly severe. The symptoms of systemic congestion may be present in patients with shock if RVF occurs secondary to LVF. The symptoms of elevated central venous pressure, with jugular venous distention, hepatomegaly, and peripheral edema, may be evident.

Physical Signs

The physical signs apparent in the shock state are generally minimal. A ventricular gallop (S3) occurs frequently because of the severe LVF, with rapid ventricular filling. The heart sounds are often muffled, reflecting diminished contractility [2]. Heart enlargement may be evident on chest roentgenogram [21]. Exhibit 10.3 summarizes the common symptoms and physical signs that occur in cardiogenic shock.

EXHIBIT 10.3
Clinical Manifestations of Cardiogenic Shock

Symptoms	*Physical Signs*
Restlessness	Pulmonary rales
Confusion	Cheyne-Stokes respirations
Cool, moist skin	Tachycardia
Cyanosis	Dysrhythmias
Dyspnea	Muffled heart sounds
Decreased urine output < 20 cc/hr for 2 consecutive hr	Ventricular gallop (S3)
Lowered blood pressure (30 mm Hg drop from basal level)	
Narrow pulse pressure	

LABORATORY FINDINGS

Prior to treatment, serum electrolyte levels are generally normal in patients with cardiac failure. Diuretics, digitalis, and sodium restriction, however, often result in hyponatremia and hypokalemia. The hyponatremia is usually dilutional and managed by fluid restriction. Potassium supplements are frequently required in patients treated with thiazides or loop diuretics such as spironolactone and furosemide, particularly if digitalis therapy is used in combination with these diuretics.

Blood urea nitrogen and creatinine levels may be elevated in cardiac failure. These changes are a result of reductions in renal blood flow and glomerular filtration rate secondary to the diminished cardiac output occurring in heart failure.

Considerable hepatomegaly may result in elevation of the liver enzyme levels, particularly the serum glutamic oxaloacetic transaminase (SGOT) concentration.

The chest roentgenogram may demonstrate two features useful in diagnosing cardiac failure. The size of the heart provides information on chamber dilatation, and the lung fields will demonstrate evidence of pulmonary congestion. The earliest radiographic abnormality is prominence of congested upper lobe pulmonary veins. Severe pulmonary congestion results in alveolar pulmonary edema, which will appear as hazy mediastinal margins and lung fields with soft, patchy infiltrates [31].

Arterial blood gas analysis is useful in monitoring the patient's response to therapy. It may also help in distinguishing between LVF and chronic obstructive lung disease as a cause of dyspnea. In LVF, hypoxemia occurs with a normal or slightly decreased CO_2 tension and mild alkalosis. Patients with chronic obstructive pulmonary disease usually demonstrate hypoxemia with an increase in the CO_2 tension and respiratory alkalosis or an increase in serum bicarbonate levels [31].

MANAGEMENT OF CARDIAC FAILURE _____

Therapeutic Outcomes

The management of cardiac failure, be it right- or left-sided failure or cardiogenic shock, is directed toward four key therapeutic outcomes: (1) removal or control of the underlying or precipitating cause of the failure, (2) improvement in the myocardial contractility, (3) reduction in myocardial workload, and (4) reduction in sodium and water retention. These goals are listed in more detail in Exhibit 10.4. Generally, the underlying causative factors are difficult to remove. Therefore, the thrust of medical and nursing management is directed toward symptom management. The goals of therapy are to improve contractility and cardiac output, reduce the myocardial demand for O_2 (decreased MVO_2), and control the fluid or volume status of the patient.

Improvement in Myocardial Contractility
Myocardial contractility can be enhanced by various pharmacological agents with positive inotropic properties. Cardiac glycosides augment contractility, increase stroke volume, and raise cardiac output.

Digitalis. Digitalis is an important cardiac glycoside; it has been used for nearly 200 years and is still one of the most valuable agents in treating cardiac failure [7]. The nurse who administers digitalis must know the drug action, the average dose, and the signs of toxicity. Digitalis has both an inotropic and a chronotropic action, which increases the force of contraction and slows the heart rate. Therefore, the heart will beat more efficiently and will empty more completely. An enlarged and dilated heart will actually decrease in size when adequate amounts of digitalis are administered. Cardiac output improves because there is better contractility, and consequently stroke volume improves as well.

The average dose of digitalis depends on the preparation used. It must be given first in a loading dose in order to attain a therapeutic blood level, and in a daily maintenance dose thereafter. There are many conditions capable of potentiating the effects of digitalis. Precaution must be taken in administering the drug to elderly patients, who seem to tolerate the drug poorly. In severe heart disease, only a narrow range separates a therapeutic level of digitalis and a toxic level. The dosage may need to be reduced or monitored very closely. A low serum potassium level potentiates the action of digitalis and may lead to toxicity even with normal dosages. Serum potassium level should be monitored carefully in patients receiving digitalis therapy, particularly with the concomitant administration of diuretics. Other conditions in which patients may be more susceptible to digitalis toxicity are listed in Exhibit 10.5.

Digitalis toxicity may cause a wide variety of cardiac and noncardiac symptoms. Gastrointestinal symptoms are usually evident first and include nausea, vomiting, and anorexia. The cardiac symptoms are usually various dysrhythmias, which fall into two principal categories. The first category includes dysrhythmias of ventricular irritability, which most likely are due to hypokalemia. The second category of dysrhythmias involves atrioventricular (AV) conduction abnormalities caused by increased refractoriness at the AV

EXHIBIT 10.4
Therapeutic Outcomes in the Management of Cardiac Failure

1. Remove or control the underlying or precipitating cause

2. Improve myocardial contractility through
   a. Cardiac glycosides
   b. Sympathomimetic therapy

3. Reduce myocardial workload through
   a. Rest
   b. Vasodilator therapy (preload–afterload reduction)
   c. Intra-aortic balloon counterpulsation

4. Reduce sodium and water retention through
   a. Dietary control
   b. Diuretic therapy

EXHIBIT 10.5
Conditions Increasing Susceptibility to Digitalis Toxicity

Severe heart disease

Old age

Thyroid disease

Sinoatrial and atrioventricular node block

Mitral stenosis

Acute myocardial infarction

High-output failure

Hypoxic states

Electrolyte disturbances

Renal insufficiency

Multiple drug therapy

Wolff-Parkinson-White syndrome

Adapted from Gazes, P. C., *Clinical Cardiology* (2nd ed.). Copyright © 1983 by Year Book Medical Publishers, Inc., Chicago. Used with permission.

node. The dysrhythmias commonly produced are atrial fibrillation, second- and third-degree heart block, and paroxysmal atrial tachycardia with block [22].

In general, patients on maintenance doses of digitalis who have a regular rhythm should be suspected of digitalis toxicity if any irregularity in rhythm appears. Patients whose usual rhythm is irregular should be suspected of digitalis toxicity whenever short or prolonged runs of a regular rhythm interrupt the normally irregular rhythm [1]. Neurological symptoms may also occur, although usually later. Such symptoms as blurred vision, halos around lights, color vision disturbances, and drowsiness have been reported.

Patient teaching is a large part of the nurse's responsibility. Digitalis is a drug that the patient will probably take for a long time. It is important that the patient understand the action of the drug and, most important, the signs of digitalis toxicity.

Sympathomimetic agents. Sympathomimetic drug therapy is useful in managing certain forms of heart failure and cardiogenic shock. Sympathomimetic drugs exert a positive inotropic effect that can increase stroke volume, raise cardiac output, and thus be hemodynamically beneficial. Dobutamine and dopamine are two examples of drugs with this type of effect.

Dobutamine is a synthetic catecholamine. It acts directly on the beta 1 receptors of the heart to increase myocardial contractility and cardiac output selectively without significantly changing heart rate and blood pressure [23]. Dobutamine is an excellent agent for managing low-output cardiac failure that is refractory to other therapies.

Dopamine is a naturally occurring catecholamine with both alpha and beta effects. At the lower dosage range (less than 10 μg/kg per minute), dopamine has a predominantly beta effect. Contractility is enhanced, with some increase in heart rate. The cardiac output will increase as a result of the improved contractility. Dopamine also produces vasodilatation of the renal and mesenteric vessels in the lower dosage range. As the dosage is increased, the alpha effects become prominent. At doses of more than 20 μg/kg per minute, only the alpha effects of vasoconstriction occur. Considerable vasoconstriction may increase the impedance to left ventricular ejection (afterload), which increases cardiac workload. In patients with both pulmonary congestion and hypoperfusion, dopamine therapy may be combined with vasodilator administration to reduce the impedance to left ventricular ejection.

Nursing considerations for both dobutamine and dopamine are discussed in Chapter 14.

Reduction in Myocardial Workload

One of the best methods of decreasing the work of the myocardium is to provide the patient with adequate amounts of physical and emotional rest. Each patient must be assessed as to activity tolerance and sleep and rest patterns. Nursing care should be planned to permit uninterrupted periods for sleep and rest. Sedation is useful in allaying apprehension and fear.

A relatively new approach to the management of heart failure is vasodilator therapy. When ventricular failure occurs, an increase in both arterial and venous tone is evident, caused by action of the autonomic nervous system. An increase in the arterial vascular tone distributes blood to the more vital organs and maintains arterial pressure in the face of a falling cardiac output. These beneficial effects, however, add to the cardiac workload by increasing the impedance to left ventricular ejection. If arterial vascular tone is reduced, afterload is reduced, along with cardiac workload. Vasodilator drugs that are capable of reducing the arterial vascular tone are therefore useful in managing heart failure. These agents must be used cautiously to avoid a dramatic vasodilatory effect, which may result in hypotension.

Although most agents have some effect on both arterial and venous tone, certain vasodilator agents are capable of reducing the venous tone, predominantly. Agents that work primarily on the venous tone reduce the blood return

TABLE 10.2
Vasodilators: Chief Sites of Action

Drug	Arterial	Venous	Combination
Nitroglycerin		X	
Nitroprusside			X
Hydralazine	X		
Nifedipine	X		
Isosorbide dinitrate		X	
Prazosin hydrochloride			X
Captopril			X

to the right side of the heart by increasing the venous capacitance peripherally. The reduced venous return is effective in controlling the symptoms of pulmonary congestion by lowering the LVEDP.

Nitroglycerin and nitroprusside are two agents commonly employed to decrease both preload and afterload. Nitroglycerin has predominantly a venous effect, manifested in an increase in venous capacitance and a reduction in LVEDP. Nitroprusside is a potent arterial dilator with some venous effects. Both agents should be administered in small doses initially. Dosage should then be titrated according to the hemodynamic response, which is evaluated by assessing heart rate, blood pressure, pulmonary capillary pressure, cardiac output, and systemic vascular resistance. The goal is an increase in the cardiac output and a decrease in both systemic vascular resistance and pulmonary capillary pressure, with maintenance of an adequate blood pressure. If hypotension is a problem, drug administration may have to be discontinued or an inotropic–vasopressor agent added. When the clinical and hemodynamic improvements are maintained for 24 to 48 hours, oral vasodilator therapy should be substituted. Table 10.2 lists other vasodilator agents and their predominant effects.

The intra-aortic balloon pump (IABP), a mechanical method of reducing myocardial workload, is useful in the short-term management of severe reversible, cardiac failure and cardiogenic shock. The IABP reduces left ventricular workload and improves coronary artery perfusion. The goals of IABP therapy are to improve cardiac output, to increase O_2 supply to the myocardium, and to decrease the myocardial O_2 requirements [21] (see Chapter 13).

Reduction in Sodium and Water Retention
Sodium in any form exacerbates the symptoms of cardiac failure. Control of dietary sodium intake is essential in the management of cardiac failure. The degree of sodium restriction will vary with the severity of the condition; elimination of salt in food preparation and at the table is generally sufficient, however.

Diuretics are used in the treatment of heart failure when dietary therapy alone is inadequate. By preventing the reabsorption of sodium and water in the renal tubule, they promote a reduction in total fluid volume and thus relieve the symptoms of congestion, both systemically and in the lungs. Furosemide and ethacrynic acid are potent loop diuretics with a rapid onset of action. Because of their rapidity of action, they are effective in acute conditions warranting rapid diuresis. Potassium depletion, however, is likely to occur, because potassium is excreted along with the sodium.

The nurse who administers diuretics must evaluate daily weights, measure fluid intake and output frequently, and monitor for complications of potassium depletion. Potassium supplements are frequently ordered along with diuretic therapy unless a potassium-sparing diuretic is used.

When the cardiac failure occurs suddenly, as in pulmonary edema, there is a need for an immediate reduction in fluid returning to the heart. Prior to the advent of rapid-acting diuretics and vasodilators, rotating tourniquets were the treatment of choice in this situation. They occasionally are used today by emergency personnel in nonhospital settings. The tourniquets are applied to each extremity, with three of them tightened. They retain and reduce the circulating blood volume by 1,500 ml [22]. The tourniquets should be rotated every 5 minutes, so that no one extremity has a tourniquet on for longer than 15 minutes. The pulse distal to the tourniquet must be checked to ensure arterial blood flow in the extremity. The rotating tourniquets should be removed one at a time at 15 minute intervals.

Nursing Assessment

A nursing assessment is an essential component of the nursing process, allowing problems to be identified accurately and a plan of care to be developed that is appropriate to the patient's needs. Data can be collected directly from the patient, or from family members or others close to the patient if the patient's condition does not permit a complete assessment at the time.

Immediate assessment of physical and hemodynamic variables is essential in order to obtain baseline data that will guide management and enable the nurse to monitor the patient's progress. The following variables should be assessed:

1. Patient history
2. Temperature, pulse, and respiration
3. Blood pressure and mean arterial pressure (arterial line preferred)
4. Hemodynamic variables
   a. Pulmonary artery diastolic pressure
   b. Pulmonary capillary wedge pressure
   c. Cardiac output and cardiac index
   d. Systemic vascular resistance
5. Electrocardiographic monitoring for:
   a. Dysrhythmias
   b. Ischemic changes
   c. Drug and electrolyte effects
   d. Intraventricular conduction abnormalities
6. Intake and output: Foley catheter for hourly urine measurements; daily weights
7. Level of consciousness

8. Presence of chest pain
9. Signs and symptoms of pulmonary congestion
10. Signs and symptoms of systemic congestion
11. Extra heart sounds or murmurs (auscultation)
12. Presence of rales, rhonchi, or wheezes (auscultation of lung fields); chest roentgenogram and arterial blood gas levels
13. All available laboratory data
14. Response to therapy (continuous assessment)

Plan of Care

Comprehensive nursing care plans for the patient in cardiac failure and cardiogenic shock are presented in Tables 10.3 and 10.4, respectively.

TABLE 10.3
Nursing Care Plan for the Patient in Cardiac Failure

Problem/Outcome	Intervention
1. Problem: Pulmonary congestion due to elevated left ventricular pressures Outcome: Symptoms of pulmonary congestion will not appear	a. Position patient for maximum comfort b. Administer oxygen therapy as ordered c. Monitor symptoms of pulmonary congestion; report and record progress d. Auscultate lungs for presence of rales e. Administer prescribed medication; monitor effects and progress f. Monitor hemodynamic variables PAD, PCWP, and CO/CI as indicated by the clinical severity of the failure g. Evaluate laboratory data; blood gases, electrolytes h. Assess fluid status by daily weight, intake and output; urine specific gravity.
2. Problem: Decreased activity tolerance due to lower cardiac output and pulmonary congestion Outcome: No complications of bedrest; patient verbalizes comfort; patient completes activities prior to signs of intolerance	a. Assess activity tolerance b. Maintain ordered activity level c. Plan rest periods between all activities d. While patient confined to bed, change position every 2 hrs; provide skin care with position changes e. Increase activity as ordered; monitor BP, HR, and RR before and after each activity to assess tolerance
3. Problem: Potential for further cardiac decompensation Outcome: Blood pressure within normal limits	a. Monitor for hypotension b. Assess pulse for rate, regularity, tachycardia, a pulsus alternans, and peripheral pulse deficit c. Monitor for signs and symptoms of increasing failure

TABLE 10.3 *(continued)*

Problem/Outcome	Intervention
	d. Observe for symptoms of decreased perfusion: restlessness, cool skin, diaphoresis, confusion
	e. Administer inotropic and other drug therapy as ordered; monitor for effects; record and report progress
4. Problem: Potential for dysrhythmias due to ischemia, hypoxia, or electrolyte imbalances Outcome: Patient shows regular sinus rhythm (or patient's normal heart rhythm)	a. Monitor ECG continuously b. Recognize and report all dysrhythmias c. Treat dysrhythmias by unit protocols d. Monitor serum electrolyte levels e. Emergency equipment available: defibrillator, code cart
5. Problem: Potential sleep pattern disturbance due to environment and treatment plan Outcome: Usual sleep patterns maintained	a. Assess usual sleep patterns b. Plan care around usual sleep time if possible c. Schedule medications to allow for the fewest number of interruptions during the night d. Inform the patient of all expected awakenings
6. Problem: Potential for anxiety Outcome: Patient verbalizes fears and concerns; patient verbalizes understanding of condition	a. Allow patient to verbalize feelings b. Give explanations of treatment c. Involve the patient in the plan of care d. Involve the family in the treatment plan

PAD = pulmonary artery diastolic pressure; PCWP = pulmonary capillary wedge pressure; CO/CI = cardiac output/cardiac index; BP = blood pressure; HR = heart rate; RR = respiratory rate; ECG = electrocardiogram.

TABLE 10.4
Nursing Care Plan for the Patient in Cardiogenic Shock

Problem/Outcome	Intervention
1. Problem: Hypoperfusion due to inadequate cardic output, hypoxia, and acidosis Outcome: BP > 90 mm Hg; mean arterial pressure > 65 mm Hg; urine output > 20 cc/hr; skin warm, dry; sensorium clear; CI > 2.21/min/m²	a. Monitor BP and mean arterial pressure b. Monitor CI; use as guide in tailoring drug therapy c. Administer and titrate inotropic and sympathomimetic drugs to maintain BP d. Assess for signs of peripheral hypoperfusion: skin cool, clammy, cyanotic e. Monitor urine output; report output under 20 cc/hr f. Administer diuretic therapy as ordered; monitor electrolyte levels g. Monitor for side effects of drug therapy

TABLE 10.4 *(continued)*

Problem/Outcome	Intervention
2. Problem: Pulmonary congestion due to increased LVEDP and volume Outcome: No dyspnea; arterial blood gas values normal; LVEDP 15–20 mm Hg	a. Position patient for maximum comfort b. Auscultate lungs for presence, worsening, or improvement of pulmonary congestion c. Evaluate arterial blood gas values d. Administer oxygen therapy as ordered; mechanical ventilation may be necessary to promote optimal oxygenation e. Monitor PAD and PCWP (best reflections of LVEDP) f. Administer diuretics and vasodilators as ordered; monitor closely for adverse effects on BP
3. Problem: Dysrhythmias due to ongoing ischemia, electrolyte imbalances, acidosis Outcome: Heart rhythm remains stable	a. Monitor ECG continuously b. Recognize, report, and treat dysrhythmias per unit protocol; assess effect of the dysrhythmia on the patient's clinical status c. Correct factors precipitating dysrhythmias if possible
4. Problem: Chest pain due to myocardial ischemia Outcome: Patient is pain free	a. Assess for the presence, duration, characteristic, location, and radiation of the pain b. Treat pain promptly with the smallest amount of narcotic necessary to relieve the pain; administer O_2 c. Observe closely for signs of respiratory depression; change in BP or P
5. Problem: Potential for patient and family anxiety due to fear of death, severity of illness Outcome: Patient/family able to verbalize fears; patient/family able to verbalize understanding of the plan of treatment; patient/family able to visit and be supportive	a. Maintain quiet therapeutic environment b. Explain all equipment and procedures to the patient and family c. Provide frequent information and contact with the family d. Encourage the patient and family to express their fears and concerns e. Determine if clergy is desired by the patient or family

LVEDP = left ventricular end-diastolic pressure; other abbreviations as in Table 10.3.

CASE STUDIES

CASE 1

A 75-year-old woman is awakened in the night with chest pain and severe shortness of breath. After taking nitroglycerin three times without relief, she calls for an ambulance and is taken to the hospital emergency department, where she is found to be extremely dyspneic, cyanotic, and diaphoretic, and to be complaining of chest pain. Her blood pressure is elevated (180/100 mm Hg), her pulse is 140 beats per minute, and her respiratory rate is 30 per minute. On physical examination, she is found to have an S3 gallop at the apex and moist rales, with inspiratory and expiratory wheezes in both lung fields. Initial therapy consists of nitroglycerin sublingually, morphine and furosemide intravenously, and O_2 therapy via nasal cannula; rotating tourniquets are applied. The electrocardiogram is unchanged from a previous tracing, which showed considerable left ventricular hypertrophy. Initial arterial blood gas values are abnormal, with a pH of 7.12, a pCO_2 of 45 mm Hg, a pO_2 of 60 mm Hg, and a total CO_2 level of 11 mEq/L. She improves on the provided therapy and is transferred to the coronary care unit for further observation and treatment.

1. Discuss the major therapeutic outcomes to consider in the management of this patient's condition.

2. What are the supporting signs and symptoms indicating acute LVF (pulmonary edema)?

3. Why does pulmonary edema occur more frequently at night?

4. List the major nursing implications to consider with the use of rotating tourniquets.

5. What nursing measures will be helpful in the initial management of the patient's dyspnea?

CASE 2

A 62-year-old male stockbroker is stricken at his brokerage firm with sudden, severe chest pain, nausea, and diaphoresis. He is immediately transferred to the local hospital and subsequently admitted to the coronary care unit. He shows ST segment elevation in V_1 through V_6. Serum enzyme samples are drawn.

Upon arrival in the coronary care unit, his blood pressure is 90/50 mm Hg, heart rate 125 beats per minute, and respiratory rate 36 per minute. He is pale, cool, diaphoretic, and anxious. Urine output via a Foley catheter is less than 20 cc an hour. Physical examination reveals an S3 gallop and pulmonary rales in both lung fields. A pulmonary artery catheter is inserted, and initial readings are: pulmonary artery systolic pressure, 45 mm Hg; pulmonary artery diastolic pressure, 28 mm Hg; pulmonary capillary wedge pressure, 30 mm Hg; cardiac index, 2.2 L/min/m². Arterial blood gas analysis reveals: pH, 7.55; pCO_2, 31 mm Hg; pO_2, 70 mm Hg.

Initial therapy consists of O_2 at 40% via a Ventimask. Small doses of morphine sulfate are given intravenously to treat the chest pain. Furosemide, 80 mg intravenously, is administered, and a dopamine infusion is started at 5 µg/kg per minute.

One-half hour after the dopamine infusion was started, the blood pressure has improved to 106/60 mm Hg. The pulmonary artery diastolic pressure and pulmonary capillary wedge pressure, however, are still 28 to 30 mm Hg. The decision is made to add intravenous nitroprusside administration to the therapeutic regimen.

1. List four assessment findings indicative of shock or impending shock.

2. What is the physiological basis for the patient's tachycardia?

3. Discuss the major therapeutic outcomes to consider in the management of cardiogenic shock.

4. List three interventions useful in reducing the ventricular workload.

5. Discuss the nursing responsibilities associated with the administration of dopamine.

6. What is the rationale for the use of nitroprusside in the management of this patient's problem?

7. Discuss the nursing responsibilities associated with the administration of nitroprusside.

REFERENCES

1. Arbeit, S., et al. Recognizing digitalis toxicity. *Am. J. Nurs.* 77:136, 1977.

2. Braunwald, E. Clinical manifestation of heart failure. In E. Braunwald (ed.), *Heart Disease: A Textbook of Cardiovascular Medicine.* Philadelphia: Saunders, 1980.

3. Chatterjee, K., Doyle, B., and Avakian, D. Vasodilatory therapy for heart failure. *Crit. Care Q.* 4:13, 1981.

4. Dracup, K., Breu, C., and Tillisch, J. The physiological basis for combined nitroprusside-dopamine therapy in post–myocardial infarction heart failure. *Heart Lung* 10:114, 1981.

5. Foster, S. B., and Canty, K. A. Pump failure following myocardial infarction: an overview. *Heart Lung* 9:293, 1980.

6. Franciosa, J. Nitroglycerine and nitrates in congestive heart failure. *Heart Lung* 9:873, 1980.

7. Gazes, P. *Clinical Cardiology: A Bedside Approach* (2nd ed.). Chicago: Year Book, 1983.

8. Giles, T. Principles of vasodilator therapy for left ventricular congestive heart failure. *Heart Lung* 9:271, 1980.

9. Guyton, A. *Textbook of Medical Physiology* (5th ed.). Philadelphia: Saunders, 1976.

10. Haak, S. W. Intra-aortic balloon pump techniques. *Dimens. Crit. Care Nurs.* 2:196, 1983.

11. Huss, P., et al. The new inotropic drug, dobutamine. *Heart Lung* 10:121, 1981.

12. Johanson, B., et al. *Standards of Critical Care.* St. Louis: Mosby, 1981.

13. Lewis, P. S. Evaluation of the patient sustaining a right ventricular infarction and nursing implications. *Crit. Care Nurs.* 3:50, 1983.

14. Lief, P. D. Diuretics. *Am. Heart J.* 96:824, 1978.

15. Loeb, H., and Gunnar, R. Treatment of pump failure in acute myocardial infarction. *J.A.M.A.* 245:2093, 1981.

16. Mathewson, M. New uses for old drugs: vasodilators. *Crit. Care Update* 9:7, 1982.

17. Mathewson, M. Current vasodilator therapy. *Focus* 19:49, 1983.

18. McGurn, W. C. *People with Cardiac Problems: Nursing Concepts.* Philadelphia: Lippincott, 1983.

19. Michaelson, C. Bedside assessment and diagnosis of acute left ventricular failure. *Crit. Care Q.* 4:1, 1981.

20. Park, G. Cardiogenic shock. *Crit. Care Q.* 2:43, 1980.

21. Perry, A. G. Cardiogenic shock. In A. G. Perry and P. A. Potter (eds.), *Shock: Comprehensive Nursing Management.* St. Louis: Mosby, 1983.

22. Pinneo, R. *Congestive Heart Failure.* New York: Appleton-Century-Crofts, 1978.

23. Plachetka, J. Sympathomimetic pharmacology. *Crit. Care Q.* 2:27, 1980.

24. Purcell, J., and Holder, C. Intravenous nitroglycerine. *Am. J. Nurs.* 82:254, 1982.

25. Rushmer, R. F. *Cardiovascular Dynamics.* Philadelphia: Saunders, 1976.

26. Seal, A. L. *Cardiogenic Shock.* New York: Appleton-Century-Crofts, 1980.

27. Sedlock, S. Cardiac output: physiological variables and therapeutic interventions. *Crit. Care Nurs.* 1:14, 1981.

28. Shively, M. The physiological principles of intra-aortic balloon counterpulsation. *Crit. Care Nurs.* 4:83, 1981.

29. Smith, T., and Braunwald, E. The management of heart failure. In E. Braunwald (ed.), *Heart Disease: A Textbook of Cardiovascular Medicine.* Philadelphia: Saunders, 1980.

30. Sokolow, M., and McIllroy, M. B. *Clinical Cardiology.* Los Altos: Lange Medical Publications, 1979.

31. Wenger, N. K., Hurst, J. W., and McIntyre, M. D. *Cardiology for Nurses.* New York: McGraw-Hill, 1980.

CHAPTER 11

Mechanical Dysfunction of the Heart

Janet Secatore

INTRODUCTION _____

Chapters 9 and 10 addressed the major alterations in cardiac function caused by coronary artery disease and cardiac failure. There are other cardiac disorders, however, that can produce equally marked alterations in cardiac function. These include acquired valvular disorders, ventricular septal rupture, and diseases of the myocardium. Although these disorders are less prevalent than coronary artery disease, their impact on a patient and family is no less significant. It is important that the cardiac intensive care unit (CICU) nurse has an understanding of these disorders so that the immediate and potential needs of the patient and family in crisis can be met. This chapter presents a discussion of each of the disorders just mentioned. The pathophysiology, causes, subjective and objective findings, and medical and nursing interventions associated with each of these disorders are outlined.

The first two sections of this chapter review valvular disorders and ventricular septal rupture. The valvular disorders outlined are mitral stenosis, mitral insufficiency, aortic stenosis, and aortic insufficiency. Valvular disease and ventricular septal rupture produce major changes in cardiac hemodynamics because of the associated mechanical problems. In each case a valve or the septal wall is altered so that it does not function normally, thus altering cardiac function. The grossly altered hemodynamics that can result from these disorders can occur in an otherwise normal left ventricle. In most cases, once the mechanical defect has been repaired, functioning improves. Although ventricular septal rupture in an adult is usually associated with myocardial infarction, valvular disorders are not. The causes of valvular disorders (except for some cases of acute mitral and aortic insufficiency) and coronary artery disease are different.

The third section of this chapter discusses diseases of the myocardium, including cardiomyopathy, infective endocarditis and pericarditis, and cardiac tamponade. These diseases cause changes in cardiac tissue itself, thereby altering cardiac function. Except when pericarditis is related to myocardial infarction, the changes in cardiac tissue do not result from ischemia or coronary artery disease. The causes for these disorders vary extensively.

ACQUIRED VALVULAR DISORDERS _____

Mitral Stenosis

Pathophysiology

The primary problem in mitral stenosis (MS) is the impairment of blood flow from the left atrium to the left ventricle during ventricular diastole, a dysfunction caused by a narrowed mitral valvular orifice. This obstruction to flow increases the work required by the left atrium to move blood into the left ventricle. Consequently, left atrial pressure increases and left atrial hypertrophy occurs. As the condition progresses, there is a gradual increase in pulmonary venous, pulmonary arterial, and right ventricular pressures, with eventual right ventricular failure. Initially, the left ventricle is spared and, except for the decrease in volume it receives from the left atrium, continues to function normally. As mitral stenosis becomes more severe, however, cardiac output eventually begins to decrease.

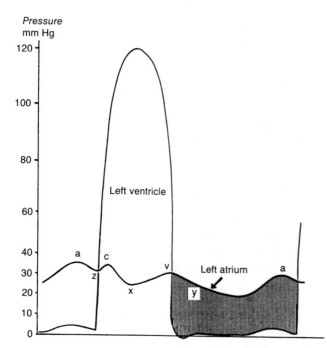

Pressure
mm Hg

FIGURE 11.1
Mitral stenosis. Shaded area represents mitral valve gradient. (Adapted from Schlant, R. C. In J. W. Hurst et al., *The Heart,* 4th ed. New York: McGraw-Hill. 1978. Used with permission.)

Normally, left atrial and left ventricular pressures are the same during ventricular diastole. As the disease progresses and the valve area decreases, a gradient develops across the mitral valve. The normal cross-sectional area of the mitral valve in an adult is 4 to 6 cm^2. As the area is reduced, a gradient as high as 20 to 40 mm Hg can occur (Figure 11.1). The size of the valve area also correlates with the symptoms exhibited. As the valve orifice narrows to approximately 2.5 cm^2, symptoms may develop with moderate exercise. During exercise, blood flow across the mitral valve must increase if the oxygen requirements of the body are to be met. A patient who is otherwise asymptomatic may develop symptoms during exercise as left atrial pressure increases in an effort to maintain left ventricular filling and cardiac output. In the patient with critical MS, the valve area is less than 1 cm^2, the gradient across the mitral valve can be 30 to 40 mm Hg, (25 mm Hg at rest), and even mild exercise may not be possible (Table 11.1).

Causation and Progresssion

The primary cause of MS is rheumatic fever, which causes inflammation of the valve leaflets. Damage to the valve is permanent, and, subsequently, the leaflets and chordae tendineae thicken, fibrose, and lose their pliability. The chordae tendineae also contract and fuse. The eventual result is a narrowed valvular orifice.

As many as 50% of the patients who evidence symptoms of MS do not report a history of rheumatic fever, but in most of these cases, rheumatic fever was probably undetected or undiagnosed [8]. Also, the relationship between MS and rheumatic fever may be difficult to establish, because the first symp-

TABLE 11.1
Hemodynamic Manifestations of Mitral Stenosis

Degree of Mitral Stenosis	At Rest	During Exercise
Mild (2.5–1.5 cm²)		
LAP	Normal	Slight ↑
Dyspnea	None	+
Cardiac output	Normal	Slight ↓
Moderate (1.5–1.0 cm²)		
LAP	↑	↑ ↑
Dyspnea	+	+ +
Cardiac output	Normal	↓
Severe (< 1.0 cm²)		
LAP	↑ ↑	↑ ↑ ↑
Dyspnea	+ +	+ + +
Cardiac output	↓	↓ ↓

LAP = left atrial pressure.

toms of MS usually appear about 20 years after the rheumatic fever. Although the disease is still common in other parts of the world, the incidence of rheumatic fever has decreased considerably in the United States in the last 30 years. It remains to be seen what effect this decreased incidence will have on the appearance of MS. Currently, MS occurs twice as frequently in women as in men.

A careful assessment of the patient with MS will reveal characteristic subjective and objective data. Both the physician and the CICU nurse must be able to identify these findings and to monitor changes in them as well. Although the objective data are more numerous, the subjective findings are usually the reason the patient seeks medical attention. Alleviation of the symptoms is the aim of treatment. Subjective and objective findings of MS are summarized in Exhibit 11.1.

Subjective Findings

As left atrial pressure increases, pulmonary venous pressure rises also, producing some degree of pulmonary congestion. The pulmonary congestion, in turn, causes dyspnea, which is the symptom most commonly associated with MS. In the early stages of the disease, dyspnea may occur only during periods of strenuous exercise, but as the disease progresses, it occurs with moderate or even mild exercise.

Normally, during exercise the flow of blood across the mitral valve increases to meet the body's demand for O_2. Because of the obstruction to flow caused by the stenotic mitral valve, however, left ventricular filling is compromised and is generally insufficient to produce the cardiac output required by the body, and fatigue results. Patients with MS often unknowingly limit their activity as a means of reducing symptoms. Unaware of the underlying problem,

EXHIBIT 11.1
Subjective and Objective Findings in Mitral Stenosis

Subjective Findings	Objective Findings
Dyspnea	On auscultation
Fatigue	Accentuation of S1
Paroxysmal nocturnal dyspnea	Opening snap
Orthopnea	Diastolic murmur
Hemoptysis	On chest roentgenogram
Systemic embolization	Left atrial enlargement
Symptoms associated with right ventricular failure	Right ventricular hypertrophy
	Congestive heart failure
	On electrocardiogram
	P mitrale
	Right axis deviation
	Atrial fibrillation
	On cardiac catheterization
	Elevated left atrial and pulmonary artery pressures
	Mitral valve gradient
	Abnormal size of valve orifice

they may characterize themselves as having little or no energy and may adopt more sedentary lifestyles and hobbies.

Other symptoms can include paroxysmal nocturnal dyspnea, orthopnea, hemoptysis, systemic embolization, chest pain, and symptoms associated with right ventricular failure.

Objective Findings

Auscultatory. The most important objective findings of MS are evident on auscultation. The three hallmark sounds are (1) accentuation of the first heart sound, (2) opening snap, and (3) rumbling diastolic murmur.

S1 occurs at the beginning of ventricular contraction, after the mitral valve is closed. Although the mechanism is not completely understood, this sound may be produced in part by the vibration in early systole of the valve leaflets and chordae tendineae. When these structures are stenosed and their mobility is decreased, they do not vibrate in quite the normal way. The fibrosis and scarring of the leaflets and chordae tendineae alter the vibratory characteristics of these structures and result in an accentuation of S1. This finding is useful in diagnosing the presence of MS, but not its severity.

An important sign of MS is the opening snap. Normally, when the mitral valve opens at the end of systole, no sound is produced. An opening snap occurs in MS in early diastole, however, and represents the sudden cessation of the opening of the valve leaflets when they reach the limits of their mobility. The opening snap is a brief, high-pitched, popping sound that is best heard with the diaphragm of the stethoscope at the lower left sternal border. The severity of MS can be correlated with the length of the interval between the second heart sound (S2) and the opening snap [8]. If the interval is short, there is a very small valve opening. A longer S2–opening snap interval indicates

II.

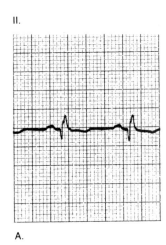

A.

V_1

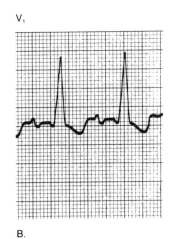

B.

FIGURE 11.2
Left atrial enlargement may produce (A) broad P waves in limb leads, (B) wide biphasic P waves in V_1, or both.

greater excursion of the leaflets and a larger valve opening. This interval should be evaluated regularly to assess the progress of the disease.

The third auscultatory abnormality associated with MS is a diastolic murmur. This harsh, rumbling, low-pitched murmur is best heard with the bell of the stethoscope at the apex. The rumbling quality of the murmur, frequently described as sounding like "wagon wheels over a dirt road," is produced as blood flows across the abnormal valve. The murmur is usually accentuated with exercise and tachycardia, as flow and turbulence over the abnormal valve increase and diastolic filling time decreases. The intensity of the murmur varies from patient to patient, and the loudness of the murmur does not generally correlate well with the severity of MS. Change in the loudness and intensity of the murmur in an individual, however, is useful in assessing the severity and progression of the condition in that patient.

Radiological. Left atrial enlargement may be evident on the chest roentgenogram, and cardiomegaly may be noted if right ventricular hypertrophy is marked. If the degree of congestive heart failure is sufficient, pulmonary venous and arterial changes may be observed as well.

Electrocardiographic. The electrocardiographic (ECG) changes observed in MS are not specific and do not correlate well with severity. The ECG can be normal in cases of severe MS. Left atrial enlargement may cause a change in the shape of the P wave. P mitrale is a common finding, representing altered atrial depolarization of the enlarged, hypertrophied chamber (Figure 11.2). Right axis deviation may occur if right ventricular hypertrophy is considerable [30]. Atrial fibrillation is the most common dysrhythmia observed and occurs in 30% to 40% of patients with MS. When it appears, the loss of atrial contraction, which normally accounts for 20% to 30% of cardiac output, combined with a decrease in diastolic filling time, can markedly decrease cardiac output.

Echocardiographic. Although echocardiography does not indicate the severity of MS, it can diagnose the condition by demonstrating abnormal leaflet movement and thickening (see Chapter 4).

Cardiac catheterization. Cardiac catheterization is not generally indicated for the young person with isolated MS. As the disease progresses, however, cardiac catheterization is necessary to determine (1) cross-sectional valve area, (2) gradient at the mitral valve, and (3) left atrial and pulmonary artery pressures. This information is crucial in deciding the timing of surgery. Cardiac catheterization also provides information about other valvular abnormalities and coronary artery anatomy.

Because the degree of symptoms exhibited is related to the exercise level, it may be necessary to exercise the patient during the procedure to provoke symptoms and demonstrate an increase in left atrial pressure. The patient can be made to pedal a bicycle against resistance or do hand-gripping exercises or leg raises.

Medical Interventions

No form of medical treatment can alter or decrease the amount of stenosis present. The medical management of MS consists of assessing, monitoring, and treating the subjective and objective findings associated with the disorder.

As the signs and symptoms of pulmonary hypertension and congestive heart failure develop, they are treated with digitalis and diuretics. If atrial fibrillation occurs, it is essential that antiarrhythmic agents be added to the regimen to restore normal sinus rhythm. Once atrial fibrillation has appeared, complications related to systemic embolization can occur. Decisions regarding anticoagulation therapy must be made on an individual basis. Antibiotic prophylaxis for some dental, gynecological, gastrointestinal, and genitourinary procedures is imperative if complications related to endocarditis are to be avoided.

As the stenosis becomes more severe, medical treatment becomes more difficult, and it is at this point that an evaluation for surgery is indicated. Commissurotomy is an option when MS is the only abnormality. This is generally an interim measure, however, and more extensive surgical procedures are required later. Mitral valve replacement is indicated when the stenosis is very severe, when considerable valvular calcification is present, or when mitral insufficiency accompanies MS. For an explanation of these procedures, see Chapter 12.

The optimal timing of mitral valve replacement is not always easy to determine. For patients with critical mitral stenosis, surgical intervention is the treatment of choice. Mildly symptomatic patients are often among those who have subconsciously modified their activities to reduce symptoms. Therefore, symptoms may not accurately reflect the severity of MS in these cases. A careful assessment of activity tolerance is necessary to determine the actual degree of MS and the need for surgery. It has been found that when surgery is performed early in this group, the results are often unexpectedly good [8].

**Mitral
Insufficiency/
Mitral
Regurgitation**

Pathophysiology

Mitral insufficiency results when there is incomplete closure of the mitral valve at the end of ventricular diastole. During ventricular systole blood is ejected into the aorta and backward through the incompetent valve into the left atrium. The regurgitation eventually compromises left ventricular functioning. Mitral insufficiency can occur chronically, acutely, or intermittently.

In chronic mitral insufficiency, left atrial dilatation is the first change, as the left atrium stretches to accommodate the regurgitant volume. This dilatation may be extensive, producing a giant left atrium visible on chest roentgenogram and palpable on physical examination. Left atrial hypertrophy eventually develops as left atrial work increases. This enlargement finally affects pulmonary venous and arterial pressures and produces symptoms of congestive heart failure. Large volumes of blood then enter the left ventricle during diastole. The consistently elevated left ventricular end-diastolic volumes eventually result in an elevation of left ventricular end-diastolic pressure (LVEDP) and the development of left ventricular hypertrophy. Long-standing left ventricular hypertrophy impairs left ventricular functioning, decreases cardiac output, and eventually produces left ventricular failure.

If mitral insufficiency is acute or intermittent and the left atrium is not dilated, rapid changes in left atrial pressure can produce a sudden onset of congestive heart failure, acute pulmonary edema, and even cardiogenic shock. A slight elevation in left atrial pressure occurs normally during ventricular systole as the mitral valve leaflets bulge slightly into the left atrium. When mitral insufficiency occurs, however, there is a marked increase in left atrial pressure when some portion of left ventricular volume is ejected into the left atrium. This increase is represented by an abnormally large V wave on the left atrial or pulmonary capillary wedge pressure tracings observed on the pressure monitor (Figures 11.3 and 11.4). This enlarged V wave is always observed in acute mitral insufficiency. When mitral insufficiency occurs intermittently, the enlarged V wave may appear intermittently as well. When present, this wave is very useful in establishing a diagnosis. Its absence, however, does not exclude mitral insufficiency. The enlarged V wave may not be present if the left atrium is so dilated that the addition of the regurgitant volume no longer alters left atrial pressure. Its absence generally indicates long-standing mitral insufficiency and a grossly dilated left atrium.

Causation and Progression

The progression of mitral insufficiency is determined by its cause. Chronic mitral insufficiency is usually the result of rheumatic fever. Complications of rheumatic fever produce progressive changes in the valve leaflets and chordae tendineae that eventually prevent complete valve closure. With each systole, the left atrium receives some portion of left ventricular stroke volume. Over time, a gradual accommodation to this increased volume is made and the left atrium dilates. During ventricular diastole the left atrium then contributes a large volume of blood to the left ventricle, which must work harder to eject the increased volume of blood. So long as the ventricle is normal, however, the

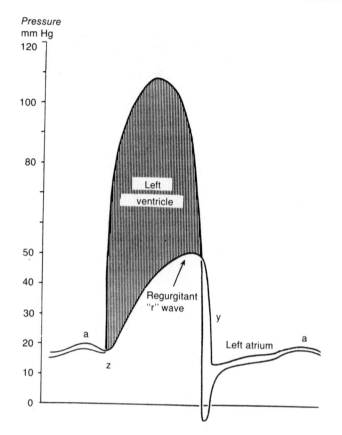

Pressure
mm Hg

FIGURE 11.3
Left atrial and left ventricular pressure tracings observed in mitral insufficiency. V wave is sometimes referred to as r wave. (Adapted from Schlant, R. C. "Altered Cardiovascular Function of Rheumatic Heart Diseases and Other Acquired Valvular Disease." In J. W. Hurst et al., *The Heart,* 4th ed. New York: McGraw-Hill, 1978. Used with permission.

increased volume increases fiber stretch, stroke volume, and, therefore, cardiac output. Left ventricular compliance gradually increases, and LVEDP, as well as left ventricular O_2 requirements, remains normal for a long time.

Acute mitral insufficiency usually occurs as a complication of a myocardial infarction or trauma that causes interference with, or rupture of, a papillary muscle or chordae tendineae. It may also occur after mitral valve replacement if a perivalvular leak develops. A valve leaflet may be "wide open" during systole, causing acute changes in left atrial and pulmonary venous pressures, changes that are generally poorly tolerated.

Intermittent mitral insufficiency usually occurs with ischemic heart disease and is referred to as papillary muscle dysfunction. When ischemia occurs in the area of a papillary muscle, the muscle function can be compromised, preventing complete valve closure. The signs and symptoms of mitral insufficiency can accompany an episode of angina but be absent when angina is relieved. Depending on the regurgitant volume and the frequency of ischemic attacks, the condition may be moderately or poorly tolerated. In addition, cardiac dilatation and cardiomyopathy may distort the left ventricle so that the functioning of one or both of the papillary muscles is interfered with, producing signs and symptoms of intermittent or chronic mitral insufficiency.

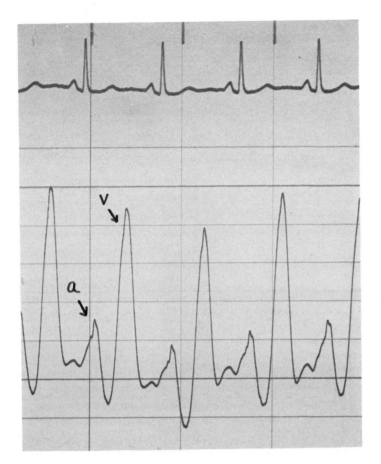

FIGURE 11.4
Pulmonary wedge pressure tracing with large V wave. Note that V wave occurs after the T wave on the ECG.

Subjective Findings

If mitral insufficiency is chronic or mild, there are few symptoms. The progressive nature of the disorder allows for gradual compensation by the left atrium and ventricle. The only subjective finding reported may be palpitations, caused by a hyperdynamic left ventricle and the ejection of large stroke volumes (Exhibit 11.2).

Because left ventricular end-diastolic volume is chronically elevated, the work required to eject large volumes eventually takes its toll. Left ventricular hypertrophy develops and eventually progresses to left ventricular failure and a decrease in cardiac output. Ultimately, the increased volumes and pressures affect the pulmonary venous and arterial systems, causing symptoms of dyspnea and orthopnea as well as episodes of pulmonary edema. These symptoms intensify and can eventually cause severe restriction of physical activity.

When mitral insufficiency is acute or intermittent, the symptoms vary in intensity depending on the amount of regurgitation occurring. If rupture of chordae tendineae or papillary muscles has produced a wide open mitral valve, the rapid changes in left atrial pressure can produce severe dyspnea and acute

EXHIBIT 11.2
Subjective and Objective Findings in Mitral Insufficiency

Subjective Findings	Objective Findings
Palpitations	Laterally displaced, hyperdynamic apex
Dyspnea	Systolic murmur
Fatigue	S3
	Left atrial enlargement
	Cardiomegaly
	Change in P wave morphology
	Atrial fibrillation
	Left ventricular hypertrophy
	V wave
	Grading of mitral insufficiency

pulmonary edema. If the problem is intermittent, the symptoms may be moderate to severe.

Objective Findings

On palpation, the apical impulse appears hyperdynamic, sustained throughout systole, and displaced laterally. This finding is generally observed in both chronic and acute mitral insufficiency. If the condition is long-standing and the left atrium is grossly dilated, it may be felt as well, occurring just before the ventricular impulse and slightly above it (Exhibit 11.2).

The auscultatory abnormalities associated with mitral insufficiency are a systolic murmur and an S3. The murmur of mitral insufficiency is holosystolic and has a high-pitched, blowing quality. It radiates to the axilla and is best heard with the diaphragm of the stethoscope at the apex. The sound is produced as the regurgitant volume moves across the mitral valve into the left atrium. The intensity of the murmur does not correlate well with the severity. A variation of mitral insufficiency may be heard when the murmur is late in systole and is preceded by a mid- or late-systolic click. The mitral valve is competent early in systole, but as left ventricular pressure increases, the leaflets balloon into the left atrium, allowing some regurgitation. The other characteristic heart sound heard on auscultation is a loud, high-pitched S3 that occurs when the large left atrial volume enters the ventricle in early diastole. This sound can be observed in chronic and acute mitral insufficiency.

Radiological. Left atrial enlargement may be visible. If left ventricular hypertrophy has occurred, cardiomegaly may be present.

Electrocardiographic. Left atrial dilatation may produce changes in the shape of the P wave. Atrial fibrillation is common, and a pattern of left ventricular hypertrophy may be observed.

EXHIBIT 11.3
Grading of Mitral Insufficiency

1+: Faint puff of dye in LA.

2+: Regurgitant jet. Moderate opacification of LA that clears quickly.

3+: No regurgitant jet. Immediate opacification of LA, as intense as that in LV.

4+   LA opacification more intense than that in LV and aorta and persisting through several systoles.

LA = left atrium; LV = left ventricle.

Echocardiographic.   Echocardiography is less useful in mitral insufficiency than it is in MS. The valve may appear to function normally even in the presence of severe regurgitation. Assessments of left atrial and ventricular enlargement and left ventricular contractility, however, can be made.

Cardiac catheterization.   Cardiac catheterization provides the most accurate means of assessing the amount of regurgitation. During left ventriculography, dye is ejected into the ventricle. Mitral insufficiency is then graded from 1+ to 4+, reflecting the amount of left ventricular volume ejected into the left atrium (Exhibit 11.3).

In acute or intermittent mitral insufficiency, cardiac catheterization is necessary to determine left ventricular hemodynamics and to assess coronary artery anatomy.

Medical Interventions

The management of mitral insufficiency is aimed at decreasing the regurgitant volume into the left atrium and increasing cardiac output. A combination of vasodilator and diuretic therapy is usually instituted for the management of chronic mitral insufficiency. A reduction in systemic resistance (afterload) increases forward flow into the aorta and decreases the amount of regurgitation to the left atrium. Diuretics reduce preload and aid in the management of pulmonary congestion. Although not as crucial in mitral insufficiency as in MS, the maintenance of normal sinus rhythm is desirable, and digitalis, quinidine, or other antiarrhythmic agents may be required. Systemic embolization is less common also, but it can occur when atrial fibrillation is present. Decisions regarding anticoagulation therapy are made on an individual basis.

If mitral insufficiency is the result of papillary muscle dysfunction, conventional therapy aimed at controlling angina should be instituted. The addition of nitrates and beta blockade may be necessary.

Mitral valvular replacement may be required on an emergency basis if acute mitral insufficiency occurs. The patient may develop cardiogenic shock if the amount of regurgitation to the left atrium is great enough to produce a considerable drop in cardiac output. The resultant rise in systemic vascular resistance, which is a normal response to the shock state, can further decrease cardiac output and increase the amount of regurgitant volume into the left atrium, causing further deterioration. Under these circumstances, the placement of pulmonary artery and peripheral arterial catheters is followed by the institution of vasodilator therapy. When pharmacological therapy is insufficient, mechanical afterload reduction can be achieved with the insertion of an intra-aortic balloon. The treatment of choice for acute mitral insufficiency is mitral valve replacement, but aggressive medical management is necessary to stabilize the patient for surgery and to provide time to determine overall cardiac function and the presence of other abnormalities.

Mitral valve replacement is necessary for patients with long-standing mitral insufficiency that no longer responds to medical therapy. Again, the timing of surgery is not always easy to determine. Although valve replacement results in symptomatic improvement in most patients, if surgery is delayed too long and left ventricular dysfunction is severe preoperatively, a return to normal or near-normal functioning may not be possible.

Aortic Stenosis

Pathophysiology

In aortic stenosis a narrowed aortic valve orifice restricts the flow of blood from the left ventricle to the aorta during ventricular systole. This obstruction to left ventricular emptying considerably increases left ventricular work and produces left ventricular hypertrophy and, eventually, left ventricular failure.

A systolic gradient between the left ventricle and the aorta develops and may reach 150 mm Hg (Figure 11.5). As the ventricle hypertrophies, normal stroke volume is maintained for a long time, because the increased pressure is distributed over a larger contractile area. Eventually, however, LVEDP remains elevated even at rest. As aortic stenosis progresses, the left ventricle fails.

Maintenance of normal sinus rhythm is particularly important, because in aortic stenosis atrial contraction contributes up to 40% of left ventricular stroke volume instead of the normal 25%. Left atrial contraction enhances left ventricular end-diastolic volume and fiber stretch, which aid effective left ven-

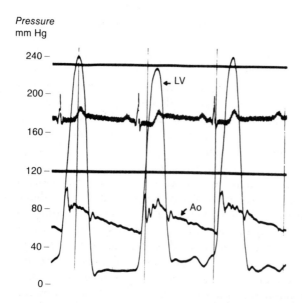

Pressure
mm Hg

240 —

200 —

160 —

120 —

80 —

40 —

0 —

← LV

Ao

FIGURE 11.5
Simultaneous left ventricular (*LV*) and aortic (*Ao*) pressures demonstrate the systolic pressure gradient observed in aortic stenosis. (From Levinson, G. E., "Aortic Stenosis." In J. E. Dalen and J. S. Alpert (eds.), *Valvular Heart Disease.* Boston: Little, Brown, 1981. Used with permission.).

EXHIBIT 11.4
Subjective and Objective Findings in Aortic Stenosis

Subjective Findings	Objective Findings
Dyspnea	Hyperdynamic apical impulse
Angina	Harsh, rumbling holosystolic murmur
Syncope (effort)	Decreased S2
	Early ejection click
	S4
	Cardiomegaly; valve calcification
	Left ventricular hypertrophy
	Abnormal systolic gradient
	Reduced cross-sectional valve area

tricular emptying. Left atrial pressure rises to accomplish this emptying. A pressure elevation to 30 to 35 mm Hg may occur during systole, but pulmonary edema does not usually occur until the mean left atrial pressure rises above 25 mm Hg [30].

Causation and Progression

Rheumatic fever is a common cause of aortic stenosis and often occurs in conjunction with a congenital bicuspid valve. Rheumatic calcific and fibrotic changes result in decreased leaflet pliability and mobility, as well as a narrowed valve area. Other causes of aortic stenosis include a congenital bicuspid or unicuspid valve, infective endocarditis, and the normal aging process, which produces calcification of the leaflets. Progression is gradual and can be undetected for years.

Subjective Findings

In the early stages of aortic stenosis, subjective findings are absent, but the lack of symptoms does not preclude the presence of considerable stenosis. Symptoms usually occur when the area of the valve orifice has been reduced from the normal 2.6 to 3.5 cm^2 to the critical range below 0.7 cm^2. The symptoms most commonly associated with aortic stenosis are dyspnea, angina, and syncope (Exhibit 11.4).

The most serious finding in aortic stenosis is left ventricular hypertrophy. It eventually produces left atrial hypertrophy and an increase in pulmonary venous pressure. Dyspnea occurs first with exertion but eventually occurs even at rest.

Angina results not from coronary artery disease but, rather, from an imbalance between myocardial O$_2$ supply and demand. The hypertrophied left ventricle requires more O$_2$ than even normal coronary arteries can supply. The concomitant development of coronary artery disease is a serious problem, however.

Effort syncope is the third symptom associated with aortic stenosis. As the name implies, this syncope occurs during exercise. There is an abrupt decrease in cardiac output that is not mediated by other compensatory mechanisms. The appearance of this symptom is an ominous sign and is associated with a high mortality [5].

Objective Findings

A sustained, heaving apical impulse is revealed on palpation. Often atrial systole can be felt as well.

On auscultation the characteristic finding is a harsh, rumbling holosystolic murmur, which results from the movement of blood across the valve during systole. It is best heard with the bell of the stethoscope in the second intercostal space to the right of the sternum. Radiation to the neck and apex is common. The intensity of the murmur is variable, but generally, the louder and longer the murmur, the more severe the stenosis.

Other auscultatory findings include a decreased S2, an early ejection click, and an S4. The delayed closure of the aortic valve, caused by prolonged left ventricular ejection time, and calcification of the valve combine to soften S2. An early ejection click, representing leaflet movement, may be heard if the stenosis is not too severe. Loss of this early ejection click represents a decrease in leaflet mobility and increased stenosis. An S4 occurring late in diastole is frequently observed and represents the "atrial kick."

Radiological.   Cardiomegaly may be present but is not diagnostic for aortic stenosis. Although they do not correlate well with the degree of stenosis, calcification at the aortic valve and poststenotic dilatation may be evident.

Electrocardiographic.   Left ventricular hypertrophy is generally observed. Left bundle branch block and nonspecific intraventricular conduction defects may occur as well.

Echocardiographic.   Echocardiography is not diagnostic for aortic stenosis. Thickened valve leaflets may be observed, but the severity of aortic stenosis cannot be determined with this tool.

Cardiac catheterization.   Cardiac catheterization is necessary to determine cross-sectional valve area and to measure the systolic pressure gradient. There are technical difficulties associated with this procedure, however. Introduction of a catheter into the left ventricle can be very difficult and somewhat dangerous. If the aortic valve cannot be crossed, a transseptal approach to the left ventricle from the right ventricle can be attempted. Coronary artery anatomy can be assessed also. Because angina is frequently associated with aortic stenosis, it is critical that the angina's cause be determined.

Medical Interventions

The most important aspects of medical management are the immediate recognition of symptoms and the initiation of treatment until valve replacement can be performed. The possibility of rapid deterioration or sudden death compels some physicians to recommend surgery, in the absence of symptoms, if on cardiac catheterization critical aortic stenosis and a systolic gradient greater than 50 mm Hg are present [30]. If surgery is deferred, treatment is instituted to relieve dyspnea and angina.

Aortic Insufficiency/ Aortic Regurgitation

Pathophysiology
In aortic insufficiency the aortic valve does not close completely at the end of ventricular systole. As the pressure in the left ventricle drops abruptly, some portion of the cardiac output returns to the left ventricle. At the end of diastole, the ventricle must then eject this increased volume with the subsequent systole. The basic hemodynamic alterations in aortic insufficiency result from left ventricular volume overload and accompanying dilatation. The severity of the condition depends on the area of the regurgitant orifice and the pressure gradient between the left ventricle and the aorta.

Left ventricular compliance increases as the ventricle dilates. This increased compliance accounts for an increase in stroke volume and the maintenance of normal cardiac output. Eventually, left ventricular failure develops which may limit further regurgitation: As cardiac output decreases, left ventricular end-diastolic volume and pressure rise, decreasing the gradient between the left ventricle and the aorta and reducing the amount of regurgitation.

LVEDP may rise enough to cause premature closure of the mitral valve. The cost to the left atrium is an increased pressure, which can lead to pulmonary venous pressure changes.

Finally, peripheral vasodilatation decreases afterload by increasing forward flow and decreasing the amount of regurgitation. Patients with aortic insufficiency can tolerate moderate exercise, because the accompanying peripheral vasodilatation actually improves their condition by decreasing the amount of regurgitation to the left ventricle.

Causation and Progression
Aortic insufficiency can occur chronically or acutely. Rheumatic fever produces the same changes in the aortic valve that it does in the mitral valve. Other causes of aortic insufficiency are syphilitic aortitis (less common now), myxomatous degeneration of the leaflets, and bicuspid valves. Acute aortic insufficiency can occur as the result of infective endocarditis, dissecting aortic aneurysm, aortic trauma, or postoperative perivalvular leak.

Subjective Findings
The subjective findings associated with aortic insufficiency can be quite noticeable (Exhibit 11.5). Palpitations are most commonly noted first and result from a forceful left ventricular contraction. The patient may complain of dizziness and become aware of pulsations as well as throbbings in the neck. Headaches are common as well. There is a gradual decrease in exercise tolerance, and as the condition progresses, dyspnea evolves into pulmonary congestion and edema. Angina is associated less commonly with aortic insufficiency than it is with aortic stenosis but can occur with normal coronary arteries. The low diastolic pressure accompanying aortic insufficiency can decrease coronary artery perfusion enough to cause an inadequacy of O_2 supply to a grossly dilated ventricle.

EXHIBIT 11.5
Subjective and Objective Findings in Aortic Insufficiency

Subjective Findings	Objective Findings
Palpitations	Hyperdynamic apex, displaced laterally
Dizziness	Aortic systolic murmur
Headaches	Aortic diastolic murmur
Neck throbbings	Apical distolic murmur (Austin Flint)
Angina	S3
	Peripheral findings[a]
	Cardiomegaly
	Left ventricular hypertrophy
	Grading of regurgitation[b]

[a]See Exhibit 11.6.   [b]See Exhibit 11.7.

Objective Findings

On palpation the apex is found to be displaced laterally and inferiorly and to have the sustained and hyperdynamic characteristics of a hyperactive left ventricle.

On auscultation a high-pitched, blowing diastolic murmur radiating to the apex can be heard, most effectively with the diaphragm at the third and fourth intercostal spaces. Before symptoms appear, this murmur may be the only indication of the disorder. As the condition progresses, the murmur becomes longer and louder and eventually can be heard all along the left sternal border. The severity of the murmur, however, does not correlate well with the severity of aortic insufficiency. With left ventricular failure and an increase in systemic vascular resistance, LVEDP rises and the systolic gradient decreases. As a result, the regurgitant volume decreases and the murmur softens. An aortic systolic murmur, observed in the absence of aortic stenosis, can often be heard as the large stroke volume is ejected. An apical diastolic murmur (Austin Flint murmur) suggestive of mitral stenosis may be heard, but the absence of an opening snap ensures that the murmur does not represent MS. Along with the systolic murmur, a systolic click may be present. Finally, because left atrial volume enters an already filled left ventricle, an S3 is common.

Some of the most noticeable physical findings associated with aortic insufficiency are observed peripherally. A bounding pulse, characterized by a wide pulse pressure, develops. Stroke volume is usually twice normal but may reach 200 to 300 ml [30]. This stroke volume markedly elevates systolic pressure. The pulse collapses, however, when as much as 80% of the stroke volume reenters the left ventricle [5]. The peripheral objective findings occurring in aortic insufficiency are summarized in Exhibit 11.6.

Radiological.   Chest roentgenographic findings are not specific to aortic insufficiency and may be normal with severe disease. Left ventricular enlargement may produce cardiomegaly, and with the development of congestive failure, pulmonary vascular changes occur.

EXHIBIT 11.6
Peripheral Objective Findings in Aortic Insufficiency

Corrigan's sign:	"Water-hammer" pulses
De Musset's sign:	Head bobbing with each systolic pulsation
Quincke's sign:	Alternating reddening and blanching of nailbeds
Duroziez's murmur:	Slight compression of large arteries, producing systolic *and* diastolic bruits
	"Pistol-shot" pulses

Electrocardiographic. The ECG commonly demonstrates left ventricular hypertrophy but can be otherwise normal. Atrial fibrillation does not usually occur unless mitral valvular disease is present.

Echocardiographic. Although it provides useful information about left ventricular function, echocardiography does not offer specific information diagnostic for aortic insufficiency.

Cardiac catheterization. Cardiac catheterization provides the most useful information regarding the amount and severity of regurgitation. After dye is ejected into the aorta, just above the aortic valve, regurgitation of blood can be visualized; aortic insufficiency is then graded from 1+ to 4+ (Exhibit 11.7). Left ventricular function, coronary artery anatomy, and the presence of other valvular abnormalities can be ascertained as well.

Medical Interventions
The most important aspect of medical management of a patient with a murmur of aortic insufficiency is careful monitoring to ensure immediate recognition of symptoms and referral for surgery. Infective endocarditis can produce a sudden deterioration of chronic aortic insufficiency, and the need for antibiotic prophylaxis must be monitored vigilantly. Aortic valve replacement is indicated when symptoms occur. Treatment, including preload and afterload reduction may be necessary until that time. In general, surgery should not be delayed. If considerable damage has already occurred, left ventricular dysfunction may persist after aortic valve replacement. In acute aortic insufficiency, large regurgitant volumes can cause rapid changes in pressure, which are

EXHIBIT 11.7
Grading of Aortic Insufficiency

1+: Slight puff of dye into LV; clears with subsequent systole
2+: Faint opacification of LV; does not clear after systole
3+: Dense opacification of LV; persists through several cycles
4+: LV opacification; more dense than aortic after one diastole

LV = left ventricle.

poorly tolerated, and acute decompensation can occur. In this instance, immediate surgical intervention may be necessary.

Nursing Interventions

The role of the nurse in managing patients with valvular disorders incorporates (1) the delivery of skilled nursing care, (2) collaboration with other members of the health care team, and (3) patient and family teaching. These functions are called upon at all stages of the disease, from chronic to acute, and in all settings, from the community to the intensive care unit. The extent of the nurse's involvement in each of these functions may depend, however, on the severity of the patient's condition. Regardless of the setting, patient and family needs can be identified only after a comprehensive nursing assessment, including the taking of a nursing history and a physical assessment.

In the CICU setting, however, a comprehensive nursing assessment may have to be deferred until a patient's condition can be stabilized. Under these circumstances, the CICU nurse must be able to assess and meet a patient's most critical needs quickly. The CICU nurse must develop an organized and consistent approach to a critically ill patient so that findings are not overlooked or obtained haphazardly. As soon as possible, a more complete assessment should be obtained. This comprehensive assessment then becomes the basis for:

1. Identifying the subjective and objective findings associated with the disorder
2. Determining the degree of severity represented by these findings
3. Evaluating patient and family needs for teaching and support
4. Establishing a baseline against which the effectiveness of medical and nursing interventions can be evaluated

The accurate assessment of a patient's needs and an ability to anticipate changes, interpret subjective and objective data, and assess the effectiveness of medical and nursing interventions are important aspects of the CICU nurse's role. The ECG must be carefully monitored for the development of rhythm and rate changes. Also, the auscultatory manifestations of valvular disorders should be monitored. If the patient's condition warrants it, pulmonary artery and capillary wedge pressures must be monitored and interpreted. Correct interpretation of the measurements obtained is essential. For example, the CICU nurse must be aware of the significance of the enlarged V wave observed in mitral insufficiency. When the heart and lungs are normal, pulmonary artery diastolic and pulmonary capillary wedge pressures reflect left atrial pressure, which in turn reflects LVEDP. The pressure between the left ventricle and the pulmonary artery equilibrates at 4 to 12 mm Hg. When MS is present, however, left atrial pressure no longer reflects LVEDP. Left atrial pressure can rise to 40 to 50 mm Hg if the stenosis is severe. Because of this gradient, an assessment of left ventricular functioning cannot be made on the basis of pulmonary artery diastolic or wedge pressures.

Other subjective and objective findings must be monitored closely as well. For example, activity tolerance is an easily observed variable. Also, if aortic insufficiency occurs as a result of infective endocarditis, for example, objective peripheral signs may develop and progress rapidly. As the health team member who usually has the most contact with a patient, the CICU nurse is in the best position to recognize these signs as they occur. Careful monitoring of the subjective and objective data associated with these disorders allows the CICU nurse to intervene when necessary and effectively communicate with the rest of the CICU team.

Teaching can take many forms, including teaching the patient and family about (1) the disease process itself, (2) the subjective and objective findings associated with it, (3) the management of symptoms, (4) the avoidance of complications, (5) medical treatment interventions, and (6) the probable future course. For example, because MS occurs gradually, patients may modify their activity patterns over time in order to reduce the symptoms of dyspnea and fatigue. The nurse must be skilled at eliciting information about the severity of the symptoms and about the impact that they have on the lifestyle and activities of the patient and family. Also, the nurse needs to determine how much the patient and family know about the disease and its treatment, and what kinds of fears or anxieties they may have about them. Finally, the patient and family must be adequately prepared for procedures, medical and surgical, when indicated.

Table 11.2 presents an example of an approach the CICU nurse could use to obtain information from a patient or family regarding MS. A similar format could be used in the case of other valvular disorders. The nursing assessment should be an effective tool for demonstrating the problems or potential problems that can result from these disorders.

Thus, the nursing management of a patient with a valvular disorder consists of (1) monitoring subjective and objective data, (2) assessing the patient and family needs resulting from the disorder, and (3) developing and implementing with the patient and family strategies aimed at meeting those needs. The short-term goals for a patient with an acute valvular disorder would likely include monitoring objective data, titrating medication and fluids based on those data, providing the patient and family with emotional support, and preparing them for surgery. For the less acutely ill patient, goals may include assisting the patient and family in (1) learning more about the disorder and its impact on them, (2) modifying activity patterns to maximize functioning, minimize fatigue, and avoid symptoms, and (3) understanding the necessity for antibiotic prophylaxis.

VENTRICULAR SEPTAL RUPTURE

Pathophysiology

When the ventricular septum ruptures, two left ventricular outflow tracts are created, and the right ventricle competes with the aorta for left ventricular stroke volume. With each ventricular contraction, blood is shunted from the left ventricle to the right ventricle, and, depending on the size of the defect, a considerable decrease in cardiac output can result. The amount shunted to the right ventricle can be two, three, or even four times the amount ejected into the aorta. The right ventricle suffers immediate volume and pressure overload, which is generally poorly tolerated.

TABLE 11.2
Approach to a Patient with Mitral Stenosis

Problem	Goal	Assessment	Intervention
Dyspnea Fatigue	Develop activity patterns that accomplish patient goals and manage symptoms	Determine amount of physical limitation When do you feel SOB or fatigue? How long have you had the problem? Has it changed? How? Do you enjoy physical activity? Why? Why not? What do you do to ease SOB or fatigue? Determine normal patterns of lifestyle Tell me about your morning routine. Do you do your own housework? What is your typical day at work like? Do you take medications? When?	Short term Plan care with patient to allow him or her as much control as possible Schedule activities to prevent exertion Promote periods of rest and sleep Monitor patient's need for assistance, and provide it when necessary Long term With patient and family, begin to plan alterations in daily patterns aimed at alleviating symptoms Plan the coordination of medications and activity when possible
Lack of knowledge about disease	Increase patient and family knowledge about disease, complications, and treatments	Determine level of knowledge about MS Do you know what MS is? Can you tell me what you think it is? Do you know what causes it? What complications can occur? Do you know what the treatment is?	Provide as much information as patient and family can understand Explain treatment and procedures Do pre-op teaching if indicated
Potential for fear and anxiety	Decrease fear and anxiety about disease and its implications	Assess fears about illness, death, and surgery Do you generally talk about fears you may have? Are you a little afraid of having surgery? Most patients are. Do you think it will change your life? We generally tell patients about everything we are going to be doing. Does that make you feel more or less comfortable?	Provide support and information aimed at decreasing anxiety Begin more extensive patient and family teaching about disease and complications Discuss need for antibiotic prophylaxis Begin to prepare patient and family for surgery

MS = mitral stenosis, SOB = shortness of breath.

Causation and Progression
With the exception of congenitally occurring defects, ventricular septal rupture (VSR) occurs as a result of an acute anterior or inferior myocardial infarction. Rather than being one discrete hole, the defect is more characteristically described as "swiss cheese." VSR can occur within the first 24 hours of a myocardial infarction but can appear as late as ten days to two weeks afterward. The severity of the condition is related to the size of the defect and the amount of shunting from the high-pressure left ventricle to the low-pressure right ventricle.

Subjective Findings
The symptoms observed with VSR range from mild right-sided failure, pulmonary congestion, and fatigue to severe dyspnea, chest pain, and syncope. The degree of symptoms is based on the amount of left-to-right shunt and the extent of the decrease in cardiac output.

Objective Findings
The auscultatory hallmark of VSR is a loud, high-pitched holosystolic murmur heard best with the diaphragm at the lower left sternal border. The murmur occurs as blood flows through the defect to the right ventricle during systole. An S3 occurs commonly as well. If the amount of shunting is considerable, signs of cardiogenic shock may be evident.

Radiological.   The chest roentgenogram may demonstrate cardiomegaly and the pulmonary changes associated with congestive heart failure.

Electrocardiographic.   The ECG will show evidence of a recent anterior or inferior myocardial infarction. Atrioventricular conduction disturbances and bundle branch block patterns may be present.

Echocardiographic.   Contrast echocardiography may be useful in determining blood flow patterns and the presence of a shunt.

Pulmonary artery catheter.   In combination with the clinical picture and the presence of appropriate physical findings, the diagnosis of VSR can be made from information obtained during the insertion of a pulmonary artery catheter. As the catheter is passed through the right atrium and ventricle, O_2 saturation levels in the blood from each chamber are measured. The presence of a step-up, or an abnormal rise, in O_2 saturation from the right atrium to the right ventricle is diagnostic of VSR. If the tricuspid valve is competent, the only way for the O_2 saturation of blood in the right ventricle to be higher than that in the right atrium is via a communication with the left ventricle (Table 11.3). The placement of a pulmonary artery catheter can be accomplished easily at the bedside.

Cardiac catheterization.   This procedure is still necessary to assess the degree of shunting and to determine the location of the defect. Overall cardiac hemo-

TABLE 11.3
Oxygen Saturation Step-Up with Ventricular Septal Defect

Structure	O₂ Saturation Level (%)	
	With Ventricular Septal Defect	Normal
Superior vena cava	69	70–75
Right atrium	71	70–75
Right ventricle	89	70–75
Pulmonary artery	85	70–75
Femoral artery	95	98

dynamics can be assessed, and because VSR occurs as a complication of an acute myocardial infarction, coronary artery anatomy can be examined as well.

Medical Interventions

The treatment for VSR is surgical repair. Ideally, surgery is delayed for as long as the patient's condition permits so that some healing and fibrosis will have occurred at the site of the rupture. This time allows the area to stabilize so that a patch can be securely sutured over the area of perforation. Thus, the aim of medical management is to maintain the patient until surgical intervention can be performed.

The use of both arterial and venous vasodilators may be necessary. Isosorbide dinitrate or intravenously administered nitroglycerin for preload reduction, and sodium nitroprusside for afterload reduction, are both useful. Afterload reduction is the key to successful medical management. With a decrease in systemic vascular resistance, ejection of blood to the systemic circulation is enhanced, reducing the amount of shunting to the right ventricle. Intra-aortic balloon pumping can be effective if adequate afterload reduction cannot be achieved pharmacologically. Considerable hemodynamic and clinical stabilization can occur, allowing time for healing to begin at the site of rupture.

Nursing Interventions

The patient with VSR may present in cardiogenic shock and will therefore require maximum medical and nursing management. Accurate assessment of patient needs, continual monitoring of subjective and objective findings, and the interpretation and evaluation of treatment interventions are important aspects of the CICU nurse's role.

Continuous intra-arterial and pulmonary artery pressure monitoring and the careful titration of a combination of preload- and afterload-reducing agents will be required to stabilize the condition of a critically ill patient. In addition, the CICU nurse must be prepared for and assist in the placement of a pulmonary artery catheter. It should be remembered that thermodilution cardiac output determinations are unreliable in the presence of VSR. This technique measures right ventricular cardiac output, which, under normal circumstances, is the same as left ventricular cardiac output. Left-to-right shunting with VSR, however, falsely elevates the thermodilution cardiac output and renders such determinations useless in assessing left ventricular output.

When more traditional treatment modalities are inadequate, an intra-aortic balloon may further reduce afterload and improve cardiac output. This technique will be discussed in greater detail in Chapter 13. Balloon timing must be readjusted and evaluated frequently to ensure maximal hemodynamic benefit from this mode of therapy. The monitoring of pedal pulses to assess distal blood flow and the monitoring of coagulation status to prevent the destruction of platelets, as well as the careful positioning of the patient, become important nursing considerations.

In addition to the considerable physical support needed by these patients, emotional support for the patient and family is a part of nursing management. A long CICU stay can be accompanied by problems of sensory deprivation, sleep disturbance, and anxiety. Careful management of these problems, with the patient allowed as much control over his or her care as possible, is an important nursing goal.

Virtually all these patients eventually require cardiac surgery. Physical and emotional preparation is important in the preoperative phase. Nursing management is aimed at meeting the learning needs of the patient and family regarding surgery and providing them with as much information as they can absorb at the time so that postoperative management will be simplified.

DISEASES OF THE MYOCARDIUM

Cardiomyopathy is an abnormality of the heart muscle itself, characterized by the presence of congestive heart failure, cardiomegaly, and dysrhythmias in the absence of other conditions such as valvular disease, hypertension, ischemic heart disease, and congenital and pulmonary abnormalities [12]. Cardiomyopathies are classified as congestive, restrictive, or hypertrophic, depending on physiological findings. They can occur acutely or chronically. The cause is often difficult to determine, and progression is variable. The CICU patient with cardiomyopathy may have an acute or end-stage disease or may have cardiomyopathy complicating other cardiac problems.

Congestive Cardiomyopathy

Pathophysiology

The problems encountered in congestive cardiomyopathy are those of cardiac failures. Characteristically, the heart is dilated. Both ventricles are involved, and although the valves themselves are normal, functional valvular abnormalities can occur if left ventricular distortion resulting from dilatation interferes with their functioning. As the left ventricle fails, cardiac output drops, producing an increase in afterload and thereby further impairing left ventricular functioning. The increase in LVEDP produces changes in pulmonary venous, pulmonary arterial, and right ventricular pressures. The result is severe cardiac dysfunction and biventricular failure.

Subjective Findings
Symptoms vary in intensity and generally include dyspnea, orthopnea, fatigue, and other symptoms of congestive heart failure.

Objective Findings
Right-sided failure is evidenced by an elevated jugular venous pressure. Hepatomegaly and peripheral edema may be present as well. On palpation the apex may be found to be hypodynamic and displaced laterally. On auscultation an S3 is usually heard and an S4 may be audible as well. If ventricular distortion has produced functional valvular disorders, murmurs of mitral or tricuspid insufficiency may be heard. If heart failure produces a marked drop in cardiac output, systemic vascular resistance may rise, further impairing left ventricular functioning.

Radiological.   Cardiomegaly, pulmonary congestion, and edema may be evident on the chest roentgenogram.

Electrocardiographic.   The ECG is invariably abnormal, with changes reflecting left ventricular hypertrophy and, less commonly, left atrial enlargement. Forms of atrioventricular and bundle branch block patterns may appear because of distortion and fibrosis of the structures of the conduction system. Nonspecific ST and T wave changes may occur because of altered depolarization, and dysrhythmias may appear at any time.

Echocardiographic.   Although echocardiography is not diagnostic for congestive cardiomyopathy, it may demonstrate increased left ventricular volumes, decreased wall motion, and changes in septal mobility.

Cardiac catheterization.   This procedure provides information about left ventricular function and helps rule out coronary artery disease as a cause of heart failure. An evaluation of mitral valve functioning can be made as well. In conjunction with cardiac catheterization, a right ventricular endomyocardial biopsy may provide confirmation of the diagnosis of congestive cardiomyopathy.

Medical Interventions
The management of congestive cardiomyopathy is dictated by symptoms. Patients may require bed rest or restricted activity for a prolonged period, while the conventional treatment for congestive heart failure is employed. Anticoagulants may be necessary if the patient is confined strictly to bed or has marked lower extremity edema, or if pulmonary or systemic embolization occurs. Because of its myocardial depressant action, alcohol ingestion is forbidden. Vasodilators are added as the condition progresses. As cardiac failure worsens, the patient will require more sophisticated management. The CICU provides the setting in which invasive hemodynamic monitoring and complicated pharmacological management are possible. Cardiomyopathy is among the most common diagnoses for referral for cardiac transplantation.

Restrictive Cardiomyopathy

Pathophysiology

Restrictive is the least common type of cardiomyopathy; it occurs when there is a marked reduction in left ventricular cavity size. Such reduction can occur when necrosis and fibrosis of myocardial tissue produces severe left ventricular hypertrophy, or when an overgrowth of fibrous tissue actually extends into the ventricular cavity, obliterating it. The restriction to ventricular diastolic filling stems from within the ventricles. The myocardium becomes thickened, rigid, and noncompliant. Pulmonary hypertension often occurs as well. The cause of restrictive cardiomyopathy is usually unknown but can often be related to prolonged eosinophilia and amyloidosis, which cause fibrotic changes in endocardial and myocardial tissue.

Findings

The clinical findings associated with restrictive cardiomyopathy progress to the signs and symptoms of congestive heart failure. On chest roentgenogram an enlarged cardiac silhouette and evidence of pulmonary congestion may be evident. The ECG is not specific for restrictive cardiomyopathy but may demonstrate low voltage and changes in the shape of the P wave when atrial enlargement is present. Cardiac catheterization provides information about cardiac hemodynamics and helps differentiate restrictive cardiomyopathy from constrictive pericarditis. Right ventricular endomyocardial biopsy may demonstrate the presence of abnormal endomyocardial tissue.

Hypertrophic Cardiomyopathy

Pathophysiology

Hypertrophic cardiomyopathy (HCM) is characterized by a hypertrophied, but not dilated, left ventricle. The septum is usually hypertrophied disproportionately to the other ventricular walls, and septal or mitral valve leaflet movement may cause a physical muscular obstruction to left ventricular outflow. This condition was formerly called idiopathic hypertrophic subaortic stenosis. A nonobstructive form of HCM has been clearly identified, however, and is actually more common. Therefore, the designation of HCM is more appropriate.

Systolic and diastolic hemodynamic abnormalities are observed in HCM. The left ventricle is hyperdynamic and has a high ejection fraction. In some instances the cavity is obliterated during systole. Left ventricular hypertrophy decreases compliance and results in an increased LVEDP. LVEDP causes an increase in left atrial pressure, as the left atrium works to fill the ventricle adequately.

Causation and Progression

The cause of HCM is generally unknown, but the condition appears to be transmitted genetically. Symptoms are usually present in early adulthood, but the progression of the disorder varies considerably depending on the degree of hypertrophy and the status of left ventricular functioning. Frequently, males with the disorder have particularly muscular, athletic builds.

Subjective Findings

Patients with HCM show a wide range of symptoms. An increased left ventricular filling pressure can cause pulmonary venous hypertension and dyspnea. Exertional dyspnea is the most common symptom associated with HCM. Other symptoms include fatigue, angina, dizziness, syncope, and even sudden death. Prognosis is grim when syncope and dyspnea occur at rest.

Objective Findings

On palpation the apical impulse is found to be hyperdynamic and displaced laterally. Also, if left atrial hypertrophy has developed, a presystolic left atrial contraction can be felt. Carotid pulses are bounding, because of rapid left ventricular ejection. They may have a bifid quality, which is caused by the slowing of ventricular ejection late in systole. In contrast, the carotid pulse in aortic stenosis is sustained, without a bifid quality.

Auscultation reveals a midsystolic ejection murmur best heard at the lower left sternal border and apex. Its location also helps differentiate it from the murmur of aortic stenosis. Maneuvers such as the Valsalva maneuver and the administration of nitroglycerin and amyl nitrite tend to increase the outflow obstruction and decrease the murmur. Maneuvers that decrease outflow obstruction such as hand gripping and squatting, and such agents as phenylephrine increase the murmur. An S3 and an S4 are commonly audible. A murmur of mitral insufficiency may be heard if forceful left ventricular contraction causes some regurgitation into the left atrium.

Radiological.   Left ventricular hypertrophy is evident, but it is not specific for HCM and its severity correlates poorly with the degree of disability.

Electrocardiographic.   The ECG reflects left ventricular hypertrophy. Another characteristic finding is the presence of deep Q waves in leads II, III, aV_F, and V_4 through V_6. These represent the slowed spread of depolarization through the thickened septum. In addition, ECG findings characteristic of Wolff-Parkinson-White syndrome may be observed.

Echocardiographic.   Echocardiography is the most useful diagnostic procedure and can confirm the diagnosis of HCM. This technique readily demonstrates increased wall thickness and septal hypertrophy. Also, septal motion and abnormal systolic anterior movement of the anterior mitral valve leaflet can be observed. Echocardiography can be used to follow a patient's progress and to screen other members of his or her family for the disorder.

Cardiac catheterization.   Catheterization is no longer necessary to establish the diagnosis of HCM. It is helpful, however in assessing the level of obstruction, left ventricular hemodynamics, and coronary artery anatomy, especially if surgical treatment is being contemplated.

Medical Interventions

Prompt recognition of symptoms and proper diagnosis of the disorder are essential for successful management of HCM. Prophylactic measures include the avoidance of strenuous exercise, and antibiotic prophylaxis to prevent the development of infective endocarditis.

Beta blockade is usually instituted and increases ventricular compliance. By blocking sympathetic input to the left ventricle and therefore decreasing the strength of contraction, left ventricular outflow obstruction is decreased. Verapamil has been used effectively also, and it may prove to be more desirable because it does not produce fatigue [17, 26].

Angina associated with HCM does not usually result from coronary artery disease. The coronary arteries are usually normal, but during exercise the O_2 requirement of the left ventricle is so great that the supply is inadequate and chest pain results. Angina is often atypical and does not respond to nitroglycerin. Propranolol can also aid in preventing chest pain by decreasing heart rate and, therefore, O_2 demand.

Aggressive management of atrial fibrillation is essential. With the development of atrial fibrillation, there is a loss of the "atrial kick" and a decrease in diastolic filling time. In the noncompliant left ventricle, left atrial contraction substantially augments left ventricular diastolic filling, and a loss of this "atrial kick" can be catastrophic, causing acute deterioration. If left ventricular outflow is obstructed, digitalis administration should be avoided; it can exacerbate the problem by increasing contractility and, therefore, the obstruction. Quinidine or propranolol, or both, may be more useful.

The surgical management of HCM involves the resection of a portion of the hypertrophied septum, although surgical treatment is not indicated for the nonobstructive form of the disorder. This intervention provides symptomatic relief in most patients [5]. The major complications include VSR, interference with mitral valve functioning, and conduction disturbances. Surgery has been proposed for the asymptomatic patient with high outflow pressures in an effort to prevent sudden death. For much the same reason, aortic valve replacement is usually recommended for asymptomatic patients with high transvalvular gradients. Clinical investigation of the efficacy of surgery in asymptomatic patients continues [5].

Nursing Interventions

Nursing management of a patient with a cardiomyopathy will depend on the severity of the patient's condition and the prognosis. While the patient is hospitalized, the nurse must carefully monitor the signs and symptoms associated with the disease. In the CICU setting this management can become very difficult, because pharmacological therapy is frequently altered and titrated based on the moment-to-moment changes in the patient's condition. At the same time, the nurse can assess the patient and family needs for support upon discharge and can begin to contact referral agencies when indicated. Often, the principal nursing goal is to assist the patient and family to cope with the significant impact this disease can have on their lifestyle. The social and financial assistance required by a family may be considerable. Anxiety related to these matters can be markedly reduced if careful and complete discharge plans are formulated and implemented. These patients may ultimately be referred for cardiac transplantation, depending on their age and overall health status.

**Infective
Endocarditis**

Pathophysiology

Endocarditis occurs when there is a direct infection of the endocardium or of a natural or prosthetic heart valve. Because the organisms responsible for endocarditis include not only bacteria, but also viruses, fungi, and rickettsiae, the previous classification of the disease as "bacterial" endocarditis has been replaced with the more accurate designation of "infective" endocarditis. In addition, the terms *acute* and *subacute* endocarditis have become less useful. They refer to the expected course of the disease and the clinical presentation [1].

The endothelial lining of a valve leaflet, one of the heart chambers, or the lining of a blood vessel becomes damaged by the development of vegetations. These consist of irregular masses of platelets and fibrin to which infecting organisms become attached [12]. The organism proliferates and is difficult or impossible for the host to eliminate. Vegetations are most commonly found on the low-pressure or atrial and ventricular surfaces in the presence of mitral and aortic insufficiency, respectively, and on the ventricular and aortic surfaces in mitral or aortic stenosis [1, 29]. Damage to the involved valve can be extensive, and severe insufficiency can result. Although both right-side and left-side heart valves can be affected, the condition is more common on the left, and the mitral valve is more frequently affected than the aortic valve [1].

Causation and Progression

The development of infective endocarditis is generally associated with congenital or acquired heart disease, such as bicuspid valves, VSR, or rheumatic heart disease. In each case the abnormal valve surface attracts platelets and fibrin, and vegetations develop. Subsequent bacteremias deposit organisms, which become imbedded in the vegetations and produce the subjective and objective findings associated with infective endocarditis. Other causes include cardiac surgery (especially prosthetic valve surgery), parenteral drug administration and abuse, and the placement of intravascular foreign bodies, such as pacemakers and intravenous lines. Infective endocarditis following prosthetic valve surgery takes two forms. Early endocarditis occurs within two months of surgery; late endocarditis is that occurring after that time. Other differences between the two forms include usual infecting organism and the mortality. *Staphylococcus aureus* is the organism most commonly associated with early endocarditis; *Streptococcus* is associated with late endocarditis. The mortality of early endocarditis is approximately 80%, whereas that of late endocarditis is somewhat lower, 25% to 40% [19].

Bacteria normally enter the bloodstream from many sources. An asymptomatic bacteremia commonly occurs after tonsillectomy, dental surgery, and even tooth brushing. Bacteremias may also follow simple procedures of the gastrointestinal and genitourinary tracts. In addition, bacteria can be introduced at the time of cardiac surgery, with the placement of foreign bodies such as pacemakers and heart valves, and via intravenous catheters and drugs. Under normal circumstances the body overcomes the bacteremia. When a vegetation becomes infected, however, its avascular nature prevents the body's normal defenses from reaching the organism, and the organism proliferates.

Bacteria then enter the circulation as the blood comes in contact with the infected vegetation.

The progression and prognosis of infective endocarditis depend on the speed of isolation and the success of treatment of the involved organism, the presence or absence of embolic complications, and the amount of valvular injury that has occurred.

Subjective Findings

The most common symptom associated with infective endocarditis is fever. Depending on the organism involved, the fever can be either insidious or dramatic and accompanied by rigor and sweating. *Staphylococcus* is associated with a more dramatic infectious process. *Streptococcus* usually produces a more moderate response. Other possible subjective findings include joint pain, abdominal pain caused by splenomegaly, fatigue, anorexia, and weight loss [1, 6, 12].

Objective Findings

Cardiac involvement depends on the location of the lesion and the amount of valvular dysfunction. The development of a new murmur of mitral or aortic insufficiency, or a change in an existing one, is a reliable sign. Cardiac dysfunction can range from minimal to severe, if chordae tendineae rupture or cusp perforation occurs. Other findings associated with infective endocarditis include anemia, petechiae, clubbing of the fingers and toes, Janeway lesions, Osler's nodes, and Roth's spots [1, 6, 12]. Janeway lesions are small, erythematous, partially hemorrhagic, painless lesions that may develop on the fingers, toes, earlobes, and the tip of the nose. They may be caused by small emboli that occlude terminal arteries, producing small areas of gangrene [12]. Osler's nodes commonly occur in the pads of the fingers and are red, papular, painful, subcutaneous nodules [12]. Roth's spots are retinal hemorrhages with pale centers, seen in the optic fundus [1]. Embolic complications may occur as well. Neurological changes may occur if emboli travel to the brain. Emboli that move to the kidneys, spleen and intestines, and peripheral extremities can cause hematuria, abdominal pain, and peripheral vascular insufficiency, respectively.

Echocardiography may demonstrate valvular vegetations. It may also be useful in monitoring a change in vegetation size and the effectiveness of antibiotic treatment.

The most definitive finding in infectious endocarditis is the identification of the causative organism in the blood. Aseptic methods to obtain bacterial, fungal, or rickettsial cultures and titers must be used. Strict adherence to sterile technique is necessary to prevent contamination of the specimen at the time of venipuncture. Several cultures from various sites should be obtained. Blood should never be obtained from an indwelling catheter, and the specimens should be placed in appropriate media immediately. Other laboratory findings include an elevated eosinophil sedimentation rate, an elevated white blood count, and anemia.

Medical Interventions

The aim of specific antibiotic therapy is to eliminate the organism from the blood and to sterilize the vegetations. These goals necessitate long-term parenteral administration of antibiotics. The achievement of bacteriocidal levels in the blood is necessary to ensure sterilization of the vegetations, and these levels should be checked regularly throughout the course of therapy. When antibiotic therapy is stopped, specimens for blood cultures should be drawn and the temperature monitored carefully for any sign of reinfection. The remainder of medical treatment involves the concurrent management of complications and the prevention of further bacteremias.

The correct role of surgery in the treatment of the patient with infective endocarditis is still disputed [1, 12]. Surgical valve replacement is generally considered, however, in several instances: (1) for severe fungal infections, (2) when valvular dysfunction is severe, (3) if infection persists despite ostensibly adequate therapy, (4) when repeated systemic embolization occurs, and (5) if relapse occurs.

Long-term treatment goals include educating the patient and family regarding antibiotic prophylaxis and preventative measures, and screening other family members for the presence of predisposing factors, such as a congenitally occurring bicuspid valve.

Nursing Interventions

The patient with infective endocarditis presents the nurse with several challenges. First, the lengthy course of therapy necessitates a long hospitalization, frequently six to eight weeks. Related potential problems include depression, anxiety, boredom, and social and financial difficulties. Primary nursing provides the continuity that allows the nurse to coordinate the patient's care, identify problems as they arise, and develop strategies to meet them.

Second, successful antibiotic treatment requires careful management of intravenous administration sites. Careful monitoring of catheter sites for patient comfort and the development of localized infections, such as phlebitis, are important aspects of the nurse's role. Current recommendations are that parenteral intravenous sites be changed every 48 hours [14]. For the patient with infective endocarditis, this in itself presents a source of discomfort. Sites should be inspected daily for signs of local infection, and sites should be rotated to preserve tissue and muscle integrity and to ensure their potential for reuse later in the course of treatment.

The potential development of antibiotic drug toxicity or hospital-acquired infections is a third nursing concern. The nurse must be aware of the possible side effects associated with the prescribed antibiotic therapy and must carefully assess the patient for the appearance of these effects.

Fourth, the patient must be closely monitored for the development of valvular dysfunction. If complications of mitral or aortic insufficiency occur, the patient may require transfer to the CICU for closer observation. The patient's condition can deteriorate rapidly, necessitating surgical valve replacement. The nurse must be able to (1) identify and monitor the subjective and objective findings associated with the valvular disorder, (2) interpret information from sophisticated invasive monitoring devices, (3) assist the patient and family in coping with the increased anxiety and fear they may experience, and (4) begin preoperative teaching when surgery is imminent.

Teaching is a fifth primary nursing function. After the nurse has made an assessment of the needs of the patient and family regarding knowledge of the disease and its implications, the nurse should develop a teaching plan, with the goal of providing enough information to prevent reinfection in the future. The need for antibiotic prophylaxis for some dental, gastrointestinal, and genitourinary procedures must be stressed. Careful observation of otherwise simple cuts, bruises, and infections is also important. In addition, appropriate referrals for medical and nursing follow-up in the community can be arranged. In sum, the patient and family must be made aware of the potentially severe problems that can arise when signs and symptoms are not properly treated.

PERICARDITIS

Pericarditis is a general term that refers to an inflammation of the pericardium. Pericarditis can be classified in several ways, including early (acute) or late (Dressler's syndrome), and with or without effusion and constriction. Regardless of the cause, upon injury, pericardial cells are altered and an inflammatory process ensues. Numerous causes of pericarditis have been identified, and the clinical manifestations, progression, and prognosis of the condition are related to the cause. Pericarditis may be the primary problem or may develop as a complication of another process. Exhibit 11.8 lists the current, commonly recognized causes of pericarditis [13, 20, 27, 28].

Constrictive Pericarditis

This form of pericarditis is relatively rare and is characterized by calcified, fibrous tissue in the pericardium, which severely restricts the systolic and diastolic movement of the heart. The decline in incidence of constrictive pericarditis is related to the decline in its principal cause — tuberculosis. The clinical manifestations of constrictive pericarditis are dyspnea, hepatomegaly, pleuritic pain, cough, jugular venous distention, and low ECG voltage. On auscultation a pericardial "knock" can be appreciated. This loud, characteristic sound occurs between S2 and S3 and represents the sudden cessation of rapid ventric-

EXHIBIT 11.8
Common Causes of Pericarditis

Infections: viral, bacterial, fungal, and parasitic

Connective tissue disorders: lupus, polyarteritis nodosa, rheumatoid arthritis, rheumatic fever, drugs

Myocardial infarction: early and late

Cardiotomy

Trauma: penetrating and nonpenetrating wounds, ruptured aortic aneurysm, or other causes of hemorrhage into pericardium

Uremia

Neoplasm

Radiation exposure

ular filling that occurs when the heart reaches the limits of its mobility [10]. Classic constrictive pericarditis usually develops gradually, as do the clinical findings.

The diagnosis of constrictive pericarditis is difficult to establish, because ECG, radiological, echocardiographic, and cardiac catheterization findings cannot be specifically related to the condition. The diagnosis can sometimes be made, however, as such other causes as congestive heart failure, cirrhosis of the liver, and superior vena caval obstruction are ruled out. Because involvement of the myocardium is almost inevitable, a distinction between constrictive pericarditis and restrictive cardiomyopathy is extremely difficult to make. The former diagnosis is more likely when there is a low pulmonary artery pressure, equalization of diastolic pressure throughout the heart, and a high right ventricular diastolic pressure [27].

The treatment of constrictive pericarditis is surgical resection of the fibrosed pericardium. Pericardectomy is usually lengthy and technically difficult and is associated with a 5% to 10% mortality [3]. The procedure becomes necessary, however, when cardiac movement is severely restricted.

Acute Pericarditis without Effusion

Unlike constrictive pericarditis, acute pericarditis is not a slow, progressive disorder but, rather, one that develops as a result of an infectious process, a myocardial infarction or cardiac surgery, trauma, malignancy, or other primary processes such as uremia and lupus erythematosis. Early pericarditis usually refers to the form that occurs as an early complication of a myocardial infarction. Subjective and objective findings usually appear within two to three days following infarct. In late pericarditis, or Dressler's syndrome, subjective and objective findings do not occur until three to six weeks after a myocardial infarction and persist for a longer time. In the latter case the cause is not irritation but, rather, an autoimmune response [27]. Late pericarditis can also occur after cardiac surgery, presumably for the same reason.

Subjective Findings
The most characteristic finding is persistent substernal chest pain, varying in intensity from a dull ache to severe pain, the latter mimicking a myocardial infarction. The pain is usually exacerbated by coughing and inspiration and is often alleviated by leaning forward. The patient may also be febrile, but depending on the cause, the fever may have preceded the pericarditis.

Objective Findings
The most characteristic finding associated with pericarditis is a scratchy pericardial friction rub. This sound may be persistent or intermittent, however, and may be present for several hours to several days. The key to its distinction from a pleuritic rub is its presence when respiration is held.

Radiological.   Roentgenographic findings are not specific in pericarditis and may simply reflect changes related to the underlying disease process.

Electrocardiographic.   The ECG undergoes characteristic changes. Initially, ST and T wave elevations are noted in all leads but aV_R and V_1. Over the course of a few days to several weeks, the T waves return to baseline and become inverted. Eventually, T waves return to normal. When this process occurs rapidly, the combination of ECG changes and the patient's symptoms calls for careful observation of serum creatinine phosphokinase levels to rule out a myocardial infarction. The ECG does not evolve to develop Q waves, but in the initial stages of presentation, differentiation from an acute myocardial infarction may be difficult.

Echocardiographic. Echocardiography is not particularly useful in establishing the diagnosis of pericarditis. Once the pericardium has healed, there may be evidence of a thickened pericardium. Echocardiography is much more useful when an effusion is present (see the discussion of pericarditis with effusion that follows).

Medical Interventions

The treatment of any pericarditis depends on the severity of symptoms and the degree of cardiac involvement. The identification and treatment of the underlying process or disorder may alleviate the condition. In general, combinations of salicylates, analgesics, indomethacin, and corticosteroids will successfully manage the symptoms reported in pericarditis.

Pericarditis with Effusion

This condition develops when the inflammatory process is accompanied by an accumulation of fluid or exudate in the pericardial sac. This sac normally contains from 10 to 30 ml of straw-colored fluid that lubricates the space between the layers of pericardium and allows for movement of the heart during systole and diastole.

The characteristic friction rub will be present but, perhaps, muffled, and the patient will experience chest pain. The ECG may demonstrate low voltage in addition to other changes, depending on the size and location of the effusion. If the effusion is great, the patient may also experience dyspnea and orthopnea. The roentgenogram may reveal an enlarged cardiac silhouette, but the distinction between cardiomegaly and an effusion may be difficult to make. Currently, echocardiography is extremely useful; it can confirm both the presence and the location of an effusion and can be used to direct catheter placement when pericardiocentesis is required.

The severity of the condition is related less to the amount of effusion than to the rate of accumulation of the fluid. The pericardium resists rapid stretching but can be stretched gradually to accommodate volumes as great as 2 to 3 L. Pericardiocentesis should be done to evacuate an effusion; the procedure may produce temporary or permanent relief. Analysis of specimens from the pericardium can provide therapeutic information regarding infectious agents and malignancies.

Cardiac Tamponade

As the accumulation of fluid in the pericardium increases, pressure increases as well, compromising diastolic filling and eventually affecting left ventricular stroke volume. Initially, cardiac output and blood pressure are maintained by the development of a tachycardia and an increase in systemic vascular resistance. Cardiac tamponade occurs when these compensatory mechanisms fail, causing an acute, rapid deterioration in cardiac output and necessitating immediate emergency treatment. The patient may show signs and symptoms of cardiogenic shock. An enlarged cardiac silhouette, a narrowed pulse pressure, and pulsus paradoxus (a decline in systolic blood pressure of 10 mm Hg or more on inspiration) are usually present. On inspiration, a lowered intrathoracic pressure allows increased right ventricular stretch and contraction. Relaxation of the pulmonary vasculature on inspiration, however, decreases blood flow to the left side of the heart, thus decreasing left ventricular filling and cardiac output. Also, the septum may bulge slightly into the left ventricle, further compromising left ventricular filling [27]. Monitoring of chamber pressures demonstrates an equalization or narrowing of LVEDP, wedge, and right ventricular pressures. Emergency support of blood pressure with volume, inotropic agents, and catecholamines will be necessary while the patient is being prepared for pericardial tap or operation.

The decision to perform a tap or surgery may depend on the facilities available and the experience of the physicians involved [3]. A pericardial tap can be performed quickly but requires a skilled cardiologist and echocardiographic and cardiac catheterization facilities. If surgery is selected as the appropriate treatment, symptomatic relief can usually be achieved with the evacuation of small amounts of fluid, thus stabilizing the patient's condition until surgery can be performed. The major complication of a tap is inadvertent puncture of the heart. Resection of a portion of the pericardium, a "pericardial window," allows fluid to drain freely into the pleural space and may be necessary if repeated pericardiocentesis is required.

Nursing Interventions

Although the prognosis for most cases of pericarditis is excellent, the discomfort the condition can produce should not be minimized. Especially for the patient who is recovering from a myocardial infarction, the reoccurrence of chest pain can be frightening and anxiety producing. The CICU nurse should carefully investigate any complaints of pain. The character of the pain and its relationship to movement, along with the presence of a rub, will help differentiate pericarditis from angina and possible reinfarction. Also, once pericarditis has been identified, appropriate analgesic and anti-inflammatory treatment can be initiated. Pericarditis occurs as a complication in about 15% of patients who have a myocardial infarction, so the CICU nurse must be aware of the associated clinical findings [20, 27]. In addition to maximizing comfort and providing emotional support, the CICU nurse must carefully observe the patient for the development of complications such as tamponade by continually monitoring chamber pressures (via a pulmonary artery catheter), blood pressure, and cardiac output. As the CICU team member who spends the most time with the patient, the nurse is in the best position to recognize early signs of catastrophic events, thus preventing or minimizing the risk to the patient.

SUMMARY _____

> The CICU nurse must be equipped with the knowledge required to provide patients and their families with skilled nursing care, with the aim of restoring a maximum level of health, and to collaborate effectively with other health care professionals.

STUDY QUESTIONS _____

1. What is the normal cross-sectional area of the mitral valve in an adult?

2. Critical mitral stenosis is defined as a valve area _____ .

3. What are the subjective findings most commonly associated with mitral stenosis?

4. Name the three auscultatory hallmarks associated with mitral stenosis.

5. When mitral stenosis is present, left atrial pressure is _____ (equal to, greater than, lower than) LVEDP?

6. The intermittent appearance of a V wave on a pulmonary capillary wedge pressure tracing usually suggests the presence of:
   a. long-standing mitral regurgitation
   b. papillary muscle rupture
   c. papillary muscle dysfunction

7. What is the normal cross-sectional area of the aortic valve in an adult?

8. Critical aortic stenosis is defined as a valve area _____ .

9. Name the three most common subjective findings associated with aortic stenosis.

10. In aortic stenosis, the contribution of left atrial contraction to left ventricular stroke volume approaches:
    a. 30%
    b. 40%
    c. 50%

11. Echocardiography is most useful in diagnosing which valvular disorder?

12. Match the primary hemodynamic alteration with its disorder.
    a. Mitral stenosis   _____ Left ventricular hypertrophy
    b. Mitral insufficiency   _____ Left atrial hypertrophy
    c. Aortic stenosis   _____ Left ventricular dilatation
    d. Aortic insufficiency   _____ Left atrial dilatation

13. The use of the intra-aortic balloon is contraindicated in which valvular abnormality?
    a. Mitral stenosis
    b. Mitral insufficiency
    c. Aortic stenosis
    d. Aortic insufficiency
    e. None of the above

14. How can the insertion of a pulmonary artery catheter assist in diagnosing the presence of VSR?

15. The key to successful medical management of VSR is:
    a. maintenance of normal sinus rhythm
    b. preload reduction
    c. afterload reduction
    d. control of angina

16. Name the classifications of cardiomyopathies.

17. Which cardiomyopathy is least common?

18. Which cardiomyopathy appears to be transmitted genetically?

19. Which valve is most frequently infected in infective endocarditis?

20. Infective endocarditis occurring after prosthetic valve surgery usually takes two forms, early and late. To which form does each of the following statements relate?
    a. It occurs within two months of surgery.
    b. It occurs two months or more after surgery.
    c. Mortality is 25% to 40%.
    d. Mortality is 80%.
    e. *Streptococcus* is the most common causative organism.
    f. *Staphylococcus* is the most common causative organism.

21. Match the name of the finding with its manifestation.
    a. Roth's spots   _____ Painful, papular,
    b. Janeway lesions   subcutaneous nodules in
    c. Osler's nodes   pads of fingers
                             _____ Retinal hemorrhages
                             _____ Painless, erythematous,
                                   partially hemorrhagic
                                   lesions on fingers, toes,
                                   earlobes, and nose

22. What is the most common subjective finding associated with pericarditis?

23. What is the most characteristic objective finding associated with pericarditis?

24. When pericarditis with effusion occurs, the severity of a patient's condition can be related to:
    a. the amount of the accumulation
    b. the rate of the accumulation

25. True or False: The causes of early and later pericarditis are presumably the same.

REFERENCES

1. Barry, J., and Gump, D. Endocarditis: an overview. *Heart Lung* 11:138, 1982.

2. Baumgartner, W. A., et al. Cardiac homotransplantation. *Curr. Probl. Surg.* 16:1, 1979.

3. Bonchek, L., and Brooks, H. *Office Management of Medical and Surgical Heart Disease.* Boston: Little, Brown, 1981.

4. Borow, R. M., et al. End systolic volume as a predictor of postoperative left ventricular performance in volume overload from valvular regurgitation. *Am. J. Med.* 68:655, 1980.

5. Chesler, E. *Schirer's Clinical Cardiology.* Bristol, England: John Wright and Sons, 1981, pp. 214–232, 252–264.

6. Christopherson, D. J., and Sivarajan, E. S. Infective endocarditis. In S. L. Underhill, et al. (eds.) *Cardiac Nursing*. Philadelphia: Lippincott, 1982.

7. Committee on Prevention of Rheumatic Fever and Bacterial Endocarditis of the AHA. Prevention of bacterial endocarditis. *Circulation* 56:139, 1977.

8. Crawley, I. S., Morris, D. C., and Silverman, B. D. Valvular heart disease. In J. W. Hurst, et al. (eds.), *The Heart* (4th ed.). New York: McGraw-Hill, 1978.

9. Dracup, K. A. Unraveling the mysteries of cardiomyopathy. *Nurs. 79* 9:84, 1979.

10. Fowler, N. O. Constrictive pericarditis: new aspects. *Am. J. Cardiol.* 50:1014, 1982.

11. Fuster, V., et al. Natural history of idiopathic dilated cardiomyopathy. *Am. J. Cardiol.* 47:525, 1981.

12. Goldberger, E. *Textbook of Clinical Cardiology*. St. Louis: Mosby, 1982.

13. Goldman, M. J. Pericarditis. *West. J. Med.* 123:467, 1975.

14. Goldmann, D. A., et al. Guidelines for infection control in intravenous therapy. *Ann. Intern. Med.* 79:848, 1973.

15. Goodwin, F., and Oakley, C. M. The cardiomyopathies. *Br. Heart J.* 34:545, 1974.

16. Guzman, L. Nursing management of the parenteral drug abuser with infective endocarditis. *Heart Lung* 10:289, 1981.

17. Kaltenbach, M., et al. Treatment of HOC with verapamil. *Br. Heart J.* 42:35, 1979.

18. Kay, J. H. Emergency operation for complications of myocardial infarction. *Heart Lung* 11:40, 1982.

19. Kluge, R. M. Infections of prosthetic cardiac valves and arterial grafts. *Heart Lung* 11:146, 1982.

20. Moore, S. J. Pericarditis after acute myocardial infarction: manifestations and nursing implications. *Heart Lung* 8:551, 1979.

21. O'Rourke, R. A., and Crawford, M. H. Timing of valve replacement in patients with aortic regurgitation. *Circulation* 61:493, 1980.

22. Rackley, C. E., et al. Mitral valve disease. In J. W. Hurst (ed.), *The Heart* (5th ed.). New York: McGraw-Hill, 1982, pp. 892–927.

23. Rackley, C. E., et al. Aortic valve disease. In J. W. Hurst (ed.), *The Heart* (5th ed.). New York: McGraw-Hill, 1982. pp. 863–892.

24. Sanderson, R. G., and Kurth, C. L. *The Cardiac Patient: A Comprehensive Approach* (2nd ed.). Philadelphia: Saunders, 1983.

25. Schlant, R. C. Altered cardiovascular function of rheumatic heart disease and other acquired valvular disease. In J. W. Hurst (ed.), *The Heart* (4th ed.). New York: McGraw-Hill, 1978.

26. Shabetai, R. The diagnosis and treatment of pericardial effusion. *Cardiovasc. Med.* 6:125, 1981.

27. Sokolow, M., and McIlroy, M. B. *Clinical Cardiology* (3rd ed.). Los Altos: Lange Medical Publications, 1981.

28. Spodick, D. H. Differential diagnosis of acute pericarditis. *Prog. Cardiovasc. Dis.* 14:192, 1971.

29. Trobaugh, G. Cardiomyopathies. In S. L. Underhill et al, *Cardiac Nursing*. Philadelphia: Lippincott, 1982.

30. Underhill, S. L. Valvular disorders. In S. L. Underhill et al., *Cardiac Nursing*. Philadelphia: Lippincott, 1982.

PART IV

Clinical Management of the Cardiac Patient

CHAPTER 12 ———————————————————

Cardiac Surgery

Kathleen Ahern Gould

INTRODUCTION

Cardiac surgery has become a feasible treatment alternative for many forms of severe cardiac disease. Open heart surgery is indicated to treat progressive cardiac disease, to repair or replace diseased valves, or to bypass obstructed coronary arteries. Surgery may also be the treatment of choice for repairing congenital cardiac defects or traumatic injury. The decline in surgical mortality over the past decade can be attributed largely to the improved surgical techniques and the many advances in perioperative patient management.

Nurses are called upon as a resource for the patient, family, and other members of the health care team as the possibility of surgery is explored for each patient. They are continually challenged to remain informed in a rapidly changing field while retaining a personal approach amidst the technological equipment so prevalent in critical care units today.

The public has become more aware of cardiac surgery as an alternative therapy through media coverage of those who emerge from medical centers across the country to resume jobs and their previous lifestyles. Such attention motivates a certain number of people to explore with their physicians the possibility of surgery for the treatment of their cardiac disease.

CORONARY ARTERY BYPASS GRAFTING

Patient Selection

In the past decade numerous studies have been conducted concerning patient selection for coronary artery bypass grafting (CABG). It remains a controversial issue. The latest study results [7, 8] indicate that CABG is a life-prolonging intervention only for the patient with an obstruction of the left main coronary artery who would otherwise risk sudden death. In other patients, even those with multivessel disease, the surgery may offer relief of symptoms but has not been shown to prolong life. The most important result of the surgical procedure is the reduction in the frequency and severity of anginal pain. A reduction in pain that had been refractory to medical management is reported in 80% to 90% of patients [5]. Complete relief of angina has been reported in as many as 70% of the patients studied. In contrast, substantial relief of angina with medical therapy occurs in only 25% of patients [4, 7].

The number of CABGs performed increased from 24,000 in 1971 to 159,000 in 1981 [7, 8]. The determination that CABG is the treatment of choice for coronary artery disease (CAD) in the individual patient is made following a thorough evaluation of the patient's condition. This evaluation is based on an extensive history, including a description of the effects of the disease on the patient's daily activities, as well as objective data such as a resting electrocardiogram (ECG), exercise tolerance testing, and echocardiogram. These data are evaluated along with detailed information obtained from cardiac catheterization.

Cardiac catheterization provides accurate measurements of left ventricular function and the extent of coronary artery obstruction. During cardiac catheterization, actual visualization of the coronary arteries is possible using radiographic dye. The dye outlines the lumen of the arteries, revealing obstructions and the collateral circulation.

"Significant disease" is defined as occlusion in a single vessel greater than 70%. Left ventricular function is evaluated by determining the ejection fraction (EF) and the hemodynamic capabilities of the ventricular muscle. An EF of less than 30% has been associated with an increase in mortality [17]. An EF of less than 30% is not an absolute contraindication for surgery, however. In some individual instances it is believed that surgery may lead to an improvement in the patient's left ventricular function.

After reviewing the coronary arteriogram, the surgical team determines whether the obstructions can be treated surgically. In the ideal case, the lesion or obstruction occurs at the proximal end of the vessel and the vessel receives adequate blood flow below the obstruction. Diffusely diseased vessels with poor distal flow may not be amenable to bypass or may be at high risk for clot formation postoperatively. Whether early occlusion of a coronary artery graft occurs depends primarily on the size of the coronary artery distal to the obstruction and the myocardium it perfuses. A distal coronary artery with poor flow (less than 1.5 mm in diameter) is associated with an 80% early occlusion rate [17]. Other causes of early graft occlusion include thrombosis and mechanical failure of the vein graft, such as kinking or tearing at the suture line.

If surgery is offered to the patient, the members of the health care team may be called upon to present more detailed information regarding the disease itself or the survival rate following surgery. The most recent studies have shown consistently low mortalities of 0.7%, 1.0%, and 1.5% in patients with single, double, and triple bypass procedures, respectively, and an average mortality of 1.1% [8].

With the advent of percutaneous transluminal angioplasty (PCTA) and improvement in pharmacological interventions, surgery is no longer the only choice for relief of symptoms of CAD. The patient must be informed of all the options before a final decision is made. The nurse must be aware of these choices to be able to assist and counsel the patient and family as they make their decision.

The CASS Study

A major recent study has compared the efficacy of medical and surgical treatment of CAD. The Coronary Artery Surgery Study (CASS) was a randomized, controlled, clinical trial that evaluated surgical versus medical treatment for 780 patients with stable ischemic heart disease over a four-year period. The study excluded patients with left main artery disease, because studies had already indicated improved survival rates for these patients.

The purpose of the CASS was to determine the survival data as well as the quality of life in each group of patients studied. Quantity of life is analyzed in a fairly straightforward and objective manner by viewing survival statistics. Quality of life is highly subjective and may be very difficult to analyze. The CASS investigators proposed that improved quality of life is indicated by improved functional status, relief of cardiac-related symptoms, and a return to gainful employment and recreational activity. Conversely, diminished quality of life may be indicated by the need for ancillary supportive treatment (such as extensive drug therapy), recurrent hospitalization, and the need for lifestyle modification [7].

The CASS survival data showed excellent survival rates in both the patient groups—those assigned to receive medical therapy, and those assigned to receive surgical therapy. The similar survival rates in the two groups led the investigators to conclude that patients similar to those enrolled in this trial can safely defer bypass surgery until symptoms worsen to the point at which surgical palliation is necessary [8].

The study also demonstrated that for patients who are asymptomatic after infarction or who have chronic, stable angina, elective CABG does not prolong life to any greater extent than does conventional medical therapy. Surgery, however, may improve quality of life through reduction in chest pain, improvement in both subjective and objective indicators of activity level, and reduction in the need for daily drug therapy [7].

The CASS study did report, however, that no significant effect of treatment on employment or recreational status was shown in either the medical or surgical group. Investigators reported an increased frequency of hospitalization in the surgical group, owing to the initial hospitalization for the surgery itself.

Thus, it appears that patients who are asymptomatic after infarction or who have mild, chronic, stable angina should be managed initially with appropriate medical therapy to prevent or control ischemic symptoms. If the patient's symptoms worsen or if the patient becomes dissatisfied with any lifestyle limitations, CABG may be performed electively with the reasonable expectation that it will improve the quality of life [7].

VALVULAR SURGERY

Surgical intervention for valvular disease began in 1940, when Baily and Harkin introduced the technique of closed mitral commissurotomy. Because of the symptomatic improvement noted by patients after commissurotomy, interest was generated in the development of valve prostheses. Today, valvular repairs account for about 10% of all cardiac surgical procedures in the United States annually [3].

Replacement of the cardiac valves may be indicated for any valvular dysfunction resulting from stenosis or regurgitation. Valvular disease appears to affect the valves in the left side of the heart more commonly, resulting eventually in signs and symptoms of left-sided heart failure. Dysfunction of the aortic or mitral valves can also lead to right-sided failure, however, secondary to pulmonary congestion. (Chapter 11 provides a detailed discussion of valvular disease.)

Once the patient evidences symptoms of valvular dysfunction, hemodynamic function is thoroughly evaluated. Initially, medical therapy may afford the patient adequate control of symptoms. Because valve disease is a slow, progressive disorder, however, almost all patients require surgery at some point in the course of their disease. Surgery is recommended for patients who are hemodynamically stable, because the preoperative condition influences the chances for survival: The longer the patient is hemodynamically decompensated preoperatively, the greater the postoperative risk. Therefore, the correct time for surgical intervention must be evaluated individually.

Patient Selection   The patient's hemodynamic status and level of ventricular function, the presence or absence of atrial fibrillation and cardiomegaly, the cardiac surgical history, and the number of episodes of congestive heart failure must all be considered in determining the feasibility of surgery. Left ventricular function, as well as associated medical disorders and overall cardiovascular condition, are important factors in determining postoperative mortality.

Valve Selection   In 1952 Hafnagel implanted a caged-ball device in a patient with aortic insufficiency. In 1953 Gibbon introduced the technique of cardiopulmonary bypass making feasible a direct surgical approach to all cardiac valves. Direct visibility allowed for restoration, debridement, and mobilization of diseased valves, as well as an improved technique for prosthetic replacement. The development of the various prosthetic devices used today followed.

In 1960 Starr and Edwards introduced an improved caged-ball valve prosthesis, leading to the first successful valve replacement. Since then a variety of innovative valve designs have been introduced that attempt to mimic the natural heart valve both structurally and functionally.

Mechanical and biological tissue valves are presently available, allowing the physician to choose the type of valve that is better for the patient's disease state and lifestyle (Figure 12.1). Mechanical valves have proved to be extremely durable because of the metal, plastic, and Dacron components. The valves vary in design, allowing for choices in size and desired performance characteristics.

Biological tissue valves have received increased interest since 1970; their use has been hampered, however, by their limited availability. These valves are obtained from two sources: animal heart tissue (xenographs) and human heart valves taken from cadaver donors (homographs).

Inherent in the use of tissue or biological valves is the risk that they will be altered by the techniques of harvesting, handling, shipping, and preservation. Studies have shown improper handling to cause preimplantation changes that may affect the durability of the valve. Degradation or calcification, with stiffening of the leaflets, has been noted to begin to occur five years after insertion. Patients with altered metabolism may be predisposed to early calcification. Homograft valves present problems in availability and sizing as well as introducing the risk of host-versus-graft disease and rejection.

The selection of the proper valve depends on the anatomical characteristics of the patient, the extent of disease, the medical history, the patient's age and lifestyle, and the surgeon's preference. The ideal valve should fulfill the following criteria:

1. *Hemodynamic properties.*   There should be minimal obstruction to flow when the valve is open and no regurgitation when it is closed [37]. Turbulence may cause internal proliferation of thrombi and hemolysis.

2. *Minimal thrombogenicity.*   As thrombi accumulate on the cage or sewing ring, they may occlude the valve orifice or lead to systemic embolization.

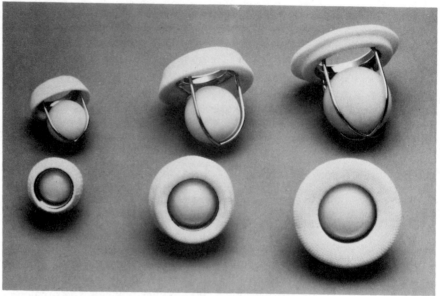

A.

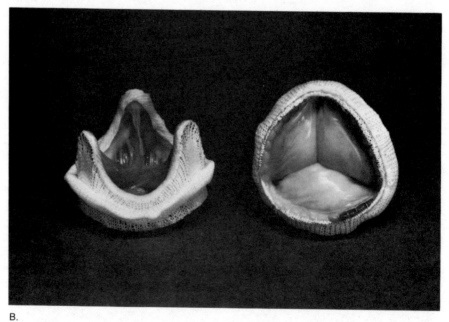

B.

FIGURE 12.1
Cardiac valves. (A) Mechanical valve (Starr-Edwards). (B) Biological tissue valve
(Carpentier-Edwards). (Used with permission of American Edwards Laboratories.)

3. *Durability.*   The prosthetic valve should last the patient's lifetime. Degeneration or calcification are two causes of postoperative valve failure.

4. *Insertibility.*   The valve should be easy to insert. A valve that requires a complicated insertion technique prolongs the operative period and endangers the patient.

5. *Minimal audibility.*   The patient should not be aware of the valve sound produced during closure. Quieter models have been designed that are audible only with a stethoscope [40].

Postoperative management of the cardiac patient will be discussed later in this chapter.

ADDITIONAL INDICATIONS FOR CARDIAC SURGERY

Congenital Defects   The many advances in cardiac surgery have enabled children who previously had poor prognoses to live into adulthood. Congenital disorders may change anatomically and physiologically throughout childhood and may evolve into clinically significant disorders in adulthood. Congenital disorders requiring surgery in adulthood include septal defects and Ebstein's anomaly.

Septal defects may occur in utero yet not require repair until early adulthood, depending on the degree of hemodynamic compromise. The goal in these cases is to offer surgical repair prior to the development of detrimental effects on the pulmonary vascular system. Cyanosis and biventricular enlargement are usually evident with high pulmonary vascular pressures. Surgical intervention is then warranted.

Atrial septal defect (ASD), an abnormal opening in the atrial septum, allows blood to flow between the atria. Predominantly a left-to-right shunt occurs, because left-sided pressures are normally greater than right-sided pressures. The condition is well tolerated in infancy and early childhood, but in young adulthood mild fatigue and dyspnea occur with exercise. Surgical treatment may offer a complete cure. It is almost always possible to close the defect by direct suture, or with a synthetic graft in the case of a larger defect [28].

Ebstein's anomaly is a downward displacement of portions of the tricuspid valve into the right ventricle. Mechanically, portions of the right ventricle become part of the right atrium. The right ventricle appears very small, the right atrium very large, and the tricuspid valve incompetent. This anomaly is usually compatible with an active life into the third decade, when surgical intervention is required [6].

Chest Trauma   Cardiac surgery may be a life-saving intervention in cases of both blunt and penetrating chest trauma, but the mortality is extremely high following serious cardiac injury. The advent of trauma centers and paramedical support care at the accident scene has greatly increased the numbers of patients surviving to reach a medical center.

Patients with penetrating heart wounds can be categorized into three general groups: (1) those who have received extensive lacerations or large-caliber gunshot wounds; (2) those with small wounds of the heart caused by ice picks, knives, or other small agents; and (3) those with associated serious injuries in the chest and elsewhere in the body that may contribute to death. The immediate cause of death may be rapid blood loss, cardiac tamponade, or injury to the conduction system.

Cardiac Tumors

Cardiac surgery is often the treatment of choice for primary tumors within the heart and mediastinum. Surgery is indicated for benign tumors that are discovered following the development of a variety of signs and symptoms. More than 75% of all primary lesions found in the heart are benign. Such tumors may arise from any of the myocardial layers. Half of these are myxomas; the second most common type is the rhabdomyoma [28]. Myxomas arise from the endocardium on the left side of the heart and occupy the left atrium in most cases. They are most common in women between the ages of 30 and 60 years. Common symptoms include syncopal episodes with position changes; these result from sudden changes in cardiac output. Signs of valvular stenosis or insufficiency may be evident if the tumor is obstructing flow across a valve orifice. Thrombosis, embolization, and hemodynamic dysfunction are potential complications of intracardiac tumors. Removal of a benign lesion will greatly improve the patient's prognosis.

Primary malignant tumors of the heart are rare. Symptomatic treatment for metastatic or inoperable tumors may include pacemaker insertion and pharmacological support for symptoms of congestive failure. Other palliative measures, such as pericardiocentesis, may be offered.

CARDIAC TRANSPLANTATION

The first human heart transplant was performed in 1968 by Christiaan N. Barnard of South Africa. Since that time, considerable improvements have been made in the technique and in the management of patients. After almost two decades of research and experience, cardiac transplantation can now be considered a reasonable and therapeutic treatment to extend life in selected individuals [32]. Patients selected for cardiac transplantation have advanced end-stage cardiac disease for which the standard forms of medical and surgical treatment may have already been found nonbeneficial. Additional primary selection criteria include (1) irremediable, terminal cardiac disease with less than 10% likelihood of survival for six months, (2) patient age of 50 years or younger, and (3) normal function or reversible dysfunction of liver and kidney [32]. The numerous contraindications include insulin-dependent diabetes mellitus, active infection, peptic ulcer disease, peripheral vascular or cerebrovascular disease, mental deficiency, and inadequate external psychosocial support [32].

The primary variable restricting the number of cardiac transplantations is the limited availability of suitable donors. The clinical criteria for donor matching are not absolute, but it is suggested that donors be males between the ages of 15 and 35 and females between the ages of 15 and 40 without prior history of severe or chronic liver or heart disease [29]. When a donor does become available, all potential recipients are cross-matched against the donor.

If more than one recipient is appropriate, the candidate with the shortest predicted survival time is selected [35]. Improved methods for procurement of donor hearts are attributable to efforts by local and national organ banks, which provide information to the public as well as giving support to families and hospital personnel.

After a comprehensive evaluation of 227 cardiac transplant patients at Stanford, Pennock and colleagues [32] determined the major causes of death to be infection, acute rejection, graft arteriosclerosis, and malignancy. Despite these problems, the survival rates are improving and are reported to be 63%, 55%, 51%, 44%, and 39% at one, two, three, four, and five years after operation, respectively [32]. Although the in-hospital recovery period is long (approximately two months), individuals experience an improvement in their quality of life and many return to full-time employment.

PATIENT MANAGEMENT

Preoperative Nursing Management

Preoperative preparation begins as soon as surgery is considered. The nurse serves as a resource and teacher for both the patient and the family as they begin to prepare for the upcoming operation. This can be a busy and confusing time for an already frightened patient.

The nurse evaluates the patient's readiness to learn and his or her knowledge regarding the surgical procedure. A teaching plan can then be developed based on the individual needs of the patient. The nurse may conclude that certain patients are not receptive to teaching and need only the reassurance that they will be well cared for and carefully monitored.

The nursing staff — or, ideally, the primary nurse — often serves as the coordinator of care for the multidisciplinary team. A preoperative teaching schedule is used with a multidisciplinary approach including all members of the medical team who will be directly involved in preparing the patient for the procedure. The patient will receive information from the surgeon, respiratory therapist, intensive care nurses, anesthesiologist, and physical therapist. Other individuals, such as the nutritionist and psychiatrist, may also be introduced at this time.

The formation of a multidisciplinary preoperative committee has been found to be a very effective strategy to coordinate preoperative teaching. The goal of this approach is twofold: (1) to provide each member of the preoperative team with an awareness of the roles and procedures of each discipline, thereby providing a cross reference for each caregiver who is involved with the patient; and (2) to minimize the amount of time taken by each discipline during preoperative teaching sessions and to maximize the information received from each discipline. A preoperative committee is helpful in determining how each discipline will interact with the patient and his or her family. A common goal is defined: to provide the patient and family with accurate information regarding the preoperative preparation required and the postoperative course. Many caregivers believe that the patient who has the benefit of a thorough preoperative teaching program will have a more relaxed, uncomplicated course [9].

Prior to visiting the patient, the team should carefully review the patient's social and medical history. This enables the nurse and others to assess what previous teaching has been done and how much the patient knows about the disease or the proposed surgery.

Each discipline involved with the patient records information on a patient education flow sheet kept in the patient record. The flow sheet serves as a guide to each caregiver visiting the patient and documents content that has been discussed, family involvement, and the patient's response to the teaching session (Exhibit 12.1).

The patient's questions may vary from one extreme to another. One patient may want to know every detail, whereas another patient may want to know only that he or she will be well cared for. The questions may request reinforcement of information provided by others. The nursing staff should consider (1) that the patient and family may be at different levels of understanding and need constant clarification and explanation; (2) that each patient may display periods of curiosity, fear, and rejection of information provided; (3) that each patient should be approached as an individual with a unique learning style and level of understanding and interpreting information; and (4) that some patients do not want detailed information, which would only increase their anxiety. It may be helpful for the patient and family to view pictures of the physical setup of the cardiac care unit or specific pieces of equipment, such as the ventilator.

Ideally, most of the patient teaching is done two or three days before the day of surgery. By the morning of the operation, the patient should be adequately prepared without being unduly frightened or overwhelmed by the preoperative preparation. The family members should also be adequately prepared and secure in their feelings. They should be informed of what to expect when seeing the patient postoperatively.

A preoperative order sheet is helpful in providing routine preoperative care other than teaching: laboratory work, medications, and preoperative activity (Exhibit 12.2). All patients are ready for the operating room when laboratory values are within normal limits and routine preoperative care is completed. The physician and patient then share the responsibility for providing informed patient consent to the surgical procedure.

Intraoperative Management

An understanding of intraoperative management is essential for preoperative preparation and postoperative nursing management. The intraoperative management of the cardiac surgical patient has undergone many changes over the past decade. The decline in surgical mortality has resulted from improvements

---

EXHIBIT 12.1
Patient Education Flow Sheet for Cardiothoracic Patients

I. *Preoperative teaching*   Comments

Discuss the immediate preoperative routine:
A. Overview of teaching personnel
B. Surgical prep, showers, and shave

EXHIBIT 12.1 *(continued)*

    C. Eating and drinking prohibition
    D. Preoperative medications

    Describe the preoperative events:
    A. Disposition of valuables
    B. Religious counseling
    C. Family involvement
    D. Smoking prohibition

Date   Signature

II. *Anesthesiologist visit*

Comments

    Review patient history; explain preoperative
    events following premedication:
    A. Insertion of intravenous lines and monitoring
       equipment
    B. Insertion of endotracheal tube
    C. Wake-up phase

Date   Signature

III. *Respiratory therapist and chest physiotherapist visit*

Comments

    Demonstrate the techniques used in coughing
    and deep breathing during splinting of the
    surgical site.

    Explain the importance of postural drainage and
    percussion.

    Demonstrate the incentive spirometer and
    request return demonstration from patient.

Date   Signature

IV. *Surgical intensive care nurse visit*

Comments

    Describe the immediate postoperative course,
    allowing for patient and family questions:
    A. Arrival in CICU
    B. Nurse-to-patient ratio
    C. Medication available for pain
    D. Clearing of secretions from endotracheal
       tube
    E. Monitoring devices and alarms
    F. Fluid balance: intravenous lines, daily
       weights, urinary catheter, fluid restrictions
    G. Methods of communication while intubated
    H. For family members: patient status reports,
       primary nurse contact, visiting hours,
       telephone communication
    I. Discharge from CICU
    J. CICU itself (provide photos or site visit)

Date   Signature

EXHIBIT 12.2
Diagnostic Studies Completed Preoperatively

Vital signs:	BP: right arm, left arm		Temperature
	Pulse	Respirations	Weight
ECG:	Rate	Rhythm	Axis
	Stress test report		
Chest roentgenograms:	PA and lateral views		

Pulmonary function tests and arterial blood gas analysis

Catheterization data

LABORATORY DATA

Routine studies
  HCT
  Hemoglobin
  WBC, diff.

Urine:	Specific gravity	WBC	RBC	Bacteria
	Albumin	Bile	Glucose	Acetone

Stool guaiac test
Hinton test

Electrolytes:	Na	K$^+$	C1	CO_2

Blood sugar

Blood bank specimen:	Type and cross match

Bleeding studies
  Platelet count
  Prothrombin time
  Partial thromboplastin time
  Euglobulin clot lytes
  Fibrinogen

Renal studies	*Liver studies*
BUN	Bilirubin
Creatine	Alk. phos.
24-hr creatine clearance	SGOT
Urine culture	LDH
	Total protein and albumin

in patient selection, cardiac anesthesia, patient monitoring, cardiopulmonary bypass techniques, and valvular prosthetic devices. Improved methods of myocardial preservation may be responsible for the decreased incidence of intraoperative and perioperative myocardial infarction and for the increased maintenance of optimal myocardial functioning during and after surgery.

Upon arriving in the operative area, the patient will be identified by the operating room nurse and anesthesia personnel. Monitoring devices, inserted percutaneously, include an arterial line to monitor mean arterial blood pressure continuously and a thermodilution pulmonary artery catheter, which is used postoperatively to obtain left-sided pressure and cardiac output values. Additional intravenous catheters are used as needed for crystalloid and colloid replacement as well as for the administration of anesthetic agents. A Foley catheter allows for close monitoring of urine output, and a nasogastric tube is inserted to decompress the stomach, thereby minimizing the risk of aspiration. Rectal and esophageal probes may be inserted for continuous temperature monitoring during the procedure. Cardiac monitoring is accomplished by means of electrodes placed on the back or extremities, leaving the chest free for surgical access. The patient is intubated to maintain adequate oxygenation and ventilation throughout the procedure. At the time of intubation, a topical anesthetic, sprayed on the back of the throat, may be used to decrease sensation and localized swelling.

Cardiac anesthesia is instituted slowly while the patient's vital functions are monitored. Generally, all inhalation agents act as myocardial depressants, including halothane, which is used most often in cardiac surgery for low-risk patients. Halothane is very effective in minimal concentrations and is not associated with ventricular irritability. Narcotic anesthesia is preferred because of the lack of myocardial depression. Morphine is used, because it causes vasodilatation and may be useful in controlling systemic vascular resistance. A balanced combination of fentanyl (Sublimaze) and pancuronium bromide (Pavulon), a muscle relaxant, may be used throughout the operative procedure. Adjuncts to anesthesia or additional medications such as vasopressors or inotropic agents are given by the anesthesia team as needed [4].

A medial sternotomy incision is used in the majority of adult cardiothoracic patients. This approach offers adequate exposure of the heart and minimizes incisional pain during the postoperative period.

Intraoperatively, atrial and ventricular pacing wires are attached to the epicardium and brought out through the chest wall for possible use in the immediate postoperative period. Mediastinal and chest tubes are placed to facilitate postoperative drainage of the incision area.

In high-risk patients femoral cannulation for cardiopulmonary perfusion may begin as the chest is opened, although most surgeons prefer direct arterial cannulation into the ascending aorta. The venous cannulas are placed in the right atrium through the vena cava. Two cannulas are beneficial in controlling venous return to the oxygenator (Figure 12.2). Regardless of the type of cardiac surgery, the goals of cardiopulmonary bypass include [13]:

1. *Diversion of blood.* Suction and pumping allow the surgeon a bloodless field for greater visibility, removal of venous blood for cell washing and oxygenation and return of blood to the ascending aorta, and control of both venous and arterial flows.

2. *Control of blood temperature.* Blood temperature can be regulated for systemic cooling or rewarming during removal from cardiopulmonary bypass. During the operative period, the patient is cooled to a temperature of 28 to 30°C to slow systemic metabolism and reduce O_2 demands.

3. *Autotransfusion.* Blood obtained from the operative field and venous cannulas may be washed and preserved by means of a cell saver for use at a later time in the operation or in the immediate postoperative

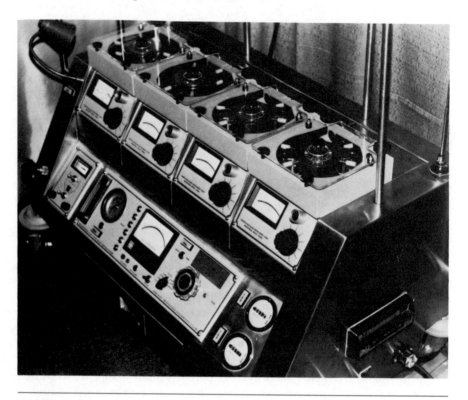

FIGURE 12.2
Cardiopulmonary bypass machine. (From Cardiovascular Instrument Corporation, Wakefield, Mass. Used with permission.)

period. This procedure eliminates the risk of a blood reaction from the use of banked blood.

4. *Additional pharmacological support.*   Pharmacological agents may be added to the arterial flow to enhance acid-base balance or to produce desired hemodynamic effects.

At the start of a CABG procedure, a surgical team may harvest the saphenous vein from either lower extremity for use as a vein graft. The vein is lifted out in one segment for the surgeon to examine, repair, and resect to provide the desired length of vein graft required for each bypass. Segmental or sequential grafts may be used in an effort to maximize the use of the available vein grafts. The surgeon may choose to perform direct aortocoronary artery bypass with a graft or to use the left internal mammary artery for a distal anastomosis site (Figures 12.3 and 12.4).

During open heart surgery all efforts are made to decrease mechanical or chemical myocardial damage, that is, to preserve the myocardium. The goals of myocardial preservation are (1) to maintain a quiet operative field with no myocardial movement and thus allow for decreased metabolic demands as well as operative accessibility, (2) to decrease myocardial injury by reducing O_2 requirements at the cellular level, and (3) to prevent anaerobic metabolism

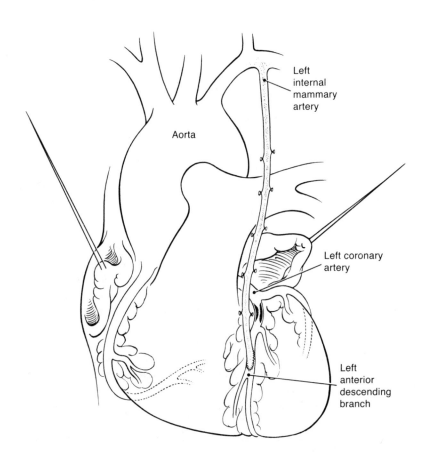

FIGURE 12.3
Single coronary bypass in which the left internal mammary artery has been used to bypass the obstruction. (From Phipps, W. J., Long, B. C., and Woods, N. F. *Medical-Surgical Nursing: Concepts and Clinical Practice,* 2nd ed. St. Louis: Mosby, 1983. Used with permission.)

Left internal mammary artery

Aorta

Left coronary artery

Left anterior descending branch

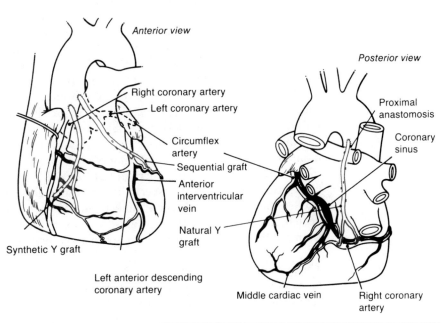

Anterior view

Posterior view

Right coronary artery

Left coronary artery

Circumflex artery

Sequential graft

Anterior interventricular vein

Natural Y graft

Synthetic Y graft

Left anterior descending coronary artery

Proximal anastomosis

Coronary sinus

Middle cardiac vein

Right coronary artery

FIGURE 12.4
Vein grafts, obtained usually from the saphenous vein in the leg, are sutured to the aorta and to the coronary artery distal to the obstruction.

leading to acidosis and tissue death. These goals are achieved by use of a hypothermic, pharmacological fluid called cardioplegic solution. This fluid may vary in composition from institution to institution but commonly contains some type of hyperosmolar solution to enhance substrate passage to the myofibrils, potassium to induce systolic arrest, a buffering solution of tromethamine or bicarbonate to counteract any acidosis, and a dextrose component to provide cellular nutrients. Other additives, such as calcium or insulin, may be found in some cardioplegic solutions. The solution is kept at approximately 4°C and infused as needed while the perfusionist records cardiac tissue temperatures through a myocardial probe attached to the heart tissue by the surgeon.

When myocardial protection is established, the aorta is cross clamped, and full bypass is maintained while the surgical team reconstructs the diseased areas. The cross-clamp time is noted on the operative records as an indicator of the period of time myocardial preservation must be maintained, because the heart receives virtually no perfusion of oxygenated blood during the procedure. The cross-clamp time is determined by the amount of time necessary to replace, repair, or reconstruct the diseased or damaged myocardium.

The total pump time is considered to be the period of time during which blood is removed from the patient and circulated through the heart-lung machine, ending when the final volume of blood is returned to the patient. At that point the venous cannulas are clamped and the aortic return cannula is prepared for removal. Once normal circulation is complete, the heart rhythm is restored, either by defibrillation or spontaneously once the cardioplegic solution has been washed out and the patient is rewarmed. At this time the patient is considered "off pump." In some instances the patient requires inotropic agents to enhance myocardial functioning. In severe cases, when myocardial contractility is diminished considerably, the intra-aortic balloon pump may be used to assist the patient being weaned or removed from bypass.

During this period, the heart muscle may become irritable after pumping is resumed if rewarming has occurred too rapidly. This irritability occurs because the core body rewarms first (as in all induced or accidental hypothermic rewarming cycles) and cool or cold blood may return rapidly to the heart as vasodilatation takes place. For this reason, rewarming techniques are carefully monitored and extend for 6 to 12 hours postoperatively. The patient may return to the CICU with a temperature of 92 to 97°F. Each institution should have written guidelines that specify interventions at various temperatures, including the use of hypothermia blankets or simply covering the patient with a heated bath blanket. The nurse must anticipate the vasodilatation resulting from rewarming and monitor it closely to avoid hypotension.

Postoperative Management

The postoperative management of the cardiac surgical patient is intensive, with many disciplines participating. The primary nurse recognizes the patient's self-care deficits and acts as the patient advocate in overcoming many potential complications during the postoperative period. In the initial postoperative period, the focus may be on maintaining optimal hemodynamic and physiological functioning of the cardiopulmonary and other body systems.

Prior to receiving the postoperative cardiac patient, the surgical intensive care unit or recovery room prepares to meet all possible needs. All emergency equipment, including pacemakers, code carts, ECG machine, and defibrillator, is checked on each shift. For patients who have undergone open heart surgery, the sterile internal defibrillator paddles are checked as well as the open chest cart, which includes sterile equipment such as wire cutters that may be needed if open chest resuscitation becomes necessary. It is essential that the area or cubicle that receives the patient be checked for the availability and functioning of all equipment, including suction regulator, O_2 outlets, and intravenous controllers.

To ensure proper preparation of each patient's room, a standard list of equipment and emergency drugs is made available. Additional supplies that must be gathered are listed in Table 12.1. This set-up serves to prepare the nurse for complications that may occur in the immediate postoperative period, thereby saving valuable time in obtaining emergency medications or equipment. Because the immediate postoperative period is one of physiological transition for the patient, when major complications may occur rapidly, the nursing team must be prepared to intervene immediately.

All efforts are made to facilitate the transition from the operative suite to the CICU with a minimum of risk to the patient. Ideally, the two areas are in close proximity so that transport time is limited to only a few minutes. The patient will be monitored with portable equipment by the anesthesia team until the CICU nurse assumes responsibility.

Communication between the operating room personnel and the CICU nurse is essential to inform the receiving unit of the patient's anticipated time of arrival and about any special requirements, such as intravenous medication administration and special equipment. One CICU nurse is assigned to each patient who has undergone open heart surgery, but upon admission to the unit, a second nurse is usually needed to assist with the set-up of lines, chest tubes and monitoring equipment and the preparation of emergency drugs or equipment.

Specific information about the operation is provided to the primary nurse by the surgical team and anesthesia personnel. Important factors that may affect postoperative management are communicated, such as preoperative and intraoperative hemodynamics and intraoperative complications. The nurse also receives information regarding any of the technical aspects of the surgical procedure that may produce complications in the postoperative period. A report of the operative fluid and blood loss levels and the amounts replaced is obtained. Continuing orders for fluid and electrolyte replacement are determined by the physician. The nurse continues the total patient assessment to determine priorities of care, to identify problems, and to initiate a plan of care for a successful outcome.

When the patient is admitted to the CICU, and frequently thereafter, a systematic head-to-toe assessment should be conducted to allow the nurse to establish baseline information. Priorities are established based on the patient's physiological status. Close monitoring of the levels of all intravascular fluids, vasopressors, and vasodilating agents is essential during this transition period.

TABLE 12.1
Equipment Needed in Caring for Patients Following Open Heart Surgery

Equipment	Rationale
Transducers, precalibrated and primed	Immediate reliability
CICU bed with K-thermia blanket on: K-thermia machine on standby	Patient may require immediate warming because of hypothermic state induced in OR
IV poles on bed	
Cardiac monitor and leads	

Cubicle

Recheck module for 4 working suction setups; include 1 straight connector, Hoffman clamp	1 for endotracheal suction 1 for gastric suction 1 for chest tube suction 1 backup
	Patient may arrive with multiple chest tubes; provisions should be made so that all may be connected as soon as possible to facilitate drainage and prevent tamponade

Recheck for fully stocked bedside unit. Include:
    Extra syringes of various sizes
    Extra needles and prep kits
    Heparinized syringes
    Stopcock covers
	The nurse should anticipate all requirements, eliminating any need to leave the patient unattended

Thermometer	
Cardiac output computer	
Four 250 cc bottles of 5% dextrose + ¼ normal saline solution or solution ordered	Small bottles for KVO lines
Ventilator and Ambu-bag	

Medications on Hand

Potassium chloride drip on IV control pump	Maintenance potassium therapy may begin immediately
Dopamine or sodium nitroprusside with IV solution	
Lidocaine bolus	Vasopressors should be available *in the room*, where the nurse may mix them if required, so the patient is not left unattended

Emergency Equipment

Pacemaker equipment at bedside ECG Code cart Chest cart Defibrillator Sterile paddles (all checked prior to admission)	The nurse accepting the patient should ensure that a pacemaker and emergency equipment are immediately available and in working order

TABLE 12.1 *(continued)*

Documentation of Data

Weight card

Flow sheet, nurses' notes

Doctors' order sheets

Prestamped blood tubes (red, blue, and purple)

Prestamped lab slips

Prestamped doctors' order sheets, and PT consult sheet

All supplies are prestamped and readily available so that the nurse need not leave the patient area

---

CICU = cardiac intensive care unit; K-thermia = hypo/hyperthermia; OR = operating room; IV = intravenous; KVO = keep vein open (the slowest rate for an IV); ECG = electrocardiogram; PT = physical therapy.

Nursing care during this time must include the following:

1. Regulation of the levels of all medications, blood products, and crystalloids being infused.
2. Assessment of cardiac rate and rhythm, or cardiac pacing status.
3. Hemodynamic assessment of blood pressure; mean arterial pressure; pulmonary artery systolic, diastolic, and mean pressures; pulmonary artery wedge pressure; central venous pressure; left arterial pressure; cardiac output and index; and continuous mixed venous O_2 saturation levels.
4. Management of respiratory support systems, including O_2 delivery and mechanical ventilator settings, and evaluation of bilateral breath sounds to determine proper endotrachial tube placement.
5. Neurological assessment relative to anesthetic agents, pupillary response, level of consciousness, and movement of extremities.
6. Fluid balance including hourly urine output, nasogastric fluid, chest tube drainage (amount, color, and consistency), and any overt bleeding or drainage from incisional areas.
7. Immediate blood studies upon arrival in the CICU: electrolyte levels, prothrombin time, partial thromboplastin time, platelet count, enzyme levels, blood urea nitrogen, creatinine, serum calcium levels, as well as arterial and mixed venous blood gas analysis.

The nursing care plan assists the nurse in monitoring the patient's postoperative course and planning interventions that ensure optimal care and prevention of complications. Table 12.2 presents a nursing care plan for the postoperative cardiac patient. Management within the first 24 to 48 hours is relatively standard regardless of the exact surgical procedure performed.

TABLE 12.2
Nursing Care Plan for a Patient Following Open Heart Surgery

Diagnosis	Nursing Action
Potential for cardiac dysrhythmias	
Sinus tachycardia due to hypovolemia or hyperthermia	Closely monitor patient's ECG for presence of dysrhythmias

Atrial dysrhythmias may be due to atrial distention, increased pulmonary vascular congestion, or mechanical irritation from intracardiac monitoring lines; may include:
    Premature atrial contractions
    Atrial flutter
    Atrial fibrillation
	Maintain proper fluid balance
	Monitor electrolytes, especially potassium, continuously to maintain adequate serum levels
	Assess ABGs to ensure adequate oxygenation

AV blocks may be due to hypothermia, edema, or injury in the area surrounding the AV node; may include 1st-, 2nd-, or 3rd-degree block	
Ventricular dysrhythmias may result from a lowered fibrillatory threshold caused by anesthetic agents or cardiopulmonary bypass, potassium depletion due to cell-saver washout, or increased urine output, hypoxia, or mechanical irritation from monitoring lines or artificial valves	
Potential for respiratory failure	
Ineffective ventilation due to mechanical obstruction, mechanical failure, excessive secretions, atelectasis, pulmonary hypertension, pulmonary edema, bronchospasm, immobility	Constantly assess patient's pulmonary status by observing chest movement, respiratory rate, respiratory pattern; listening for bilateral breath sounds; monitoring mechanical ventilator settings, PO_2, tidal volume; assessing ABG's, chest film; evaluating pulmonary secretions
	Reposition patient every 2 hr to enhance air exchange; promote rest and compliance with mechanical ventilation to facilitate weaning and extubation
	Initiate bronchodilator treatments and chest physical therapy to promote airway clearance
	After extubation, encourage coughing and deep breathing every 2–4 hr
	Promote lung expansion exercises with incentive spirometer devices
	Assist patient to get out of bed in a chair
Potential for infection within the pulmonary system due to inhibition of normal respiratory functioning, such as cleaning, filtering, and humidifying air, resulting from intubation; atelectasis; incomplete reexpansion of lungs; formation of sputum; nosocomial infection	Monitor patient's temperature and WBC Note the color and consistency of sputum Maintain sterile two-glove technique for nasotracheal or endotracheal suctioning Document patient's response to pulmonary therapy and medications provided for pulmonary support
Potential for fluid volume deficit	
Vasodilatation due to rewarming after cardiopulmonary bypass	Rewarm *slowly* with topical blankets or hyperthermia blankets
Vasodilatation due to loss of regulatory mechanisms, catecholamine depletion	Monitor temperature constantly Assess BP and P every 15 min

TABLE 12.2 *(continued)*

Diagnosis	Nursing Action
Vasodilatation due to excessive medication administration	Replace fluids as needed
	Titrate fluids, vasopressors, and vasodilators according to BP and mean arterial pressure
	Calculate systemic vascular resistance, and correlate with clinical findings
	Titrate vasopressor drugs in accordance with systemic vascular resistance, cardiac output, and clinical assessment of cardiovascular response
Actual fluid deficit	
Hemorrhage due to:	Draw and monitor coagulation studies initially and daily or p.r.n. if bleeding is suspected
Disseminated intravascular coagulation	
Depletion of coagulation factors	Replace blood products as ordered by physician, and monitor for adverse reactions
Depletion of platelets; adherence to IABP, hemolysis secondary to valve dysfunction	Check chest tube drainage frequently for amount, color, consistency, and obstruction due to clot formation
Surgical/mechanical failure of suture lines, graft anastomosis cannulation sites	Prepare for and perform collection and autotransfusion of chest tube drainage
	Prepare patient and equipment for portable support if transport is necessary for reexploration of chest in operating room
Hypovolemia related to excessive urinary output and/or nasogastric drainage or decreased fluid replacement	Continuously regulate IV fluid administration, including volume contributed by medication and blood products
	Monitor urinary output and NG drainage every hour
Alteration in cardiac output	
Hypotension due to: Hypovolemia Vasodilatation Low-output syndrome Abnormal heart rate or rhythm Hemorrhage	Monitor BP, P, pulmonary artery pressures, central venous pressure, cardiac output, cardiac rhythm; maintain pressures according to unit protocol, physician preference, and patient's optimal hemodynamic performance
	Maintain MAP at 70–90 mm Hg (to prevent graft collapse in CABG patients)
	Monitor intake and output every hour
	Titrate IV medications according to the patient's hemodynamic response
Hypertension due to peripheral vasoconstriction secondary to hypothermia or medication effect	Monitor BP, MAP, SVR every hour
	Maintain MAP at 70–90 mm Hg to prevent rupture of bypass grafts or leaks at the suture lines
Complications altering cardiac output: Cardiac tamponade Hemorrhage into chest cavity Failure secondary to perivalvular leak, prosthetic rupture, ruptured papillary muscle, valvular dysfunction	Monitor CVP, PAD, cardiac output, P, BP, clinical findings
Potential for infection	
From the following sources: Lungs Urinary tract	Monitor temperature, heart rate, and WBC for signs of infection
	Maintain strict aseptic technique when suctioning patient

TABLE 12.2   *(continued)*

Diagnosis	Nursing Action
Incisions Skin Intravascular catheters Gastrointestinal tract	Ensure that ventilator tubing is changed every 24 hr
	Provide for adequate clearance of pulmonary secretions by repositioning, chest physical therapy, and suctioning every 2 hr
	Complete Foley catheter care every 8 hr
	Remove catheter as soon as possible
	Closely observe chest and graft incisions for redness, swelling, or drainage, and cover with sterile dressings according to hospital protocol
	Frequently assess condition of the skin for signs of impending breakdown
	Reposition patient frequently
	Check intravascular catheter insertion sites daily for signs of infiltration or infection
	Change catheters according to the Center for Disease Control guidelines
	Use strict sterile technique during dressing changes
	Maintain proper NG suction to prevent aspiration
	Assess bowel sounds prior to feeding patient
	Observe for signs of mesenteric ischemia related to vasopressor therapy; these symptoms may include abdominal pain, decreased or absent bowel sounds, and firm abdomen
Potential alteration in neurological status	
Due to: Anesthesia	Monitor level of consciousness, pupillary response, movement of extremities
Hypoxia, secondary to poor gas exchange, blood loss, anemia, inadequate ventilation	Monitor ABGs

Embolic complications (CVA)
  Intraoperative air or clot
  Pulmonary emboli
  Thrombophlebitis
	Ambulate as soon as tolerated out of bed to chair

Decreased perfusion due to decreased cardiac output, dysrhythmias, decreased MAP, BP	Monitor cardiac rate and rhythm, BP, MAP
Pain	
Due to:	Provide analgesics on a regular schedule
Incisions	Reposition the patient frequently; get the patient out of bed as soon as possible
Immobilization	
Drainage tubes and catheters	Be certain that drainage tubes are not pulled taut
Anxiety	Reassure that everything is going well
	Explain all procedures
	Reduce extraneous environmental stimulation

ECG = electrocardiogram; ABGs = arterial blood gases; AV = atrioventricular; WBC = white blood cell count; BP = blood pressure; P = pulse; IV = intravenous; IABP = intra-aortic balloon pump; NG = nasogastric; MAP = mean arterial pressure; CABG = coronary artery bypass grafting; SVR = systemic vascular resistance; CVP = central venous pressure; PAD = pulmonary artery diastolic; CVA = cerebrovascular accident.

Complications

Immediate care of the cardiac surgical patient centers on nursing observations and measures that would indicate the need for emergency treatment. Because the nurse caring for the postoperative patient constantly assesses and reevaluates the patient's status, certain policies and procedures are developed to allow the nurse to intervene in emergency situations so as to prevent further complications. These standing policies and procedures permit the nurse to deliver emergency treatments, such as antiarrhythmic drugs or defibrillation in the case of lethal dysrhythmias. Standard drug dilutions are available, although these may be adjusted to the patient's needs as allowed within physician orders.

Bleeding.   Several large chest or mediastinal tubes are placed within the chest cavity prior to the closure of the sternal incision. Their function is to facilitate drainage away from the operative site, thereby preventing an accumulation of blood in the thorax that could lead to cardiac tamponade or respiratory insufficiency. A large amount of chest drainage (50 to 75cc) may occur postoperatively even if hemostasis was achieved intraoperatively.

   The causes of postoperative bleeding are varied. Often the patient suffers from a depletion or washout of intrinsic coagulation factors when blood passes through the cell saver of the bypass machine. Other factors that may cause bleeding include suture line dehiscence at the graft site and rupture of the vein graft itself. Additional fluids or blood products may be necessary postoperatively. If the bleeding does not subside, however exploratory surgery may be considered to investigate the cause. If hemorrhage is not recognized or blood loss is not estimated accurately, hypotension, hypoperfusion, cellular ischemia, acidosis, and dysrhythmias may occur.

Hypotension.   Hypotension may be caused by hemorrhage or volume depletion as well as catecholamine depletion. Hypotension may cause systemic ischemia secondary to low cardiac output or cardiovascular collapse. In patients who have undergone CABG, short periods of hypotension may lead to vein graft occlusion, leading to myocardial ischemia and injury.

Hypertension.   Hypertension commonly occurs in the immediate postoperative period and most often is due to vasoconstriction, which results from hypothermia. During the immediate postoperative period, hypertension is closely controlled in an effort to minimize the myocardial O_2 demands of the left ventricle. Increasing left ventricular afterload may lead to cardiac failure and pulmonary hypertension. In patients who have undergone CABG, hypertension may adversely effect the vein graft, causing stress on the graft suture lines and thus leading to rupture.

Dysrhythmias.   A variety of dysrhythmias are evident postoperatively. The incidence in the postoperative cardiac patient is extremely high. Such dysrhythmias usually last for approximately 48 hours. Cardiac dysrhythmias must be recognized and treated immediately to ensure optimal hemodynamic functioning. They may also alert the caregivers to imbalances in the metabolic system or in O_2 demands of the myocardium. The dysrhythmias may be chemically or mechanically induced; the most common causes are myocardial ischemia and edema related to the surgical procedure, electrolyte imbalances such as hypokalemia, and acid-based imbalances. Treatment is usually directed toward eliminating the precipitating factor. Temporary pacing is frequently employed for one to two days during the postoperative period.

Cardiovascular collapse.   This syndrome may result from catecholamine depletion, transfusion reactions, anaphylaxis, or the presence of endotoxins. Cardiovascular support with potent vasopressors such as epinephrine, phenylephrine hydrochloride, and dopamine may be used to maintain an adequate systemic vascular pressure.

Fluid and electrolyte imbalances.   Close observation of fluid and electrolytes is an essential part of immediate postoperative care. Hypokalemia is very common in the early postoperative period following intraoperative diuresis. Ventricular irritability and digitalis toxicity may occur if hypokalemia is not corrected. Hyperventilation, resulting in respiratory alkalosis, may also contribute to a low serum potassium level.

Hyperkalemia must be avoided to prevent ECG changes that may lead to arrest. This dangerous condition may occur secondary to an inadequate urine output, the administration of large doses of potassium intravenously, or both. Seriously ill patients showing signs of acidosis may be at greater risk for hyperkalemia as potassium shifts out of the cell and into the intravascular space. The initial treatment depends on the potassium levels and the ECG changes observed. Sodium bicarbonate or dextrose and insulin solutions may be used to move potassium into the cell. All potassium supplements must be discontinued at the first sign of hyperkalemia.

Hyponatremia may result from dilutional volume replacement. Hypernatremia may result from elevation of the antidiuretic hormone and aldosterone levels following the stress of surgery. Sodium intake and fluid balance are carefully monitored throughout the postoperative period.

Acidosis.   Acidosis may lead to lethal dysrhythmias, depression of myocardial function, and increased demands on the respiratory system as compensation is attempted. Frequent arterial blood gas measurements are obtained to monitor for signs of respiratory acidosis or alkalosis. Monitoring of serum bicarbonate levels allows for the determination of metabolic acidosis or alkalosis. Bicarbonate solutions may reverse metabolic acidosis temporarily, but treatment of the causative factors, such as hypotension or low-output syndromes, is imperative.

Alkalosis.   Mild metabolic alkalosis may occur with many types of trauma or surgery. After cardiac surgery, alkalosis often is due to loss of hydrogen and chloride ions in patients requiring a nasogastric tube connected to suction. Respiratory alkalosis occurs commonly in ventilated patients and is often corrected by lowering the respiratory rate or tidal volume.

Many hospitals have developed rehabilitation programs for patients after cardiac surgery that are similar to the programs for those who have suffered myocardial infarctions (see Chapter 15). These programs allow the patient to share problems and experiences with similar patients, and reduce the feelings of isolation often experienced postoperatively. They also facilitate the development of a discharge plan and provide the patient with a continuing link to the hospital after discharge. The newly discharged patient then feels an increased sense of security and confidence.

Discharge from the hospital necessitates a careful teaching plan for the patient, which includes diet, exercise, weight and temperature monitoring, and medication protocol. An organized discharge teaching plan will direct the nurse, ensure consistency, and provide a comprehensive discharge plan.

PSYCHOLOGICAL REACTIONS TO CARDIAC SURGERY

Nursing personnel involved in the care of the cardiac surgical patient face some unique challenges in providing emotional as well as physical support. Considerable effort is put into preoperative and postoperative teaching and preparation for both the patient and family members. Many hospitals provide support groups and specialized educational sessions for cardiac patients, including cardiac surgical patients. The efforts try to deal not only with the risk associated with cardiac disease but also with the patient's response to the condition.

For many people the heart represents the center of life, the core of being. Through discussion with the patient, the nurse may identify the meaning of "the heart" to that individual. Patients are usually aware that the dysfunction of many organs or bodily systems may be life threatening but that the heartbeat is essential to life. Cessation of heart function would mean an end to life. Culturally, the heart is perceived as the center for emotions, life, and love. Many patients and families have visions of friends and relations suffering from a "bad heart." For these reasons, among others, the emotional stress of illness or surgery may be compounded if the heart is involved.

Preoperative teaching attempts to address many of the fears and issues that the patient and family may be experiencing. The educational sessions provide answers to commonly asked questions and allow the patient some appreciation of what to expect and what will be experienced in the CICU following surgery. The role of the preoperative teaching nurse includes providing information regarding preoperative and postoperative routines, clarifying myths or dispelling unwarranted fears, and providing reassurance that the patient is constantly and closely monitored during the immediate postoperative period. Patients have reported that their greatest fear is that of the unknown, and they welcome preoperative teaching because it allows them to become familiar with the perioperative care and the people providing it. Family members may also be overwhelmed by the number of consulting physicians and procedures that are encountered during the perioperative period. It is extremely helpful to patients and families if they are allowed to visit the CICU before surgery, accompanied by a nurse who will explain the various types of monitoring devices and the physical layout.

The nurse assists the patient to set realistic, achievable goals for the immediate recovery period. In the postoperative period many factors can contribute to psychological distress. A topic that received a great deal of attention in the 1960s and 1970s is a condition called "post-pump psychosis." Patients with this condition manifested depression, confusion, agitation, delirium, and sometimes paranoia in the immediate postoperative period. This so-called psychosis was attributed in part to such causes as microemboli, inadequate cerebral perfusion, and the amount of time spent connected to the bypass machine. Recent advances in surgical technique have eliminated these contributing factors, and there has been a decline in the prevalence and severity of "post-pump psychosis" [22].

The CICU environment itself, as well as the stress of surgery, can produce confusion and disorientation in the postoperative patient. The CICU environment has been modified recently in an attempt to alleviate postoperative psychological distress. Visiting hours are flexible, allowing families to take an active role in the recovery period and to alleviate the isolation that was previously experienced by the patient. CICU staff members, recognizing the effects of sleep deprivation and sensory disturbances, have made efforts to provide uninterrupted sleep-wake cycles for each patient. The physical environment has been modified to include windows, calendars, clocks, and televisions to combat the alienation from society patients frequently experienced. The length of stay has also been dramatically reduced.

The staff provides emotional support by acknowledging the emotional impact of cardiac surgery and encouraging the patient to discuss fears, questions, and emotions. The patient should be allowed to verbalize memories of the CICU or operating room so that these can be explored and do not remain to haunt the patient. Some research has shown that patients may recall events that occur during surgery. These memories will be less frightening if they are shared. The nurse must remember that patients frequently need reassurance and explanation regarding their conditions, their safety, what is expected of them, where they are, and what time it is.

SUMMARY

Cardiac surgery faces new and exciting challenges. The success of cardiac transplants has dramatically improved. Improved surgical techniques and methods of myocardial preservation can ensure greater safety for patients receiving new valves or coronary artery bypasses. Economic and ethical issues will be examined and debated as the population reviews the cost of health care and health maintenance. In 1983, 3.25 billion dollars was spent on coronary artery bypass procedures alone. Selection criteria and alternative treatments are being carefully reviewed by both patient and physician.

New drugs, prosthetic valves, and grafting materials will continue to be developed. Nursing care will continue to be determined by standards that are arrived at through nursing research and joint practice with all members of the cardiac surgical team.

CASE STUDIES

CASE 1

A 62-year-old man is currently being evaluated for possible CABG following several months of increased frequency of chest pains while at rest. Cardiac catheterization shows diffuse disease with severe lesions in four vessels excluding the left main coronary artery.

1. What other factors must be considered before cardiac surgery is suggested?
2. Outline a preoperative teaching schedule for the patient.
3. What are some of the emotions or feelings that the patient may have prior to open heart surgery?
4. If the nurse assesses that the patient and family are unusually anxious preoperatively, what intervention can be used to decrease this anxiety?

CASE 2

A patient has returned to the cardiac intensive care unit following a triple CABG. Although hemodynamically stable for the first 2 hours, she becomes hypotensive, with a heart rate of 110 bpm. The nurse notices that the chest tube drainage has dramatically increased, from 50 cc every hour to 200 cc, and the patient is showing clinical signs of shock.

1. Discuss three mechanisms that may explain the bleeding.
2. What would be the immediate treatment for the bleeding?
3. What complications may arise if treatment is not instituted?

REFERENCES

1. Abbott, N., et al. Infection related to physiologic monitoring: venous and arterial catheters. *Heart Lung* 12:28, 1983.

2. Abe, T., and Komatsu, S. Valve replacement for Ebstein's anomaly of the tricuspid valve. *Chest* 84:414, 1983.

3. Alderman, L., et al. Results of coronary artery surgery in patients with poor left ventricular function (CASS). *Circulation* 68:785, 1983.

4. Behrendt, D., and Austen, G. *Patient Care In Cardiac Surgery* (3rd ed.). Boston: Little, Brown, 1981.

5. Braunwald, E. Effects of coronary artery bypass grafting on survival. *N. Engl. J. Med.* 309:1181, 1983.

6. Canobbio, M., and Perhoff, J. Critical care of adults with congenital heart disease. *Crit. Care Q.* 4:39, 1981.

7. CASS Principal Investigators. Coronary artery surgery study (CASS): a randomized trial of coronary artery bypass surgery: "quality of life" in randomized subjects. *Circulation* 68:951, 1983.

8. CASS Principal Investigators. Coronary artery surgery study (CASS): a randomized trial of coronary artery bypass surgery: survival data. *Circulation* 68:939, 1983.

9. Cisar, N., and Morphew, F. S. Preoperative teaching: aorta-coronary bypass patients. *Focus* 10(1):21, 1983.

10. Conti, V. R. Crystalloid or blood cardioplegia with cardiac surgery. Chest 84:367, 1983.

11. Covner, A. L., and Shinn, J. A. Cardiopulmonary transplantation: initial experience. *Heart Lung* 12:131, 1983.

12. Cromwell, V., et al. Understanding the needs of your coronary bypass patient. *Nurs.'80* 10(3):34, 1980.

13. Diethrich, E. B. Myocardial preservation: a historical and biochemical review. *Advances in Cardiovascular Nursing*. Bowie, Md.: Brady, 1979.

14. Gordon, M. *Manual of Nursing Diagnosis*. New York: McGraw-Hill, 1982.

15. Gray, R. J., et al. The role of cardiac surgery in acute myocardial infarction. I. With mechanical complications. *Am. Heart J.* 106:723, 1983.

16. Gray, R. J., et al. The role of cardiac surgery in acute myocardial infarction. II. Without mechanical complications. *Am. Heart J.* 106:729, 1983.

17. Hillis, D. L., et al. *Manual of Clinical Problems in Cardiology.* Boston: Little, Brown, 1980.

18. Hollman, J., et al. Acute occlusion after percutaneous transluminal coronary angioplasty: a new approach. *Circulation* 68:725, 1983.

19. Horowitz, R. S. Aortic dissection following coronary arterial bypass graft surgery. *Chest* 80:749, 1981.

20. Hoyt, S. K. Chest trauma. *Nurs. '83* 13(5):34, 1983.

21. Hurst, J. W. *The Heart* (3rd ed.). New York: McGraw-Hill, 1974.

22. Isaacson, J., et al. Post pump psychosis. *Crit. Care Nurs.* 2(1):14, 1982.

23. Johnson, S. H. Nursing techniques for the artificial heart patient. *Dimens. Crit. Care Nurs.* 2(3):167, 1983.

24. Kay, H. J. Emergency operation for complications of myocardial infarction. *Heart Lung* 11:40, 1982.

25. Kern, L. S., and Gawlinski, A. Stage-managing coronary artery disease. *Nurs. '83* 13(4):34, 1983.

26. Kluge, R. M. Infections of prosthetic cardiac valves and arterial grafts. *Heart Lung* 11:146, 1982.

27. Leibrandt, T. Cardiovascular Disorders. *Diseases: Nurses' Reference Library.* Horsham, Pa.: Intermed Communications, 1981.

28. Netter, F. H. *The Ciba Collection of Medical Illustrations. Vol. 5, Heart.* Summitt, N. J.: Ciba Pharmaceutical Co., 1978.

29. New England Organ Bank. Procedure for Procurement of Organs and Tissues for Transplantation. Boston, Mass., 1984.

30. Ng, L. Nursing aspects of the surgical treatment of idiopathic hypertrophic subaortic stenosis. *Heart Lung* 11:364, 1982.

31. Olthof, H., et al. The definition of myocardial infarction during aorto-coronary bypass surgery. *Am. Heart J.* 106:631, 1983.

32. Pennock, J. L., et al. Cardiac transplantation in perspective for the future. *J. Thorac. Cardiovasc. Surg.* 83:168, 1982.

33. Proudfit, W. Fifteen year survival study of patients with obstructive coronary artery disease. *Circulation* 68:986, 1983.

34. Reynolds, S. F. Cardiac trauma and tamponade. *Crit. Care Q.* 4(3):27, 1981.

35. Schneider, J. Human cardiac transplantation at the University of Minnesota. *Minn. Med. U.* 67:209, 1984.

36. Seifert, P. C. Protection of the myocardium during cardiac surgery. *Heart Lung* 12:135, 1983.

37. Stanley, J. Closed mitral valvotomy: early results and long-term follow-up of 3724 consecutive patients. *Circulation* 68:891, 1983.

38. Thornby, D. C. Cardiac transplantation: nursing during the acute period. *Dimens. Crit. Care Nurs.* 2(4):213, 1983.

39. Valladares, K. B., and Lemberg, L. Severe coronary artery disease in asymptomatic patients. *Heart Lung* 12:559, 1983.

40. Waggoner, P. C. Postoperative care of the patient undergoing cardiac valve replacement: a nursing perspective. *Crit. Care Q.* 4(3):57, 1981.

41. Wann, S. L. Judging the success of mitral commissurotomy. *Chest* 84:121, 1983.

42. Watanabe, T., et al. Ruptured chordae tendineae of the tricuspid valve due to nonpenetrating trauma. *Chest* 80:751, 1981.

43. Weiland, A. P. A review of cardiac valve prostheses and their selection. *Heart Lung* 12:498, 1983.

44. Weinstein, J. R., et al. Ultrasonic assessment of the St. Jude prosthetic valve: M mode, two dimensional, and Doppler echocardiography. *Circulation* 68:897, 1983.

CHAPTER 13

Mechanical Interventions

Barbara Homer Yee

INTRODUCTION

One of the distinguishing features of a critical care unit is the availability of specialized equipment. Rapid technological advances have resulted in the development of complex equipment for the care of the critically ill patient. In addition, improvements in techniques and materials have expanded the indications for the use of these modes of therapy. With the recent numerous developments in cardiac pacemaker technology, for example, practitioners may find it difficult to stay abreast of the changes.

Mechanical devices such as defibrillators and pacemakers have saved many lives in the critical care unit when used by skilled practitioners. Nurses educated in the use of this equipment can halt life-threatening dysrhythmias, prevent severe complications, and reverse ischemic episodes or the shock cycle. This chapter will focus on three modes of therapy used most frequently in the cardiac critical care unit: precordial shock, cardiac pacemakers, and the intra-aortic balloon pump.

PRECORDIAL SHOCK

The conversion of dysrhythmias by direct-current electrical shock has become standard practice in the critical care unit. Potentially fatal atrial, junctional, and ventricular dysrhythmias can be terminated by passing an electrical current through the heart. Physiologically, the electrical discharge depolarizes the myocardium and terminates the dysrhythmia, thereby permitting the sinus node to resume functioning as the dominant pacemaker. This mode of therapy, which has been used successfully since 1956, is the definitive treatment for ventricular fibrillation and is rapidly becoming the treatment of choice for certain atrial dysrhythmias [29]. The electrical current is directed through the heart by placing metal paddles on the chest or directly on the heart during open heart surgery. Recently, automatic defibrillators, using an intracardiac catheter system, have been implanted in patients with refractory ventricular dysrhythmias. This new method of defibrillation will, it is hoped, save some individuals from sudden death caused by uncontrolled ventricular dysrhythmias.

In the critical care unit, two methods of electrical precordial shock are commonly performed, cardioversion and defibrillation. Although the physiological basis for the two is the same, the indications, energy requirements, and complications differ, thus warranting individual discussion.

Cardioversion

Cardioversion is used to convert several supraventricular dysrhythmias, particularly atrial fibrillation and atrial flutter, as well as ventricular tachycardia, to sinus rhythm. These cardiac rhythms represent organized electrical activity; therefore, the machine must be synchronized with the patient's electrocardiogram (ECG). The cardioverter has a time-delay circuit that holds the current and discharges it on the downslope of the R wave. This synchronized maneuver avoids the vulnerable period of the cardiac cycle and the possibility of precipitating ventricular fibrillation.

Cardioversion is most often an elective procedure and can be performed in any area of the hospital that has equipment for cardiac monitoring and emergency resuscitation. Preparation for the procedure may begin as early as three weeks prior to the procedure, or as late as the day before. Some cardiologists recommend anticoagulation three weeks prior to the procedure for certain patients in atrial fibrillation. This therapy is initiated to reduce the potential for embolic events after sinus rhythm is restored [14]. Serum levels of digoxin and electrolytes should be ascertained the day before cardioversion. If the values are abnormal, the procedure should be postponed until the imbalance is corrected. The risk of provoking ventricular fibrillation with synchronized cardioversion is enhanced by hypokalemia, digitalis or quinidine toxicity, and acute myocardial ischemia [29].

Nursing responsibilities prior to and during elective cardioversion vary among institutions. Generally, the physician explains the procedure to the patient and obtains written consent if necessary. It is helpful if the primary nurse is present during this conversation so that she or he is aware of exactly what the patient knows and can answer additional questions or clarify information for the patient and family. It is recommended that the patient fast for 6 to 8 hours prior to the procedure. This intervention is a safety precaution to avoid aspiration in the unlikely event that cardiopulmonary arrest occurs. In addition, an intravenous infusion is started for drug administration, and baseline vital signs, a rhythm strip, and an ECG are obtained and recorded. The twelve-lead ECG is examined, and the lead with the highest R wave amplitude is selected to be the triggering mode during synchronized cardioversion. Sedation and amnesia may be produced by administering 100 mg of phenobarbital intramuscularly an hour before the procedure, and/or diazepam, 5 mg intravenously, followed by 2.5 mg every 2 minutes [29]. It may be beneficial to have an anesthesiologist present during the procedure for patients who are sensitive or resistant to sedation. The machine and synchronizer switch are turned on, and the energy level to be delivered is selected.

The amount of energy required to convert a particular dysrhythmia varies. Studies have demonstrated that atrial flutter and ventricular tachycardia require very little energy, usually 10 to 25 joules. Atrial fibrillation, however, requires more energy, usually 100 to 150 joules [14]. Cardioversion should always be attempted with energy levels that are low at first and then, if necessary, titrated up. High-energy shocks have been associated with a certain degree of cardiac damage.

The paddles must be completely covered with conductive paste or gel, or with gauze pads soaked in normal saline solution, to prevent skin burns. The paddles are placed on the chest using either the anterolateral or anteroposterior position. The superiority of one approach over the other is currently under investigation; to date there is insufficient evidence to demonstrate any such superiority [35, 45]. If the anterolateral position is used, the anterior paddle is placed to the right of the sternum at the level of the second and third intercostal spaces and the lateral paddle is placed at the level of the cardiac apex at the midaxillary line. If the anteroposterior position is selected, the anterior paddle is positioned at the left of the sternum in the second or third intercostal space and the posterior paddle is placed at the angle of the left scapula (Figure 13.1). Paddles should not be placed over the sternum or scapula because bony tissue will impede the flow of current, decrease the effectiveness of the shock, and hinder good paddle–skin contact [29]. Prior to discharge of the shock, all personnel must "stand clear" of the bed. The paddles are held firmly (20 to 25 lb of pressure) on the chest and the discharge buttons depressed and held until the shock is delivered. The patient's cardiac rhythm is then checked to determine if sinus rhythm has been restored. If sinus rhythm has not been restored, cardioversion is repeated using higher energy levels until the underlying dysrhythmia is terminated. Once the procedure is completed, vital signs and the patient's level of consciousness are checked every 15 to 20 minutes until they are stable. In the event that ventricular fibrillation (VF) is precipitated, the synchronizer switch is immediately turned off and the patient is defibrillated.

Electrical conversion of ventricular tachycardia (VT) may be performed on an emergency basis or electively if the patient is clinically in stable condition. Lown and DeSilva recommend switching to the defibrillator mode and delivering a shock of 100 joules when VT is rapid and the QRS complex is wide and indistinguishable from the T wave [29]. In the critical care unit, if the nurse witnesses the onset of VT or VF on the cardiac monitor, a precordial thump is recommended prior to defibrillation [45].

Defibrillation

The protocol for defibrillation has been standardized by the American Heart Association [45]. Defibrillation is indicated for the treatment of VF (of less than 2 minutes' duration). In this situation, defibrillation should be performed as quickly as possible; the longer VF persists, the less likely it is to be terminated successfully with electrical shock. If the onset of VF is witnessed on the cardiac monitor, a precordial thump should be attempted.

The procedure for defibrillation is similar to that outlined for cardioversion except in a few minor respects. The paddles are covered with a conductive medium and placed on the chest in the anterolateral or anteroposterior position using 20 to 25 lb of pressure, and the patient is defibrillated with 200 to 300 joules of energy. If the first attempt at defibrillation does not successfully terminate VF, a second shock using 200 to 300 joules should be delivered immediately. This recommendation is based on evidence that transthoracic resistance decreases with successive countershocks. If the second countershock is not successful, basic life support should be continued while epinephrine and sodium bicarbonate are administered and a third countershock delivered using 360 joules [45].

Complications

A variety of complications have been reported to result from defibrillation and cardioversion, especially with repeated high-energy shocks. Although the incidence of serious complications is low, the patient should be monitored closely for dysrhythmias, hypotension, embolic episodes, cardiac enzyme level elevation, and ST segment as well as T wave changes. Skin burns may also occur if the electrodes are not adequately prepared with conductive paste or if the patient requires multiple shocks.

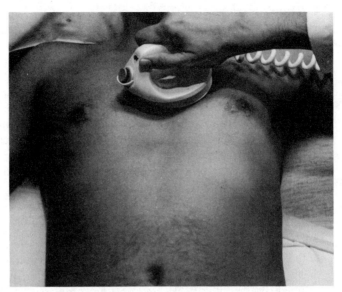

A.

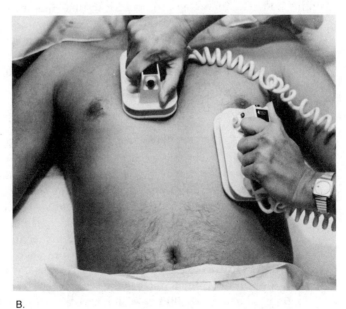

B.

FIGURE 13.1
Proper position of paddles for defibrillation. (A) Anteroposterior placement; (B) anterolateral placement.

Special Considerations in the Critical Care Unit

Electronic Equipment

Treatment of the critically ill patient often requires the use of invasive or intravascular electrical equipment such as pacemakers, the intra-aortic balloon pump, catheters attached to transducers, and ECG machines. These electronic systems are potentially vulnerable to damage from high-energy voltage delivered during external defibrillation, particularly if older equipment is being used. Most new equipment is specifically designed to be protected from electrical damage. It is therefore recommended that the critical care nurse be familiar with the defibrillation protocol in his or her particular unit prior to the occurrence of an emergency situation. In addition, after a patient undergoes defibrillation or cardioversion, the nurse should watch for possible equipment malfunction.

Orientation and Testing

When an emergency such as VF occurs, the length of time between recognition of the dysrhythmia and defibrillation is crucial. The longer VF persists, the less likely it is that electrical defibrillation will be successful. It is highly recommended that every critical care nurse be completely familiar with the equipment and procedure for defibrillation. This information should be included in an orientation program, as should instructions on routine testing of equipment on the unit. The following protocol for testing equipment is recommended by the American Heart Association. Routine maintenance checks should be performed every three months by engineering personnel. Nursing personnel should perform a full energy charge–discharge test at 50 joules every day. More frequent testing may result in increased defibrillation failure because of excessive strain placed on the operational components.

PACEMAKERS

Although cardiac pacing has been in use in the critical care unit for over 25 years, the indications have greatly expanded within the last decade. This change is largely a result of modifications in equipment design, including improvements in electrical circuitry, battery life, and leads. Today, a vast number of types of pacemakers are available. Sophisticated multiprogrammable features have been developed that allow the pacemaker to be individualized for each patient in order to optimize cardiac performance. These newer features will, no doubt, further expand the indications for pacing and increase the number of people in the United States living with pacemakers.

Approximately 202,000 procedures were performed in the United States to insert, maintain, or remove a pacemaker in 1982 [2]. Goldman and Parsonnet [23] report that approximately 100,000 new pacemakers are being implanted each year worldwide. These figures, however, do not distinguish temporary from permanent pacemakers. Temporary pacing is quite common in the critical care unit. All patients who undergo open heart surgery have two or more temporary epicardial pacing wires inserted in the operating room. Hynes and colleagues [30] reviewed the number of temporary pacemaker insertions in the CCU over a five-year period and noted that 11.3% of the pa-

EXHIBIT 13.1
Indications for Temporary Pacing

Acute myocardial infarction

  Bilateral bundle branch block
  Mobitz type II block
  Complete heart block
  Asystole

Bradycardia without myocardial infarction

  Complete heart block
  Atrioventricular block
  Asystole
  Sick sinus syndrome
  Drug toxicity

As prophylaxis during or after the following:

  Cardiac surgery
  Cardiac catheterization
  Diagnostic studies

Tachyarrhythmias:

  For overdrive suppression of atrial and ventricular tachydysrhythmias

tients admitted to the unit required temporary pacing. Of these, almost half (47%) received a permanent pacemaker before hospital discharge.

Our discussion will focus on temporary pacemakers, because this type is more commonly encountered in the critical care unit.

Indications for Use   A cardiac pacemaker is a device that delivers an electrical stimulus to the heart, causing depolarization and cardiac contraction. Normal impulse conduction through the myocardium may be temporarily or permanently altered by a variety of pathological and physiological conditions. Temporary pacemakers are most commonly used prophylactically after myocardial infarction or open heart surgery, and therapeutically for various heart blocks and bradycardias. The specific indications for temporary pacing are listed in Exhibit 13.1.

Classification   *International Pacemaker Code*   ·
In 1974 the Inter-Society Commission for Heart Disease developed a three-position code to identify the many varieties of pacemakers available [47]. Continued technological advances have necessitated expanding the code to five positions to include programmability and tachyarrhythmia functions (Table 13.1). The three-letter code is used most commonly in the clinical area, however, and is sufficient for describing most of the pacemakers in use today [39].

The code provides a shorthand description of pacemaker operation [3]. Letters in the first and second positions indicate the chambers paced and sensed, respectively. The third position describes the mode of response of the pacemaker to sensed cardiac electrical activity. With single-chamber pacing, an inhibited response means that a pacing spike is inhibited when spontaneous electrical activity is sensed. A triggered response means that the pacemaker will

TABLE 13.1
Five-Position Code for Pacemakers

Position	Characteristic Described	Code		
I	Chamber paced	V	=	ventricle
		A	=	atrium
		D	=	atrium and ventricle
II	Chamber sensed	V	=	ventricle
		A	=	atrium
		D	=	atrium and ventricle
		O	=	none
III	Mode of response	I	=	inhibited
		T	=	triggered
		D	=	atrial triggered and ventricular inhibited
		R	=	reverse
		O	=	none
IV	Programmability	P	=	programmable rate and/or output
		M	=	multiprogrammability
		O	=	none
V	Tachyarrhythmia functions	B	=	burst
		N	=	normal rate competition
		S	=	scanning
		E	=	external

From Parsonnet, V., Furman, S., and Smyth, N. P. D. A revised code for pacemaker identification. *PACE* 4:400, 1981. Used with permission.

fire an impulse in response to the patient's own electrical activity. Thus, for example, the pacing spike is delivered into the QRS complex with a VVT pacemaker and into the P wave with an AAT pacemaker. The pacemaker spike, however, is ineffective in producing further contractions because it falls during the intrinsic cardiac refractory period. With dual-chamber pacing, the inhibited or triggered response may function differently, depending on the sensing mechanism of the pacemaker. A "D" in the third position indicates that two modes of response are available: triggered and inhibited. In this case the response is determined by the timing and sequence of sensed activity. None or "O" in the third position indicates that the pacemaker does not sense any cardiac activity, a pattern occurring with fixed rate pacemakers. Reverse, or "R," indicates that the pacer fires in response to fast rhythms and thus is used to interrupt tachyarrhythmias [39].

Older Systems

The new five-position code for pacemaker identification is becoming the accepted classification system. During this period of transition, however, it is important for the nurse to understand older classification systems as well.

In the past, pacemakers have been classified in several ways:

1. By duration of use: temporary or permanent

2. By method of implantation: transthoracic, transvenous, or epicardial

3. By placement of electrodes: endocardial or epicardial

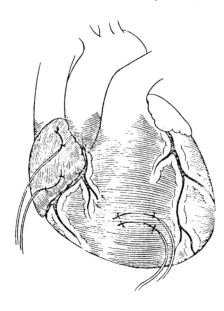

FIGURE 13.2
Epicardial pacing wires, inserted during surgery, are sutured to the right or left ventricular wall. Atrial electrodes are laid on the surface of the right atrium and secured with sutures. They must be secured sufficiently to prevent accidental dislodgment, but they must also be removable when the catgut softens. To ensure proper function, the threshold of each electrode should be tested before closure. (From Behrendt, D. M., and Austen, W. G. *Patient Care in Cardiac Surgery.* Boston: Little, Brown, 1980. Used with permission.)

4. By method of pacing: fixed rate, demand, or synchronous

5. By site of stimulation: atrial, ventricular, or atrioventricular

Methods of Temporary Pacing

Temporary cardiac pacing may be instituted during a cardiopulmonary arrest, prophylactically, or therapeutically and involve the use of one of three methods: (1) transthoracic, (2) epicardial, and (3) transvenous endocardial pacing.

Transthoracic Pacing

Transthoracic pacing is used in emergency situations during cardiopulmonary arrest when circulatory collapse prevents insertion of the wire through a vein. A pacing wire is inserted through the chest wall in the subxiphoid area into the heart. Once embedded in the ventricular wall, the wire is connected to a temporary pulse generator, and pacing is initiated. If the resuscitation effort is successful, a more stable method of pacing, such as transvenous, is initiated once the patient's condition has stabilized. The complications associated with this technique include cardiac tamponade, coronary artery laceration, and pneumothorax.

Epicardial Pacing

During cardiac surgery, when the heart is exposed, wires are attached directly to the epicardial surface of the atrium and ventricle (Figure 13.2). Frequently, two (one atrial and one ventricular) or more wires are attached, brought out through the anterior chest wall, and attached to the pulse generator if needed. Although the pacing wires are inserted as a prophylactic measure, temporary pacing is frequently needed. There is a high incidence of transient dysrhythmias and conduction disturbances after cardiac surgery, conditions that result from direct surgical trauma, cardioplegia, metabolic changes, and electrolyte imbalances. During the immediate postoperative period, pacing may also be used to increase heart rate and augment cardiac output.

The insertion site must be kept covered with a dry, sterile dressing, which is usually changed every 24 to 48 hours. Great care must be taken to prevent infection around the insertion site, because these wires provide a short, direct route to the myocardium. Although temporary pacing is usually necessary only in the first few postoperative days, the wires are left in place until the patient is in stable condition and ready for discharge. The wires are easily removed by pulling them out through the skin. After removal external or internal bleeding may occur. Thus, the nurse must observe the patient closely for signs of cardiac tamponade.

Transvenous Endocardial Pacing

Transvenous pacing is the most common type of temporary pacing and can be easily instituted at the patient's bedside. It is most frequently used in the coronary care unit for transient rhythm, rate, or conduction disturbances. The average duration of temporary pacemaker therapy is three days [30]. Before wire insertion, decisions are made regarding the area of stimulation, which is either ventricular or atrioventricular, and the mode of pacing, which is either fixed rate, demand, or sequential.

Fixed-rate pacing.   Fixed-rate, or asynchronous, pacing can be used to pace the atrium, ventricle, or both (AV sequential). This type of pacemaker delivers an electrical impulse at a preset rate regardless of the patient's intrinsic cardiac rhythm. Thus, if the rate is set at 80 bpm, the pacemaker will stimulate cardiac contraction at this rate continuously. The indications for fixed-rate pacing today are limited. It may be instituted in patients with complete heart block with consistently slow ventricular rates, or patients with normal heart rates who would benefit from an increase in heart rate (for example, to increase cardiac output in the cardiac surgical patient). The major disadvantage of fixed-rate pacing is competition between the pacemaker rhythm and the patient's own rhythm. Heart rate generally increases in response to physiological demands, even in patients with various heart blocks. Consequently, if the patient's intrinsic rate increases, competition occurs because the pacemaker has no sensing ability. Dangerous dysrhythmias, such as VT and VF, may result if the pacing stimulus occurs during the vulnerable period (T wave) of the cardiac cycle.

Demand pacing.   Demand pacing is used much more frequently than fixed-rate pacing and can also be used to pace the atrium, ventricle, or both. The electrodes used for demand pacing have the ability to sense intrinsic cardiac activity. Therefore, the pacemaker will fire only if the patient's intrinsic rate falls below the preset pacemaker rate or interval. The pacemaker circuitry is designed to function with a preset time interval. If, during that interval, no intrinsic cardiac activity is sensed, the pacemaker will fire and cause depolarization. If cardiac activity is sensed, the pacemaker is inhibited from firing and the time interval is reset. Some patients may have the newer type of QRS-synchronous, or R wave–triggered, pacemaker. This apparatus functions in the same way as a regular demand pacemaker, except the pacemaker fires into the

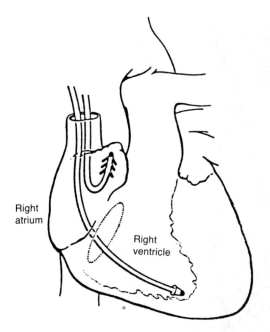

Right
atrium

Right
ventricle

FIGURE 13.3
Atrial and ventricular pacing wires in position.
(From Hawthorne, J. Indications for pacemaker
insertion: types and modes of pacing. *Prog.
Cardiovasc. Dis.* 23:393, 1981. Used with
permission.)

QRS if it senses intrinsic ventricular depolarizations. The pacemaker spike, however, does not stimulate depolarization, because the ventricle is refractory at that time. In this manner, the pacemaker function is altered from beat to beat.

Insertion

A pacing wire is inserted into the antecubital, subclavian, jugular, or femoral vein by a percutaneous stick or cutdown. Each approach has advantages and disadvantages; for example, the femoral route is associated with a high incidence of infection, and the antecubital route is frequently associated with dislodgment of the catheter tip, resulting in loss of capture. Hynes and colleagues [30] report that the lowest incidence of pacemaker-related complications occurs with the right internal jugular approach. During insertion, the tip of the catheter is monitored as to position by fluoroscopy, ECG, or both. The catheter wire is advanced into the heart and lodged in the right atrial appendage or coronary sinus for atrial pacing, or the trabeculae for ventricular pacing (Figure 13.3). The tips of the lead wires come in various designs to ensure stable contact between the electrode and the endocardium (Figure 13.4).

Electrodes are classified as unipolar or bipolar. Recall that electricity flows from a negative pole to a positive pole, or vice versa. A bipolar catheter has a negative pacing electrode at the tip and a positive sensing electrode about 1 cm proximal to the tip [28]. This type of catheter is used most frequently for temporary pacing. With a unipolar system, the intracardiac electrode is negative and the positive electrode is outside the heart. Unipolar systems are more sensitive to intrinsic cardiac activity, because there is a larger surface area between the poles. A more prominent pacer spike on the ECG also results [57]. Bipolar systems may be converted to unipolar systems when sensing problems

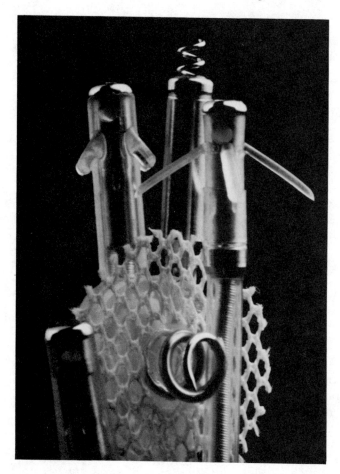

FIGURE 13.4
Several pacemaker electrodes. (Copyright ©
Medtronic, Inc., 1984. Reprinted with
permission of Medtronic, Inc.)

arise or when pacemaker spikes interfere with proper triggering of the intra-aortic balloon pump (Figure 13.5).

Operation

A pacemaker has two major components: a pulse generator and a pacing electrode or wire. The pulse generators used for temporary pacing are external, whereas those used for permanent pacing are internal. The electrical power source, consisting of batteries and electrical circuitry, is contained in the pulse generator. Temporary pacemakers use standard mercury batteries, which have a life expectancy of about one month. Usually a notation is made on the pulse generator of the date on which the batteries have been changed. Extra batteries should be readily available on the unit. The nurse should be familiar with the procedure for changing the batteries, and with the procedure for noting the date of changing. Permanent pacemakers are generally powered with lithium batteries, which have an average life span of seven to ten years.

During insertion, the electrode catheter is attached to the ECG machine by means of an alligator clamp. With this technique, the position of the tip of the electrode can be determined by the current of injury on the ECG tracing

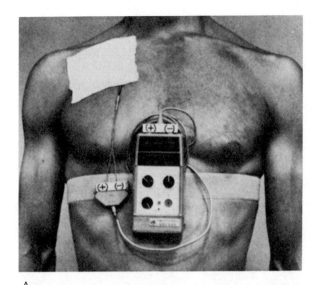

A.

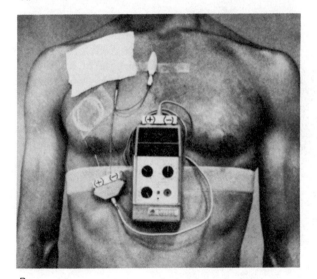

B.

FIGURE 13.5
(A) A bipolar temporary pacing system. Both lead wires, positive ($+$) and negative ($-$), are connected to the pacing cable, which is connected to the positive and negative terminals of the temporary pacemaker. (B) A unipolar temporary pacing system using a Weck electrode for grounding. The negative ($-$) lead wire is connected to the pacing cable, which follows to the negative terminal of the temporary pacemaker. The positive ($+$) lead wire is disconnected from the cable and covered to prevent any possibility of the positive pole receiving an outside electrical current. The positive ($+$) terminal of the temporary pacemaker is grounded via the pacing cable to a Weck electrode, which in this case is stitched to a subcutaneous tissue in the right side of the chest. (From Patros, R. J. Temporary ventricular pacemakers demonstrating bipolar and unipolar modes. *Heart Lung* 12:277, 1983. Used with permission.)

(Figure 13.6). Once the catheter is in the proper position, it is connected to the pulse generator, and various values are set (Figure 13.7).

Rate.   The rate dial is set to a specific value and indicates the number of times the pacemaker will pace per minute. The rate chosen will depend on the specific indication for pacing, the patient's intrinsic rate and rhythm, and the patient's hemodynamic response to various rates.

Stimulation threshold.   The stimulation threshold is evaluated immediately after wire insertion by gradually increasing the value on the output dial on the pulse generator until each pacer spike stimulates contraction. The stimulation

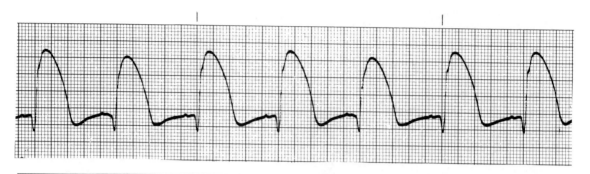

FIGURE 13.6
ECG tracing showing current of injury. Note the marked ST segment elevation; this occurs
when the catheter tip touches the endocardium.

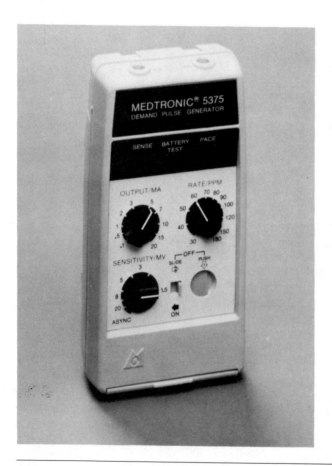

FIGURE 13.7
Values on the pulse generator are set after the pacer is inserted. See text for discussion.
(Copyright © Medtronic, Inc., 1984. Reprinted with permission of Medtronic, Inc.)

threshold (also called the capture level) indicates the amount of current, measured in milliamperes (mA), required to stimulate the chamber being paced. Generally, the lower the threshold, the better the contact between the electrodes tip and the endocardium [57]. Proper position of the catheter tip is indicated by a ventricular threshold of 0.5 to 1.5 mA, whereas a good threshold for atrial capture is approximately 1.7 mA. Because numerous factors can either decrease or increase the threshold, the milliampere level is generally set at two or three times the stimulation threshold needed for capture. If the pacemaker is on standby, the minimum milliampere level needed for capture should be checked frequently and recorded on the patient's chart.

Sensitivity. The sensitivity dial controls the level at which the sensing electrode can accurately detect or sense the patient's own atrial or ventricular activity. This dial is adjusted to allow either demand pacing or asynchronous pacing. The sensitivity is high in the demand mode and low in the asynchronous mode.

Once the rate, output, and sensitivity have been set, the catheter is sutured to the skin and the pulse generator is positioned in a secure place, determined by the insertion site. In addition, the dials on the pulse generator must be protected from accidental movement with some form of covering.

Complications

As with any mode of therapy, the chance of complications exists. Fortunately, complications related to pacemaker therapy occur relatively infrequently and rarely are fatal. In one large study of patients with temporary pacemakers [30], the complication rate was 13.7%. The number of complications increased with increasing duration of pacemaker therapy.

Various complications can occur during catheter insertion. Dysrhythmias, particularly premature ventricular contractions, VT, or VF, may result when the catheter tip irritates the endocardium. Pneumothorax, although rare, can occur with insertion via the subclavian artery. Perforation of the right ventricular wall or septum by the catheter occurs in a very small number of patients. Such an event would precipitate cardiac tamponade and is evidenced in a decreasing blood pressure, an increased pulse, a pericardial friction rub, muffled heart sounds, and a change in the polarity of the pacemaker spike [57]. Hiccoughing and abdominal twitching are other signs of possible perforation; these may also result, however, when the milliampere level is set too high on the pacemaker or the patient has a thin right ventricle, resulting in electrical stimulation of the diaphragm or abdominal muscles.

Once the catheter is inserted and pacing is initiated, additional complications can occur related to the innsertion site or pacemaker malfunction. Infection, phlebitis, thrombosis, bleeding, and hematoma may occur at the insertion site. Dislodgment of the catheter tip may result from excessive movement by the patient and is detected on the ECG.

Malfunction

The most common problems associated with temporary pacing are failure to capture, failure to pace, and failure to sense. Problems with pacing are usually detected by observing a change in the ECG or in the patient's vital signs,

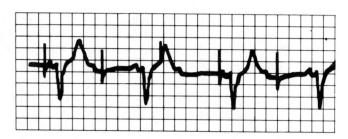

FIGURE 13.8
Failure to capture. Pacing spikes are not always followed by ventricular depolarization. Failure to sense is also evident in this rhythm strip by pacer spikes occurring after the QRS complex. (Copyright © Medtronic, Inc., 1984. Reprinted with permission of Medtronic, Inc.)

appearance, or level of consciousness. The cause of the malfunction should be determined and corrected rapidly.

Failure to Capture
Failure to capture is diagnosed from the ECG by observing pacemaker spikes that are not followed by the appropriate waveforms: either P waves for atrial pacing or QRS complexes for ventricular pacing (Figure 13.8). Failure to capture may result from a low milliampere level, an increase in the threshold needed for capture, dislodgment of the catheter wire, perforation of the myocardium, fracture of the wire, faulty connections, or battery failure. Actions that may correct the problem include increasing the milliampere level, repositioning the patient on his side, securing all connections between the pulse generator and lead wire, changing the batteries or pacemaker unit, and reversing the electrodes on the generator terminals.

Failure to Pace
Failure to pace is indicated on the ECG by the absence of pacemaker spikes or artifact (Figure 13.9). This problem occurs with battery depletion, with loose, broken, or disconnected wires, or if the sensitivity is too high. Interventions that may remedy the situation include checking the on/off switch to make sure the pacemaker has not inadvertently been shut off, changing the batteries, decreasing the sensitivity, and securing all connections between pulse generator and lead wires.

Failure to Sense
Several problems arise when a pacemaker fails to sense appropriately. These include undersensing, oversensing, and improper sensing. Undersensing results because the pulse generator receives inadequate cardiac signals, a problem that may occur if the sensitivity on the pulse generator is set too low. The solution is to increase the sensitivity. Oversensing occurs because the sensitivity is set too high or there is electrical interference. Consequently, the pacemaker senses signals that should be ignored, such as T waves and muscle twitching. The problem may be corrected by reducing the sensitivity on the pulse generator or eliminating electrical equipment that may be causing interference. Improper

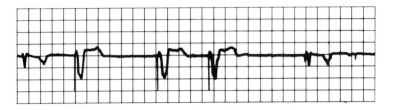

FIGURE 13.9
Failure to pace. Pacing spikes do not occur at regular intervals. (Copyright © Medtronic, Inc., 1984. Reprinted with permission of Medtronic, Inc.)

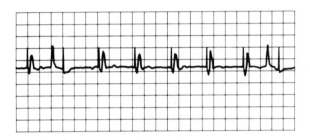

FIGURE 13.10
Failure to sense (undersensing). Note pacemaker spikes after the QRS complexes. (Copyright © Medtronic, Inc., 1984. Reprinted with permission of Medtronic, Inc.)

sensing is indicated on the ECG by pacemaker spikes occurring in inappropriate places, such as after an intrinsic QRS complex or within the T wave (Figure 13.10). This situation is dangerous because ventricular stimulation during the vulnerable period may precipitate ventricular tachycardia or fibrillation. If improper sensing is suspected, the diagnosis should be prompt and the problem corrected immediately. Improper sensing may result from a faulty sensing mechanism in the pulse generator, malposition of the catheter, or if the sensitivity is set too low.

Nursing Responsibilities

Nursing responsibilities for the care of the patient with a temporary pacemaker actually begin prior to catheter insertion. In fact, pacing is often initiated in the critical care unit, whether prophylactically or for treatment of bradyarrhythmias, because the nurse has detected changes in the patient's cardiac rate and rhythm.

Although insertion of a temporary pacemaker is usually performed under emergency or semiemergency circumstances, the nurse should prepare the patient and family as quickly as possible. The patient is informed of the purpose and action of the pacemaker, the duration of use, the insertion procedure, and the site of insertion. The use of sterile drapes during insertion is explained, particularly if the patient's face and head will be covered. Such draping is often a frightening experience, and patients are usually less anxious and more cooperative if properly prepared. Prior to insertion, the pacemaker insertion tray, pulse generator, and catheter are assembled at the bedside. Emergency equipment, although rarely used, should be on standby. Emergency drugs such as lidocaine, atropine, and isoproterenol are made available and ready for use. Finally the ECG machine is attached to the patient.

During catheter insertion, the nurse's primary concern is to watch the cardiac monitor for dysrhythmias, set the dials on the pulse generator, and provide emotional support as well as reassurance to the patient.

Once the catheter is in place, the primary goals of care are (1) to assure proper functioning of the pacemaker, (2) to assess the hemodynamic effect of pacing, (3) to prevent complications, and (4) to provide an electrically safe environment. After catheter insertion, the date, time, and location of insertion, as well as the type of wire, are noted on the nursing care plan. The mode of action, rate, stimulation threshold, and milliampere level are also recorded; the notation is updated if changes are made. Rhythm strips from the monitor are obtained frequently, assessed for proper pacemaker functioning, and placed in the patient's record. The physician will evaluate the patient's condition every day to determine the continued need for the pacemaker as well as verify proper functioning. Depending on the insertion site and the policy of the unit, certain restrictions will be placed on the patient's activity to prevent dislodgment of the catheter from the endocardial wall.

The hemodynamic effect of pacing on the patient is assessed by evaluating blood pressure, pulse, skin color and warmth, mentation, and urine output. If the patient has a thermodilution catheter in place, cardiac output and other hemodynamic variables can be measured directly and correlated with factors such as heart rate.

Another important aspect of nursing care involves prevention of potential complications. (See the previous discussion of complications.) Some complications occur during insertion and are related to technique. After insertion, two major concerns are prevention of infection at the insertion site and prevention of injury to the patient from stray electrical currents. Routine measures involve examining the insertion site for signs and symptoms of inflammation, infection, or phlebitis. Dressings over the area are changed every 24 to 48 hours. During dressing changes, extreme care must be used to prevent movement of the catheter. The patient's temperature is checked and recorded every 4 hours.

The nurse should be aware of the potential electrical hazards associated with temporary pacing and protect the patient from them. In normal individuals, the skin offers protection against small amounts of electrical current leakage. Once the skin surface is broken, however, the patient is vulnerable to electrical skin shocks. Pacemaker wires, attached directly to the heart, provide a direct low-resistance pathway for electric current. Consequently, small microshocks that are generally undetected when applied to the skin can induce VF if contact is made with the myocardium [3]. This situation has two major implications for the critical care nurse. First, specific care must be taken when handling the terminal end of the catheter wire. Rubber gloves are worn when adjusting, connecting, or disconnecting wires from the pulse generator. Temporary epicardial wires, placed in the patient after open heart surgery, are insulated with a rubber glove. Second, all equipment used in the intensive care unit by the patient and nurse must be properly grounded. Personal equipment such as electric radios, televisions, or razors are generally not permitted in the unit unless they have been checked and approved for use by the engineering department.

INTRA-AORTIC BALLOON PUMPING

The introduction of the intra-aortic balloon pump (IABP) in the late 1960s changed the treatment and outcome in cases of low cardiac output and acute myocardial infarction. When first developed, the balloon required a surgical insertion. In 1978, however, the percutaneous technique was developed, simplifying insertion. Consequently, this mode of therapy can be initiated earlier and is available to a larger population of patients.

The balloon is most often inserted into the left femoral artery and positioned in the descending thoracic aorta just distal to the left subclavian artery and proximal to the renal arteries (Figure 13.11). Once attached to the console or pump, the balloon is inflated with helium or carbon dioxide to a capacity of 40 cc. When it is timed to inflate during diastole and deflate prior to systole,

FIGURE 13.11
Balloon positioned in the descending thoracic aorta distal to the left subclavian artery and proximal to the renal arteries.

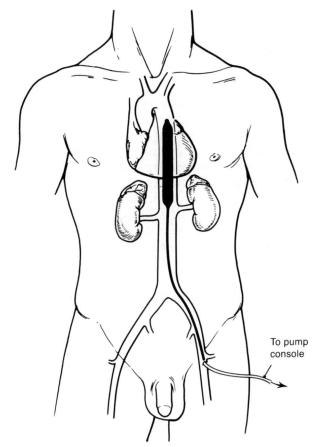

To pump console

the balloon serves two major functions: (1) it increases coronary artery perfusion pressure, and (2) it decreases myocardial workload and oxygen consumption by decreasing afterload. These hemodynamic effects are most beneficial for the following groups of patients.

Indications and Contraindications for Use

The IABP was originally developed for patients in cardiogenic shock. The indications for this mode of therapy have expanded over the years, however, because of the beneficial hemodynamic effects. In the CCU counterpulsation is most frequently used for patients with preinfarction or postinfarction angina, cardiogenic shock resulting from pump failure, and structural defects such as ventricular septal defect, mitral regurgitation, and ventricular aneurysm. This device is also used extensively with the cardiac surgical patient. It may be used preoperatively for patients with cardiogenic shock, intractable angina, severe heart failure secondary to mechanical defect, or acute myocardial infarction [32], or intraoperatively to provide pulsatile flow. Postoperatively, the balloon pump is commonly used if difficulty occurs in weaning the patient from cardiopulmonary bypass, and in cases of low-output syndrome.

The contraindications for the use of the IABP are few: aortic valve insufficiency, aortic aneurysm, and severe peripheral vascular disease.

Physiological Effects of Counterpulsation

The two major physiological effects of counterpulsation are diastolic augmentation and afterload reduction. These hemodynamic effects are a direct result of balloon inflation and deflation and depend on timing these events so that they occur in correct relation to the mechanical events of the heart.

Diastolic Augmentation

Balloon inflation is timed to occur during diastole just as the aortic valve closes. When the balloon inflates, it displaces a volume of blood equal to the balloon volume of 40 cc. The physiological effect of inflation is an elevated diastolic pressure, which in turn increases coronary artery perfusion pressure and improves systemic perfusion. Although coronary perfusion pressure is elevated by balloon pumping, variable effects on total coronary blood flow have been documented [54]. Flow through the coronary arteries may depend primarily on perfusion pressure or on autoregulation. Coronary circulation is autoregulated, meaning that blood flow is regulated automatically in response to tissue needs for O_2. Consequently, flow remains constant even though perfusion pressure varies within a range of 60 to 180 mm Hg [54, 57]. In ischemic and hypotension states, coronary perfusion is pressure dependent. Thus a rise in diastolic pressure increases flow through the coronary arteries and the amount of O_2 supplied to the myocardium.

Afterload Reduction

Balloon deflation is timed to occur just prior to aortic valve opening at the beginning of systole. When the balloon deflates, blood is redistributed from the aortic arch to the space previously occupied by the balloon, resulting in a sudden drop in aortic pressure. This drop enables the left ventricle to eject against a lower pressure (afterload reduction). The beneficial effects are decreased myocardial O_2 consumption and increased stroke volume and cardiac

TABLE 13.2
Hemodynamic Effects of the Intra-aortic Balloon Pump

Increased	Decreased
Diastolic aortic pressure	Afterload, myocardial O_2 consumption
Coronary perfusion pressure	Preload (left ventricular end-diastolic pressure)
Tissue perfusion	Left atrial pressure, pulmonary capillary wedge pressure
Cardiac output	Systolic pressure
Stroke volume	Heart rate
Ejection fraction	Systemic vascular resistance

output. In addition, the improved contractility of the myocardium results in decreased left ventricular end-diastolic pressure (preload), left atrial pressure, and pulmonary capillary wedge pressure. Effective counterpulsation also improves systemic perfusion, a change that may be evidenced clinically in an increased urinary output, improved mentation, and warm, dry skin. The hemodynamic effects of the IABP are outlined in Table 13.2.

Once balloon pumping is initiated, hemodynamic improvement is expected to occur rapidly. In one study of twenty-four patients with cardiogenic shock, marked clinical improvement was evident after 3 to 6 hours and optimal improvement occurred after 18 hours [6]. When the IABP is used in patients with preinfarction or postinfarction angina, pain is usually relieved immediately.

Triggering

Various types and models of balloon pump consoles are available today. Most pumps, however, have two or three methods of triggering or activating the pump. The ECG, the arterial waveform, or an intrinsic pump rate can be used.

In the critical care unit, the most common method of triggering the pump is via the ECG. Before the balloon is inserted, the patient's twelve-lead ECG is examined to determine the lead that maximizes the R wave and minimizes other waveforms (P, T) and artifacts. The ECG signal to the machine can be obtained directly from the patient or from the bedside monitor. Problems with triggering may arise if the patient is being paced. Older balloon consoles interpret any spike of a certain amplitude as an R wave. Consequently, the balloon may trigger twice, once off the pacer spike and once off the R wave. This problem can be resolved by selecting a lead in which the pacer spike and R wave deflections are in opposite directions. Additional problems with balloon triggering have been encountered in the clinical area since the introduction of atrioventricular sequential pacing. Newer consoles have been developed that deal with the problem of pacer spikes by changing the criteria for recognition of the R wave. Activation of the triggering circuit now depends on the amplitude and width of the R wave.

Consistent balloon pumping depends on a regular R-to-R interval. Consequently, balloon pumping may be difficult in the face of certain dysrhythmias and irregular rhythms, such as atrial fibrillation. Tachyarrhythmias may also

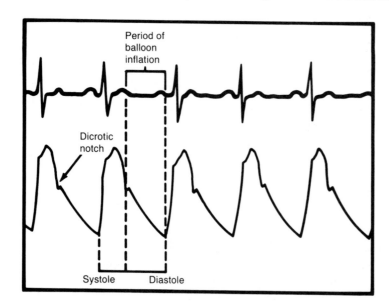

FIGURE 13.12
Arterial pressure tracing and ECG divided into systole and diastole. The dicrotic notch is considered the demarcation between systole and diastole. The balloon is inflated at the onset of diastole and deflated prior to the next systole. Points on the arterial waveform are identified to ensure accurate timing of inflation and deflation.

result in ineffective pumping, because most pumps cannot move the driving gas in and out of the balloon with sufficient speed [52].

The arterial waveform can also be used to trigger the pump. This mode may be used in the operating room during cardiac surgery during termination of cardiopulmonary bypass because electrocautery interferes with an ECG signal.

During cardiac surgery, when the patient is receiving cardiopulmonary bypass, the cardiac contraction has been stopped. Because there is no electrical or mechanical cardiac activity, neither the ECG nor the arterial waveform can be used for triggering. In this situation, balloon pumping can be used to provide pulsatile flow and the internal triggering mode used to make the balloon pump at a continuous rate. The balloon then automatically inflates and deflates at a certain rate.

Timing

To ensure maximal hemodynamic benefit from counterpulsation, the timing of the inflation–deflation sequence must be precisely correlated with the mechanical events of the heart. These events are represented on the arterial waveform and are divided into systole and diastole (Figure 13.12). Timing is set and evaluated in relation to certain points on the arterial waveform. Because there is a delay in the propagation of the waveform from the aortic root to the periphery, the onset of inflation will vary slightly, depending on which artery (aortic, radial, femoral) is being used. When timing from the aortic or radial waveform, inflation should begin just before the dicrotic notch. Inflation is earlier (about 120 msec before the dicrotic notch) with a femoral artery waveform. Deflation is timed to occur just prior to systole. Precise timing will ensure maximal hemodynamic benefit. Timing can be evaluated by examining the arterial waveform with the balloon on a 1:2 assist interval (Figure 13.13).

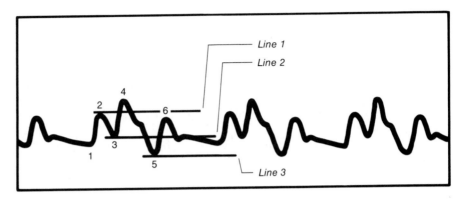

FIGURE 13.13
Several points on the arterial waveform are evaluated, with the balloon on a 1:2 assist interval, to ensure proper timing. 1 = Patients end-diastolic pressure; 2 = peak systolic pressure; 3 = dicrotic notch (balloon inflation begins here); 4 = peak diastolic pressure (augmented by balloon inflation); 5 = balloon assisted end-diastolic pressure; 6 = assisted systolic pressure. The criteria for ideal timing include the following: proper inflation begins at the dicrotic notch (line 2) and proper deflation occurs prior to the next systole. In addition, the assisted systolic pressure (6) should be lower than the peak systolic pressure (2) (line 1). The balloon assisted end-diastolic pressure (5) should be lower than the patient's end-diastolic pressure (1) (line 3). (See Figure 13.14).

Timing should be checked routinely at least every 2-4 hours or if the cardiac index decreases, the triggering mode is changed, the patient develops dysrhythmias, or there is a 20% change in the heart rate [52]. Improper timing can have severe detrimental hemodynamic effects on an already compromised myocardium.

Triggering and timing of the IABP require, then, two factors: (1) a clear ECG signal and (2) an arterial waveform. Although radial arterial lines are used frequently, an aortic arterial waveform can be obtained from the balloon catheter. In the unlikely event that an arterial line is temporarily unavailable, timing can be approximated using the ECG. Inflation is set to occur at the peak of the T wave, and deflation is set prior to the next QRS complex.

Improper Timing
Precise timing of the IABP results in two major hemodynamic benefits: diastolic augmentation and afterload reduction. Improper timing of the inflation–deflation sequence of the balloon has two consequences: (1) there will be no hemodynamic improvement (for example, there will be no increase in coronary perfusion pressure) or (2) there will be detrimental hemodynamic effects (such as an increase in afterload). These effects may occur if either balloon inflation or balloon deflation is too early or too late. These problems are portrayed in Figure 13.14.

Early inflation. Early balloon inflation increases aortic root pressure, which may force the aortic valve closed prior to complete ventricular emptying. Consequently, stroke volume and cardiac output are decreased, left ventricular end-diastolic pressure increases, afterload is increased as is myocardial O_2 consumption.

Late inflation.   When balloon inflation is late, much of the previous stroke volume is already distributed to the peripheral circulation. Consequently, the coronary arteries do not benefit from increased perfusion. In addition, the total time of increased systemic perfusion is reduced.

Early deflation.   When the balloon deflates early, the aortic root refills with blood, increasing the pressure toward normal. Thus, afterload is not reduced, nor is myocardial O_2 consumption. This situation may cause blood to flow retrograde from the coronaries or other arteries.

Late deflation.   Late balloon deflation is very detrimental to the myocardium. If the balloon remains inflated when systole begins, afterload will be increased rather than decreased. Consequently, myocardial workload, O_2 consumption, and preload will be increased. Stroke volume and cardiac output are decreased, and there is delayed opening of the aortic valve.

Complications

Complications can occur during balloon insertion, during pumping, and during and after balloon removal. The complication rate is high: 18.6% to 25% [26, 41, 44]. Although some complications are minor and easily treated, major complications such as aortic dissection and spinal cord paralysis have also been reported [41]. The benefits to the patient must outweigh the associated risks if the decision is made to use this mode of therapy.

The various complications that can occur with counterpulsation can be divided into four broad categories: (1) vascular, (2) infectious, (3) hematological, and (4) miscellaneous.

Vascular Complications

Circulatory insufficiency of the extremity distal to the insertion site is a frequent complication of IABP. It may be due to catheter obstruction of the artery, dislodgment of an atherosclerotic plaque, thrombosis, or embolization. The severity of limb ischemia varies from mild to severe and in rare cases has necessitated amputation of the limb. Thrombi may develop around the balloon if it is not inflating and deflating regularly and may result in embolization if dislodged upon balloon removal. Aortic damage, including dissection or perforation, may also occur. The aortoiliac artery may be dissected during balloon insertion, but the dissection often is not recognized clinically because the patient is asymptomatic [11, 26]. Damage to the aortic arch may result if the patient's head is elevated at an angle of more than 30 degrees, if balloon position distal to the left subclavian artery is not maintained, or if the appropriate balloon size is not chosen prior to insertion.

Infectious Complications

Wound infection at the insertion site is a frequent complication. Based on a sample of 178 patients, Macoviak [41] suggests that the incidence of wound

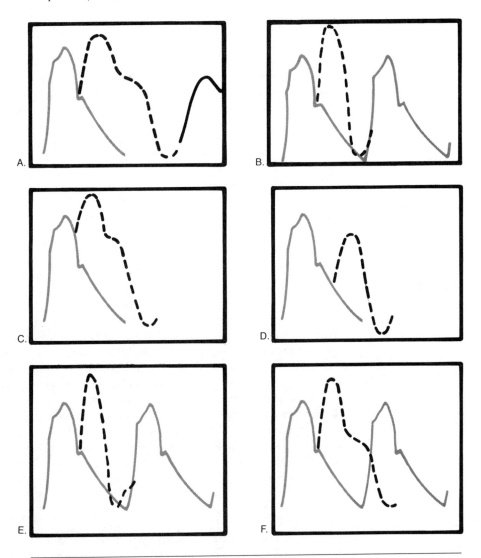

FIGURE 13.14
(A) Proper inflation; (B) proper deflation; (C) early inflation;
(D) late inflation; (E) early deflation; (F) late deflation.

infections increases as the period of IABP use lengthens. Preventative measures, therefore, must be instituted by the medical staff during insertion and by the nursing staff during pumping and until the wound heals after balloon removal. Strict aseptic technique must be maintained during insertion, dressing changes, and removal. Occlusive sterile dressings are applied over the insertion site and changed every 24 to 48 hours. In addition, some physicians advocate the use of antibiotics prophylactically.

Hemotological Complications

Thrombocytopenia and hemolysis frequently result from balloon pumping. The incidence of thrombocytopenia is closely correlated with the length of time counterpulsation is used [11]. Although hematological complications are generally mild, the possibility of persistent bleeding or anemia must be considered. It is recommended that the patient's hematocrit (Hct), hemoglobin level (Hgb), platelet count, prothrombin time (PT), and partial thromboplastin time (PTT) be evaluated on a daily basis and just prior to removal of the balloon.

Miscellaneous Complications

Additional complications occasionally seen with IABP use include balloon leak or rupture, retroperitoneal hematoma, spinal cord paralysis, and renal failure [41].

Patient Management

Responsibilities for balloon operation vary among hospitals. In some institutions, the nursing staff is responsible for total balloon operation; in others, a cardiopulmonary technician is used. Most commonly, however, a nurse and a technician share responsibilities for balloon operation. The technician's primary responsibility is generally machine operation and maintenance, whereas the nurse is in charge of patient management and balloon operation. Nursing management of the patient undergoing counterpulsation is complex. It requires a sound understanding of cardiovascular physiology and balloon operation. The nurse is expected to assess numerous vital signs, correlate and interpret the data, detect subtle changes in the patient's condition, and intervene accordingly. A nursing care plan for the patient can be divided into three major sections: (1) assessment of the patient's physical and psychological status, (2) maintenance of effective balloon pumping, and (3) prevention of complications.

Assessment

The major body systems affected by balloon pumping are the cardiovascular, respiratory, renal, and neurological systems. Assessment of the patient's cardiovascular status and hemodynamic response to counterpulsation involves monitoring several vital signs via a pulmonary artery catheter and arterial line. Vital signs are checked every 30 minutes to 1 hour and include blood pressure, balloon pressures, heart rate, left atrial pressure, pulmonary artery pressures, and cardiac output (CO) or index (CI). If the patient is on the 1:1 mode on the balloon, pressures are recorded in the following order: patient's systolic pressure, peak diastolic pressure, and balloon-assisted end-diastolic pressure (for example, 80/120/50). As previously mentioned, hemodynamic improvement is expected as outlined in Table 13.2. If there is any indication of cardiovascular deterioration, such as increasing pulmonary capillary wedge pressure (PCWP) or heart rate (HR) or decreasing CO, interventions must be planned and implemented quickly. Additional information about the cardiovascular system is obtained by evaluating skin color, warmth, and sensation and peripheral pulses, and by auscultating heart sounds.

Normal respiratory functioning, and consequently tissue oxygenation, is impaired in many critically ill patients. Tissue oxygenation may be impaired because of obstruction, decreased perfusion related to shock, and/or decreased myocardial contractility. The immobility required during balloon pumping further impairs an inadequate exchange of O_2 and CO_2. Consequently, patients frequently require supplemental O_2 or intubation with assisted ventilation. Assessment of the patient's respiratory status is performed frequently and includes observation of the pattern, rate, and rhythm of breathing; auscultation of breath sounds; and evaluation of pulmonary test values, particularly arterial blood gases. Hypoxia and metabolic acidosis are common.

In the critical care area, renal function is evaluated by measuring blood urea nitrogen and creatinine levels, hourly urine outputs, and specific gravities. These variables are monitored closely. Urinary output should be at least 20 to 30 cc per hour. Increased systemic perfusion from counterpulsation improves renal blood flow, and thus an increased urinary output is expected. Sudden decreases in output can be due to a decreased CO, dehydration, a kinked catheter, or balloon displacement, resulting in obstruction of the renal arteries.

Neurological assessment is performed routinely and used as an indicator of cerebral perfusion. Generally, mentation is improved with counterpulsation because of the increased cerebral perfusion with balloon inflation.

Maintenance of Balloon Operation

To maintain balloon pumping with the optimal hemodynamic effect, the nurse must assess the patient and the equipment. Adequate triggering of the console depends on a clear ECG signal. Consequently, patient movement must be minimized, which may require sedation, restraints, or both. The balloon catheter, generally inserted in the left groin, must be protected from kinking and possible dislodgment. If the patient is not completely coherent, such protection may be obtained by applying a loose ankle restraint or a taut sheet over the extremity.

Timing is evaluated at least every 2 to 4 hours and whenever there is a change in the patient's hemodynamic status or in the triggering mode, or a 20% change in heart rate. In the case of any of these changes, the patient is put on the 1:2 mode on the IABP and timing is evaluated from the arterial waveform as previously described. Adjusting timing precisely requires skill and a clear arterial line tracing. The insertion site of a radial arterial line should be protected from movement by immobilization of the arm on an intravenous armboard.

Prevention of Complications

Nursing care of the patient on the IABP must also be directed toward preventing complications. Four major potential complications warranting further consideration are circulatory insufficiency, infection, embolization, and bleeding.

Circulatory insufficiency.   Circulation may be impaired in several arteries because of the position of the balloon in the descending thoracic aorta and the location of the insertion site. Prior to the initiation of balloon pumping, peripheral pulses are carefully assessed. These findings can then serve as a baseline with which subsequent physical findings can be compared. The patient should be monitored frequently for possible obstruction of the left subclavian, carotid, renal, and femoral arteries. Changes in skin color and warmth, pulses, mentation, or urinary output may indicate obstruction. Leg circulation, sensation, and motion should be evaluated frequently, and abnormal findings reported. The head of the bed should not be elevated more than 30 degrees. The patient may be partially turned from side to side every hour with minimal movement at the groin insertion site.

Infection.   Patients frequently develop local wound infections at the insertion site. Strict aseptic technique must be maintained during insertion, wound care, and handling of all equipment. Occlusive dressings over the insertion site are changed every 24 to 48 hours. Dressing or wound contamination in the groin area must be prevented. The Foley catheter should be taped to the opposite leg [52]. Thorough perineal care is recommended prior to dressing changes and twice a day. In addition, the wound should be examined closely for signs of infection. The patient's temperature and white blood cell count are monitored closely. Antibiotics may be administered prophylactically.

Embolization.   The IABP increases the risk of embolization. Clots may develop on the balloon or may be dislodged during balloon insertion or removal. In addition, the patient is immobilized during counterpulsation and frequently for 24 hours after balloon removal. Several prophylactic measures are instituted to decrease the risk of this complication. Most patients are maintained on a continuous intravenous infusion of either heparin or low-molecular-weight dextran. Once the balloon is inserted, it cannot remain in position for any length of time without continually inflating and deflating. When the patient is being transported or if the electrical power source fails, the balloon is switched to battery operation. If both modes are inoperable, the balloon can be inflated and deflated manually every 5 minutes with a 50 cc Luer-Lok syringe. When the patient is being weaned from IABP, inflation and deflation must continue until the moment of balloon removal. In addition to these precautions, most manufacturers have specific guidelines to be followed during counterpulsation to avoid the development of thrombi.

Bleeding.   Bleeding may occur at the insertion site as a result of anticoagulation or upon removal. PT, PTT, Hct, Hgb, and platelet counts are monitored daily and prior to removal, and the patient is observed for signs of bleeding. Urine, stool, and gastrointestinal contents are tested for blood during balloon pumping. Mucous membranes and insertion sites of intravenous lines or any other tubes are examined for signs of blood. In addition, the balloon insertion site is inspected for bleeding, hematomas, and swelling. Retroperitoneal bleeding may occur with balloon removal and may be evidenced only in increased swelling.

Weaning and Balloon Removal

Weaning

The duration of balloon therapy varies for each individual patient. Some cardiac surgical patients in stable condition are weaned on their first postoperative day, whereas patients in cardiogenic shock may require days to weeks of counterpulsation. Most patients, however, are hemodynamically stable and can be weaned from the balloon after one to three days. The weaning process generally involves decreasing the assist frequency from 1:1 to 1:2 to 1:4 to 1:8 (depending on the type of pump used). After each change is made, the patient's hemodynamic status is monitored every 30 minutes, including CO or CI, PCWP, blood pressure, HR, and urinary output. If these variables remain stable with decreased assistance from the balloon, weaning can be continued. Weaning should not be continued if the CO, CI, blood pressure, or urinary output drops below an acceptable value, or if the PCWP or HR increases. All of these variables should be evaluated in conjunction with the appearance of the patient.

Balloon Removal

After a successful weaning period, the balloon catheter may be removed at the bedside or in the operating room. Prior to removal, the patient's PT, PTT, platelet count, and Hct are evaluated, and abnormalities corrected. The catheter and introducer sheath are removed simultaneously, firm pressure is maintained over the area for 15 to 30 minutes, and a dressing is applied. A sandbag is placed over the site for 8 to 24 hours. The groin is inspected every hour for bleeding, swelling, or hematoma formation, and distal extremity pulses are monitored. Bed rest is maintained for 24 hours.

SUMMARY

The IABP is used frequently on a short-term basis to provide circulatory assistance. When timed appropriately, the hemodynamic benefits are remarkable. Prompt relief of angina, increased coronary perfusion, and afterload reduction may interrupt the cycle of cardiogenic shock or acute myocardial ischemia.

The nurse caring for the patient on the IABP must have a firm understanding of cardiovascular physiology and thorough assessment skills, be able to interpret numerous physiological variables, and be able to operate the equipment. A skilled and knowledgeable nurse can maximize the hemodynamic benefit of counterpulsation and minimize complications.

STUDY QUESTIONS

1. What is the physiological basis of countershock?
2. What particular dysrhythmias can be terminated by cardioversion and defibrillation?
3. List the responsibilities of the nurse in preparing the patient for elective cardioversion.

4. During cardioversion, the paddles may be placed in either the anterolateral or the anteroposterior position. Where exactly are these positions on the chest?

5. List three complications of precordial shock.

6. What are the nursing responsibilities involved in the maintenance of the defibrillator in the critical care unit?

7. What is the incidence of temporary pacing in the medical and surgical cardiac patient?

8. What are the major indications for temporary cardiac pacing?

9. Using the Inter-Society Commission for Heart Disease code, explain how the following types of pacemakers function: VDD, DDD, VVI, VOO, DVI.

10. Explain briefly how transthoracic, epicardial, and transvenous pacing are instituted.

11. When initiating pacing, what three values must one set on the pulse generator?

12. List three causes for each of the following: failure to capture, failure to pace, and failure to sense. How can they be corrected?

13. Why is the patient with a temporary pacemaker at risk for electrical hazards, and what can the nurse do to avoid this risk?

14. List the indications and contraindications for IABP therapy.

15. What are the two major physiological effects of counterpulsation?

16. How is the IABP triggered, and how is it timed accurately?

17. How often and in what instances should the balloon timing be evaluated?

18. What variables should the nurse use to evaluate the hemodynamic effect of counterpulsation?

19. List the detrimental effects that can occur from each of the following: early inflation, late inflation, early deflation, late deflation.

20. What are the nursing responsibilities during weaning from the IABP?

CASE STUDY

A 55-year-old male being seen in the emergency unit presents acute retrosternal chest pain, diaphoresis, and nausea. The admitting diagnosis is probable anterior myocardial infarction with right bundle branch block and left anterior hemiblock. As the admitting nurse in CCU, you take report and discover that the physician wants to put in a pacemaker as soon as the patient is in the CCU.

1. What equipment should be gathered for a pacemaker insertion?

2. How will the physician monitor the position of the tip of the catheter?

3. What are the primary nursing responsibilities during pacemaker insertion?

4. What are the primary nursing responsibilities after insertion?

5. Because pacemaker spikes are evident on the ECG right after the QRS complex, you conclude that the pacemaker is not sensing properly. What can cause improper sensing, and what interventions can be employed to remedy the problem?

93

REFERENCES

1. Adgey, A. A., et al. Ventricular defibrillation: appropriate energy levels. *Circulation* 60:219, 1979.

2. American Heart Association, *Heart Facts* Dallas: American Heart Association, 1985.

3. Andreoli, K. G. *Comprehensive Cardiac Care* (5th ed.). St. Louis: Mosby, 1983.

4. Austen, J. L. Analysis of pacemaker malfunction and complications of temporary pacing in the coronary care unit. *Am. J. Cardiol.* 49:301, 1982.

5. Babbs, C. F. Alteration of defibrillation threshold by antiarrhythmic drugs: a theoretical framework. *Crit. Care Med.* 9:362, 1981.

6. Bardet, J., et al. Clinical and hemodynamic results of intra-aortic balloon counterpulsation and surgery for cardiogenic shock. *Am. Heart J.* 93:280, 1977.

7. Bicking, M. The patient on the intra-aortic balloon pump. *Crit. Care Nurs.* 2:50, 1982.

8. Boucher, M. J. Intra-aortic balloon counterpulsation: current practice. *Crit. Care Q.* 2:29, 1979.

9. Bregman, D. Management of patients undergoing intra-aortic balloon pumping. *Heart Lung* 3:916, 1974.

10. Britan, D., et al. Intra-aortic balloon counterpulsation in acute myocardial infarction. *Heart Lung* 10:1021, 1981.

11. Bullas, J. A. Care of the patient on the percutaneous intra-aortic counterpulsation balloon. *Crit. Care Nurs.* 2:40,1982.

12. Chrzanowski, A. L. Intra-aortic balloon pumping: concepts and patient care. *Nurs. Clin. North Am.* 13:513, 1978.

13. Cronin, K., Haagsma, J. L., and Lane, G. H. Defibrillation. *Crit. Care Nurs.* 2:32, 1982.

14. DeSilva, R. A., et al. Cardioversion and defibrillation. *Am. Heart J.* 100:881, 1980.

15. Dorr, K. S. The intra-aortic balloon pump. *Am. J. Nurs.* 75:52, 1975.

16. Eckhardt, E. Intra-aortic balloon counterpulsation in cardiogenic shock. *Heart Lung* 6:93, 1977.

17. Ehrich, D., et al. The hemodynamic response to intra-aortic balloon counterpulsation in patients with cardiogenic shock complicating acute myocardial infarction. *Am. Heart J.* 93:274, 1977.

18. Ewy, G. A. Influence of paddle-electrode location and size on success of cardioversion. *N. Engl. J. Med.* 306:174, 1982.

19. Ewy, G. A., and Taren, D. Comparison of paddle-electrode pastes used for defibrillation. *Heart Lung* 6:847, 1977.

20. Fletcher, G. F., and Murphy, P. Cardiac procedures in acute care situations. *Med. Clin. North Am.* 65:67, 1981.

21. Furman, S. Recent developments in cardiac pacing. *Heart Lung* 7:813, 1978.

22. Gascho, J. A., et al. Determinants of ventricular defibrillation in adults. *Circulation* 60:231, 1979.

23. Goldman, B. S., and Parsonnet, V. World survey on cardiac pacing. *PACE* 2:9, 1979.

24. Gould, K. A. Hemodynamic assessment of IABP timing. *Dimens. Crit. Care Nurs.* 2:205, 1983.

25. Haak, S. W. Intra-aortic balloon pump techniques. *Dimens. Crit. Care Nurs.* 2:196, 1983.

26. Hauser, A. M., et al. Percutaneous intra-aortic balloon counterpulsation. *Chest* 82:422, 1982.

27. Hawthorne, J. W. Indications for pacemaker insertion: types and modes of pacing. *Prog. Cardiovasc. Dis.* 23:393, 1981.

28. Hudak, C. M., Lohr, T., and Gallo, B. M. *Critical Care Nursing* (3rd ed.). Philadelphia: Lippincott, 1982.

29. Hurst, J. W. *The Heart* (5th ed.). New York: McGraw-Hill, 1982.

30. Hynes, J. K., Holmes, D. R., and Harrison, C. E. Five-year experience with temporary pacemaker therapy in the coronary care unit. *Mayo Clin. Proc.* 58:122, 1983.

31. Isner, J. M., et al. Complications of the intra-aortic balloon counterpulsation device: clinical and morphologic observations in 45 necropsy patients. *Am. J. Cardiol.* 45:260, 1980.

32. Kaplan, J. *Cardiac Anesthesia.* New York: Grune & Stratton, 1979.

33. Kaye, W. Invasive therapeutic techniques: emergency cardiac pacing, pericardiocentesis, intracardiac injections, and emergency treatment of tension pneumothorax. *Heart Lung* 12:300, 1983.

34. Kerber, R. E., and Sarnat, W. Factors influencing the success of ventricular defibrillation in man. *Circulation* 60:226, 1979.

35. Kerber, R. E., et al. Elective cardioversion: influence of paddle-electrode location and size on success rates and energy requirements. *N. Engl. J. Med.* 305:658, 1981.

36. Klein, L. R. Temporary AV sequential pacing. *Crit. Care Nurs.* 3:36, 1983.

37. Klein, M. D., and Levine, P. A. When should you use temporary pacemakers after an acute MI? *J. Cardiovasc. Med.* 8:429, 1983.

38. Kroncke, G. M., et al. What to do when your patient's pacemaker stops working. *Nurs' 81* 11:74, 1981.

39. Lasche, P. A. Permanent cardiac pacing: technology and follow-up. *Focus* 10:28, 1983.

40. Lefemine, A. A., et al. Results and complications of intra-aortic balloon pumping in surgical and medical patients. *Am. J. Cardiol.* 40:4l6, 1977.

41. Macoviak, J., et al. The intra-aortic balloon pump: an analysis of five years' experience. *Ann. Thorac. Surg.* 29:451, 1980.

42. Marriott, H. J., and Gozensky, C. Electrocardiogram problems created by pacemakers. *Cardiovasc. Nurs.* 12:1, 1976.

43. Matheney, L. G. Defibrillation: when and how to use it. *Nurs' 81* 11(6):69, 1981.

44. McEnany, M. T., et al. Clinical experience with intra-aortic balloon pump support in 728 patients. *Circulation* 58 (suppl. 1):1–124, 1978.

45. McIntyre, K. M., and Lewis, A. J. *Advanced Cardiac Life Support.* Dallas: American Heart Association, 1983.

46. Mirowski, M., et al. Successful conversion of out-of-hospital life-threatening arrhythmias with the implanted automatic defibrillator. *Am. Heart J.* 103:147, 1982.

47. Parsonnet, V., Furman, S., and Smyth, N. P. D. Implantable cardiac pacemakers: status report and resource guidelines. *Circulation* 50(4):A21-A35, 1974.

48. Parsonnet, V., Furman, S., and Smyth, N. P. D. A revised code for pacemaker identification. *PACE* 4:400, 1981.

49. Parsonnet, V., and Rodgers, T. The present status of programmable pacemakers. *Prog. Cardiovasc. Dis.* 23:401, 1981.

50. Patros, R. J. Temporary ventricular pacemakers demonstrating bipolar and unipolar modes. *Heart Lung* 12:277, 1983.

51. Peter, R. H. When and how to use cardioversion. *Drug Ther.* 10:23, 1980.

52. Purcell, J. A., Pippin, L., and Mitchell, M. Intra-aortic balloon pump therapy. *Am. J. Nurs.* 83:775, 1983.

53. Shilling, E. The external pacemaker: what the nurse needs to know. *Medtronic News* 12:7, 1982.

54. Shiverly, M. The physiological principles of intra-aortic balloon counterpulsation. *Crit. Care Q.* 4:83, 1981.

55. Smyth, N. P. Cardiac pacing. *Ann. Thorac. Surg.* 27:270, 1979.

56. Stack, J. M., et al. Automatic implantable defibrillator for the patient with recurrent refractory malignant ventricular arrhythmias: case report. *Heart Lung* 11:512; 1982.

57. Underhill, S. L., et al. *Cardiac Nursing.* Philadelphia: Lippincott, 1982.

58. Watkins, L., et al. Implantation of the automatic defibrillator: the subxiphoid approach. *Ann. Thorac. Surg.* 34:515, 1982.

59. Winner, J. *Pacemaker Troubleshooting Guide.* Minneapolis: Medtronic, 1981.

60. Winslow, E. H., and Marino, L. B. Temporary cardiac pacemakers. *Am. J. Nurs.* 75:586, 1975.

61. Wulff, K. S. Use of temporary epicardial electrodes for atrial pacing and monitoring. *Cardiovasc. Nurs.* 18:1, 1982.

62. Wulff, K. S. Use of atrial epicardial pacing electrodes after heart surgery. In S. L. Woods (ed.), *Cardiovascular Critical Care Nursing.* New York: Churchill Livingstone, 1983.

CHAPTER 14

Pharmacological Interventions

Laura Rossi

INTRODUCTION

Drug therapy is a cornerstone in the proper management of patients with cardiovascular disorders. During the hospitalization, the nurse assumes a primary role in treatment by ensuring the correct administration of drugs, the proper observation of drug response, and the appropriate preparation of the patient and family should drug therapy be necessary following discharge.

This chapter will present an overview of nursing responsibilities in the administration of drugs and will discuss four categories of cardiovascular drugs: those used in the treatment of cardiac emergencies, coronary artery disease, dysrhythmias, and congestive heart failure.

OVERVIEW OF NURSING RESPONSIBILITIES

Pharmacokinetics

A number of factors are known to affect the action of a particular drug, as well as the patient's response to therapy. Pharmacokinetics is the study of the metabolic processes that determine the concentration of a given drug in the body. Important concepts such as absorption, distribution, biotransformation, and elimination establish the basis for optimal drug selection in a particular situation [19].

The amount of absorption and the onset of action depend on the method of administration, the total amount of the drug administered, the solubility of the drug in body fluids, and the adequacy of circulation. The dose of the drug varies somewhat according to the route and site of administration. The intravenous dose is generally the smallest, with the usual subcutaneous and oral doses increasingly larger.

The degree to which the particular organ or tissue responds to a drug depends on the concentration of drug received by that tissue. Drug distribution occurs primarily by means of diffusion. The rate of diffusion from one fluid compartment of the body to another is directly proportional to the difference in concentration between the compartments and the resistance of a particular compartment to diffusion.

After a drug enters the bloodstream, it may become bound to plasma proteins that hold the drug in an inactive form until its release to the primary receptor in or on the effector cells. Each drug begins some biochemical transformation and elimination from cells the moment the agent is introduced into the body. This process may involve chemical inactivation, transformation into a less effective substance, or excretion from the body unchanged.

Drugs that are not stored (antibiotics, morphine, epinephrine) cannot maintain blood titers within the tissues. When degradation and excretion cause the blood titer to fall, drug action ceases. Plasma concentrations can be used to determine the specific level at which toxicity or drug failure has occurred. This level varies considerably among patients and must be evaluated within the context of the individual situation.

Elimination of drugs occurs primarily through the kidney or intestines. Drugs and their by-products are also eliminated in bile, sweat, saliva, breast milk, tears, and expired air. The rate of elimination is proportional to the drug's concentration at any given moment. The half-life refers to the amount of time required to eliminate half the drug load from the blood. It provides a useful frame of reference for timing the doses to maintain an optimal therapeutic blood level.

The loading dose is the amount of drug administered to achieve initially a given drug level. A maintenance dose is the amount of drug that is necessary to maintain this level over a certain period of time. Generally, four to five elimination half-lives are required to achieve the desired drug level if the usual maintenance dose is given.

Functional Patterns

One of the nurse's most important responsibilities in supervising the follow-up of patients receiving drugs is the ability to perceive lifestyle patterns that potentially interfere with adherence. Gordon's functional patterns [21] have been widely accepted as a comprehensive framework for evaluating patient responses to illness and treatment (Exhibit 14.1).

The category of health status perception and management refers to the patient's perception of the need for treatment and past experiences with medications. Certainly, the patient with a long history of symptomatic coronary disease and a complex medication regimen will have a somewhat different perspective from the young, asymptomatic hypertensive. Previous experience with side effects has a significant effect on the patient's decision to independently discontinue or avoid treatment when dosage titration or supervised withdrawal would have been most appropriate in averting serious consequences. Routine use of certain over-the-counter medications may provoke a variety of drug interactions that also require attention.

EXHIBIT 14.1
Functional Health Patterns Potentially Affecting Drug Regimen Adherence

Health perception/Management

Nutrition/Metabolism

Elimination

Sleep/Rest

Exercise/Activity

Sex/Reproduction

Self-concept/Self-perception

Coping/Stress tolerance

Cognition/Perception

Roles/Relationships

Values/Beliefs

The nutritional metabolic pattern is commonly altered by side effects such as nausea and vomiting. These subtle patient complaints may be attributed to a variety of other causes but frequently serve as early signs of drug toxicity. Changes in eating habits may produce electrolyte imbalances that can result in serious consequences for the cardiac patient.

Changes in the elimination pattern also alert the nurse to the possible development of drug toxicity if excretion is delayed because of liver or renal failure. Diarrhea and constipation have at times been severe enough to warrant discontinuation of a medication. Even the desired increase in fluid excretion produced by diuretics is an inconvenience that distresses many patients regardless of the time of drug administration.

Sleep and rest patterns are frequently disrupted in patients receiving cardiovascular drugs. Different preparations and dosage timings can minimize this effect. A baseline evaluation of this lifestyle pattern is important to the correct choice of drugs for the patient's cardiovascular disorder as well as appropriate intervention to resolve any preexisting sleep problem.

The exercise and activity pattern provides a description of the patient's ability to perform tasks requiring energy expenditure, including daily living practices, mobility, and recreation. This description frequently provides important information regarding the degree of the patient's illness, because cardiovascular symptoms are often produced during some type of activity and relieved by rest. After the initiation of therapy, this pattern will serve as a meaningful index for identifying improvements in the patient's overall functional capacity.

Another important area to assess is the patient's sexual and reproductive pattern, which potentially reveals the use of oral contraceptives or the existence of impotence that may be related to a particular drug regimen. Although frequently overlooked, it is an area of concern to many patients and requires careful assessment before drugs are withdrawn.

It may be difficult to determine the degree to which the patient's self-esteem and self-perception actually interfere with sexual function. Such an effect is more common than one might initially suspect, because of the common fears and misconceptions associated with cardiovascular disease and the perceived dependency on "pills" to prevent a life-threatening catastrophe.

The patient's coping and stress tolerance pattern provides further information and may substantiate impressions that stress is interfering with optimal control of angina or high blood pressure. Alternate interventions such as the teaching of relaxation techniques are frequently necessary as adjuncts to optimize pharmacological therapy.

Data revealing the patient's cognitive and perceptual pattern provide information about the patient's ability to comprehend and use information. Drug teaching requires attention to the patient's motivation and interest as well as his different learning styles and abilities. A variety of printed materials about selected drugs are available through a number of resources, including the American Heart Association, American Medical Association, and many pharmaceutical companies. Informal reinforcement of teaching at the time of drug administration familiarizes the patient with all of the medications received in addition to the ones ordered upon discharge.

The category of roles and relationships includes the patient's entire social network and his responsibilities within it. The reactions of others can affect the patient's medication-taking behavior. Consider the teacher who does not want to take nitroglycerin in front of the class or the elderly man who does not want to alarm his frail wife.

Values and beliefs also affect the patient's decision making about medication taking. Issues frequently center around the extent to which the patient will allow treatment when it interferes with his desired lifestyle.

DRUGS USED IN THE TREATMENT OF CARDIAC EMERGENCIES

Emergency administration of drugs has been described as a great concern to nurses, because the margin for error is extremely small and the potential consequences of an error are devastating [7]. The life-threatening nature of the emergency situation imposes a great deal of stress on the entire health care team. Confidence and patience are extremely important at a time when a high level of performance and skill is critical to the outcome.

Nursing Responsibilities

Although many staff members are needed in an emergency situation, the number of staff at the bedside should be kept to a minimum. One nurse and one physician should be designated to be in charge of coordinating the life-support effort. The physician assumes primary responsibility for the prescription of emergency drug treatment; the nurse assumes the responsibility for the proper preparation and administration of the drugs. These responsibilities may overlap and vary according to hospital protocol and policy.

It is extremely important for the nurse in charge to delegate certain responsibilities. One nurse generally works in a particular area to prepare drugs while another nurse is available to administer the drugs at the bedside. Ancillary staff should be available for the retrieval of intravenous (IV) controllers and pumps as well as drugs and equipment that may not be readily accessible.

Rapid and accurate selection of drugs in an emergency requires a well-organized drug cart. Routine inspection of drugs and other emergency supplies increases one's familiarity with the cart and facilitates prompt and spontaneous drug preparation. Most drugs are now available in prefilled syringes and premixed solutions, which also allows for ready access.

The expertise required for the proper emergency administration of drugs includes skill in the preparation of any necessary equipment as well as knowledge of drug action and incompatibilities. Recent studies suggest that the type of IV container and the technique used for preparing the IV admixture affect the drug concentration infused into the patient. In order to avert undesirable consequences, the following general guidelines are recommended:

1. Avoid adding any medications to a solution that is already infusing.
2. Purposefully invert the container after adding medication, and inspect it carefully before hanging it.
3. Be certain that any medication is appropriately diluted and well mixed before adding it to the infusion fluid [20].

The nurse preparing the drugs must ensure that an accurate account of the time, dose, and response of the patient is being recorded. One must be particularly alert to the rapid onset of action that follows IV administration. It is crucial that all drugs be administered slowly and carefully through the port that is closest (proximal) to the patient, with a clear flush prior to and following the administration of the drug. Clamping the main line will prevent the backflow of medication and any possible incompatibility.

Special caution must be exercised if a lack of IV access temporarily necessitates the simultaneous IV administration of more than one drug [45]. An incompatibility may occur between drugs or between a drug and a solution into which it is being placed. Therapeutic incompatibilities result when two or more drugs produce an unexpected pharmacological response in the patient. Pharmaceutical incompatibilities, which are further classified as physical or chemical, also occur. Such incompatibilities produce changes in the integrity or potency of the active ingredient that are not readily apparent.

Generally, combinations with calcium or calcium salts should be avoided because of the likelihood of precipitate formation. Simultaneous administration with total parenteral nutrition, blood, or blood products is also contraindicated. If immediate IV access is necessary, the drugs should be piggy-backed after the line has been flushed with normal saline.

The nurse at the bedside must be attentive to the ongoing assessment of the patient's progress in order to anticipate the rapidly changing needs and priorities. Taking the initiative to review the drug history with the physician also affords an opportunity to identify possible therapeutic alternatives.

Sodium Bicarbonate

Actions and Clinical Uses

Sodium bicarbonate ($NaHCO_3$) is an extracellular buffer whose metabolism is regulated primarily by the kidney, in order to maintain acid-base balance within the body. It is employed to correct metabolic acidosis, particularly during cardiopulmonary arrest. Although sodium bicarbonate does not reverse the underlying cause of the acid-base disturbance, its use is thought to enhance the patient's responsiveness to other therapeutic modalities, such as drugs and defibrillation [29].

Dosage and Administration

Arterial blood gas values and pH should guide the administration of sodium bicarbonate. These measurements provide specific cues about the extent to which ineffective ventilation is contributing to the imbalance. The initial dose is generally 1 mEq of sodium bicarbonate per kilogram of body weight. Pre-filled syringes containing 50 ml of 8.4% (50 mEq) and 7.5% (44.6 mEq) sodium bicarbonate solution are usually available. If the arrest is observed and resuscitation efforts are initiated promptly, little bicarbonate may be necessary. If the arrest was unwitnessed and arterial blood gas values and pH are unavailable, half of the initial dose may be administered empirically every 10 to 15 minutes [41].

Side Effects

The most common complication of sodium bicarbonate administration is the development of metabolic alkalosis. Serum potassium level may be lowered acutely because of the sudden shift of potassium ions intracellulary. The large sodium load in each dose may precipitate or exacerbate an episode of congestive heart failure. The potential incompatibility with other medications is also an important concern, because sodium bicarbonate is known to inactivate catecholamines and precipitate in solution.

Atropine Sulfate

Actions and Clinical Uses

Atropine is considered to be a parasympatholytic agent that reduces vagal tone by inhibiting the action of acetylcholine. These changes result in an increase in the rate of sinus node discharge and a reduction in atrioventricular (AV) node refractoriness and conduction time.

Atropine is used in the treatment of sinus bradycardia, particularly if associated with significant reduction in blood pressure or increased ventricular ectopy during acute myocardial infarction [12]. It is also useful in the presence of high degrees of AV block.

Dosage and Administration

The usual dose of atropine is 0.5 to 0.8 mg intravenously. Smaller doses are known to produce a paradoxical sinus node slowing and AV conduction delay [55]. Following the initial dose, an additional 0.3 to 0.5 mg may be given to a maximum dose of 2.0 mg unless the desired effect or an adverse reaction occurs.

The intramuscular route of administration has been used frequently in preoperative preparation; the desired cardiovascular effects generally are not achieved, however, until twice the usual intravenous dose has been administered. The onset of action is almost immediate, with action persisting for anywhere from 2 to 24 hours.

Side Effects

The side effects of atropine administration may include urinary retention and also dryness of the mouth, skin, mucous membranes, and bronchial secretions, which is what makes the drug so beneficial in preoperative preparation. Pupillary dilation, acute glaucoma, mental confusion, and delirium have also been described. During an acute myocardial infarction, there is concern that increasing the heart rate will cause further ischemia and tachydysrhythmias [39].

Calcium Chloride

Actions and Clinical Uses

Calcium ions are extremely important in generating the action potential, coupling myocardial excitation and contraction, and maintaining tone in vascular smooth muscle cells. In emergency situations it is useful because of its ability to enhance myocardial contractility and ventricular automaticity. It is particularly effective in the treatment of electromechanical dissociation, in which an orderly electrical rhythm is present without a corresponding mechanical contraction. In some situations ventricular standstill may also be responsive to the administration of calcium [9].

Dosage and Administration

Calcium chloride is generally administered as an intravenous bolus in a dose of 5 to 7 mg/kg. Prefilled syringes usually contain 10 ml of 10% solution, which contains 13.6 mEq of calcium (100 mg = 1 ml). The initial dose can be repeated at 10-minute intervals as necessary.

Although other calcium salts are available, calcium chloride is preferred because it has been shown to result in higher and more predictable plasma levels [66]. If intramuscular injection is required, calcium gluconate should be given, because it is less irritating to the subcutaneous tissue.

Side Effects

Excessive slowing of the heart rate may occur if calcium is administered too rapidly. Additional caution is warranted if the patient is receiving digitalis. The administration of calcium necessitates careful attention in order to avoid possible drug interactions, particularly with sodium bicarbonate, which will precipitate.

ADRENERGIC-STIMULATING AGENTS

Since the description of adrenergic receptors over thirty years ago, a number of perspectives on the effects of pharmacological agents on the sympathetic nervous system have evolved [70]. Drugs that stimulate the sympathetic receptors are categorized as sympathomimetic amines (agonists), which stimulate the adrenergic receptor sites, and sympatholytic agents (antagonists) which block the receptor sites. Catecholamines are all amines that serve as hormones or neurotransmitters. Endogenous or naturally occurring catecholamines, such as epinephrine and norepinephrine, are secreted by the adrenal medulla.

Any physiological effect depends on the specific adrenergic receptor sites being stimulated. Receptors have been classified as alpha and beta adrenergic and dopaminergic according to their location, physiological actions, and responsiveness to different catecholamines. Alpha receptors are located in the smooth muscle of the arterioles, where stimulation results in arteriolar constriction. They are further classified as alpha 1 and alpha 2 according to their location on the membrane of the effector cell and the sympathetic neuron.

Beta-adrenergic receptors have also been further classified, into beta 1 and beta 2 types. This categorization allows for the identification of different levels of responsiveness to drugs and facilitates appropriate prescription in the clinical situation. Beta 1 receptors are located in the heart, where stimulation will produce increases in heart rate, contractility, and AV node conduction and decreases in refractoriness. Beta 2 receptors are located in the blood vessels and lung, where stimulation produces arteriolar and bronchiolar dilation.

Dopamine receptors are located in the renal and mesenteric vascular beds. Stimulation of these receptors causes vasodilatation in these areas and results in an improvement in blood flow to the kidneys and the gastrointestinal tract.

Although sympathomimetic amines are most commonly administered for their cardiovascular effects, they may be used in other preparations, such as decongestants or appetite depressants. The effects of these agents on the central nervous system also make them very useful in the treatment of narcolepsy and parkinsonism. Nurses should have an awareness that the cardiovascular effects may be demonstrated in any persons taking these drugs.

Epinephrine

Actions and Clinical Uses
Epinephrine is an endogenous catecholamine that has been employed in the treatment of cardiac arrest for many years [34]. It possesses both alpha- and beta-stimulating actions. The drug's effect is related to the dose as well as to reflex circulatory adjustments following administration. In smaller doses, beta stimulation results in dilatation of the arterial vessels in skeletal muscles and a subsequent lowering of blood pressure. Larger doses tend to stimulate the alpha receptors, increasing peripheral resistance and blood pressure.

Generally, one expects an increase in heart rate and blood pressure and an improvement in the strength of myocardial contraction following the administration of epinephrine. It is used to stimulate spontaneous contraction during ventricular standstill and to restore contractility in pulseless idioventricular rhythms. During the resuscitation effort, epinephrine is thought to convert the fine, low-voltage ventricular fibrillation to a coarse, high-voltage ventricular fibrillation that is more amenable to defibrillation. Epinephrine is also indicated for the treatment of bronchospasm associated with anaphylaxis.

Dosage and Administration
The initial dose of epinephrine is 0.5 to 1.0 mg intravenously, which can be repeated every 5 minutes because of the drug's short duration of action. This dose is the equivalent of 5 to 10 ml of 1:10,000 solution, an amount commercially prepared in prefilled syringes. If an IV access is not readily available, epinephrine may be administered intratracheally via an endotracheal tube or directly into the heart through the fourth intercostal space [56].

Epinephrine is also available in 1 ml ampules containing 1 mg in 1:1,000 solution, which are very useful in the preparation of a continuous infusion. The infusion (usually 1 mg in 250 ml 5% dextrose in water [D_5W]) is started at a rate of 1 μg per minute and gradually increased to 3 to 4 μg per minute as necessary. Epinephrine should always be administered through a long IV catheter inserted into a deep vein. Extravasation of epinephrine into the subcutaneous tissues has been associated with necrosis of tissues.

Side Effects

Perhaps the most serious side effects result from the use of intramyocardial injection, which not only interrupts chest compression and ventilation, but also potentially causes coronary artery laceration, tamponade, and pneumothorax. The inherent stimulating effects of ephinephrine may also exacerbate ventricular dysrhythmias and precipitate myocardial ischemia because of the increased myocardial oxygen consumption. The risk of compromising renal blood flow exists because of the reflex circulatory adjustments that occur following administration. Central nervous system effects such as fear, anxiety, tension, tremor, and weakness have also been reported.

Norepinephrine

Actions and Clinical Uses

Norepinephrine (Levarterenol, Levophed) is also an endogenous catecholamine that possesses both alpha- and beta-adrenergic effects. It is different from epinephrine in that it apparently has a greater effect on the alpha receptors. Norepinephrine produces marked vasoconstriction, which promptly increases systolic and diastolic blood pressure and total peripheral resistance.

Cardiac output generally remains unchanged, although it may increase or decrease depending on the extent of the increased blood flow and the functional state of the left ventricle. As the blood pressure increases, there may be a carotid baroreceptor–mediated slowing of the heart rate. Although coronary blood flow may improve, renal, cerebral, and visceral blood flow is reduced.

The primary indications for the use of norepinephrine are hypotension and shock. Agents such as dopamine and dobutamine hydrocloride are being used more frequently because of their potential to reduce the resulting damage to the renal and mesenteric vasculature [48]. Norepinephrine may be most useful in situations in which the total peripheral vascular resistance is low.

Dosage and Administration

Norepinephrine is available in 4 mg ampules, which are used in the preparation of a continuous infusion. Two ampules in 500 ml D_5W produces a concentration of 16 μg/ml, which can be administered as the initial dose. The drug necessitates careful observation because of the rapid onset and cessation of action and the need to titrate dosage according to the patient's responses. Hemodynamic monitoring is generally used to guide therapy. A systolic blood pressure of 90 mm Hg is usually considered to be a reasonable index for titration, although this may vary according to the patient's clinical situation and physician's preference.

Side Effects

The increased contractility and left ventricular wall tension may significantly increase myocardial O_2 consumption, which presents particular difficulties in the treatment of myocardial infarction.

Extravasation of norepinephrine is known to produce ischemic necrosis and sloughing of superficial tissues at the site of injection. Therefore, it is usually recommended that norepinephrine be administered through a long IV catheter that is inserted into a deep vein. When sloughing does occur phentolamine 5 to 10 mg in 10 to 15 ml of saline solution should be infiltrated into the area of extravasation in order to decrease or prevent damage [41].

Isoproterenol

Actions and Clinical Uses

Isoproterenol (Isuprel), a synthetic sympathomimetic, acts as a beta-adrenergic stimulator with potent inotropic and chronotropic properties. Isoproterenol reduces peripheral vascular resistance and diastolic pressure, which enhances the increase in cardiac output and systolic pressure that is generally observed. Its effect in relaxing the smooth muscle of the bronchi makes it very effective as a local inhalant for patients with bronchospastic lung disease.

Clinically, isoproterenol is most frequently indicated for the treatment of hemodynamically significant bradycardia unresponsive to atropine. It is of limited usefulness in the treatment of myocardial infarction because of the resulting increases in O_2 consumption and the risk of extension or continued ischemia.

Dosage and Administration

Isoproterenol is available in 1 mg ampules, which are used to prepare a continuous infusion. Two ampules in 500 ml D_5W yields a 4 μg/ml drip. The infusion should begin at a low dosage, such as 2 to 4 μg per minute, and gradually be titrated according to the patient's heart rate and cardiac rhythm response. A heart rate response of 60 bpm may be arbitrarily considered an index for titration; this may vary in each situation, however [41]. Isoproterenol for sublingual administration (2.5 mg) is also available and may be useful when an IV line is not available.

Side Effects

Cardiac dysrhythmias frequently develop or worsen with the administration of isoproterenol. The profound stimulating effects also require that the drug be administered with great caution, particularly in the setting of an acute myocardial infarction.

The peripheral vasodilating effects of isoproterenol potentially cause hypotension if hypovolemia is present. Other circulatory changes, such as headaches, flushing, angina, tremor, dizziness, and diaphoresis, frequently occur because of the nature of the drug's effect and may be dose related.

Dopamine

Action and Clinical Uses

Dopamine (Intropin) is an endogenous catecholamine that is the immediate precursor of norepinephrine. Its cardiovascular effects result from the stimulation of alpha- and beta-adrenergic and dopaminergic receptors. The unique effect of dopamine is its ability to dilate the renal and mesenteric blood vessels. Its actions are known to vary depending on the individual patient and the dose being administered.

In the emergency setting, the primary indication for the use of dopamine is hypotension that results from cardiogenic, septic, or traumatic shock [46]. In small doses (0.5 to 2.0 μg/kg per minute) dopamine is used as a temporary measure to treat long-standing congestive heart failure that is refractory to conventional treatment with digitalis, diuretics, and oral vasodilators.

Dosage and Administration

Dopamine is available in 5 ml ampules containing 200 mg which are used in the preparation of a continuous infusion. A concentration of 800 μg/ml (400 mg in 500 ml D_5W) is commonly used for an initial infusion that may begin at a rate of 2 to 5 μg/kg per minute. The infusion is then increased and titrated until the patient's hemodynamic signs reach optimal levels.

In doses of 7 to 10 μg/kg per minute, dopamine tends to have a greater effect on the dopaminergic and beta-adrenergic receptors, which is helpful in improving contractility, cardiac output, and renal blood flow. At higher doses alpha-adrenergic effects are more apparent, with greater peripheral vasoconstriction and a higher arterial blood pressure. It is believed that when more than 20 μg/kg per minute is administered, the dilatory effect on the renal and mesenteric vessels is reversed and blood flow to these areas is compromised.

Side Effects

The most serious adverse effects of dopamine are related to the risk of cardiac dysrhythmias and increased ischemia that occurs as a result of the drug's direct stimulating effects on the heart. Tissue necrosis and sloughing may also occur with extravasation of the drug during administration.

In certain situations, such as when pheochromocytoma exists, dopamine may precipitate a serious hypertensive response and is generally contraindicated. Monomine oxidase inhibitors are also known to potentiate the effects of dopamine so that a very small proportion of the usual dose can be expected to produce a beneficial effect. As with all other vasopressors, hemodynamic monitoring and IV controllers are used to ensure safe administration.

Dobutamine

Actions and Clinical Uses

Dobutamine, (Dobutrex) is a synthetic catecholamine that acts directly on the beta receptors of the heart. As a direct beta-adrenergic agonist, it increases myocardial contractility and cardiac output. Unlike other sympathomimetics, however, it does not produce chronotropic or peripheral vasoconstricting effects [62]. This characteristic makes it extremely useful in the short-term treatment of refractory congestive heart failure, particularly in the presence of depressed ventricular function and myocardial contractility.

Dosage and Administration

A 20 ml vial containing 250 mg is reconstituted and added to 500 ml of D_5W to produce a concentration of 500 μg/ml. The infusion may be started with a small dose of 0.5 μg/kg per minute and gradually increased to the 2.5 to 10 μg/kg per minute range as necessary [26].

Side Effects

Like other agents that stimulate beta-adrenergic receptors, dobutamine may produce tachyarrhythmias. Caution should be exercised in the treatment of myocardial infarction, because it remains unclear whether dobutamine has any significant effect on infarct size [18].

DRUGS USED IN THE TREATMENT OF DYSRHYTHMIAS _____

Management of cardiac dysrhythmias is based on an understanding of the specific electrical abnormalities and the corresponding mechanical consequences. The prime deleterious effect of any dysrhythmia is generally attributable to the resulting inability of the heart to maintain adequate circulation of blood to the body. As antiarrhythmic therapy becomes more complex, it bcomes increasingly important for nurses to understand the physiological factors that serve as a basis for treatment (see Chapter 8).

Nursing Responsibilities

With the advent of various monitoring modalities, such as telemetry, trendscription, and Holter monitoring, nurses must recognize that the identification and treatment of complex dysrhythmias is not confined to the critical care unit phase of hospitalization. Nursing responsibilities will involve continuous electrocardiographic (ECG) monitoring, early emergency intervention, and the assessment of a patient's responses to the dysrhythmias as well as to drug therapy.

Specific descriptions of ECG changes and a comparison with previous ECG tracings is particularly important in documenting drug effect. The evaluation should include attention to the changes in each complex, the different leads in which the changes occur, and the relationship of the changes to the patient's symptoms, activities, and medications.

ECG monitoring should also include the measurement of all intervals. This occasionally requires that twelve-lead ECGs be obtained more frequently for a clear examination of T waves. The patient's past pattern of dysrhythmia initiation must be kept in mind. For example, did a gradual prolongation of the QRS/QT interval or an increased frequency of ventricular premature beats precede the episode of ventricular tachycardia?

It is now common practice for nurses to participate actively in the early emergency treatment of specific cardiac dysrhythmias. Nursing intervention in these situations is generally determined by hospital policy, which includes specific guidelines for emergency medication administration, defibrillation, and cardioversion.

An accurate assessment of the patient's responses also involves documentation of factors related to sympathetic nerve stimulation and acid-base imbalance that may contribute to an unpredictable cardiovascular response. Autonomic nervous system changes induced by emotional stimulation such as pain and anxiety, drugs, or endocrine disorders can lower the patient's threshold for dysrhythmia development. Knowledge of various drug actions, interactions, and toxicities is important in understanding the treatment plan, because antiarrhythmic agents can cause more severe dysrhythmias with unpredictable responses [58].

Subjective complaints of angina, fatigue, or dizziness, or symptoms of increasing cardiac failure, may be early signs of hemodynamic compromise. Skin color and the state of the sensorium can provide additional cues about the effectiveness of myocardial contraction. Correlation with the quality and regularity of peripheral pulses, vital signs, and pressure values serves as a basis for evaluating the hemodynamic response and initiating emergency treatment if called for.

The patient's symptoms of light-headedness, ataxia, confusion, palpitations, and syncope can provide markers for evaluating the need for dysrhythmia control. They can provoke a considerable amount of anxiety in the patient and family and also can increase the risk of physical injury should a serious dysrhythmia suddenly occur. At the same time, these symptoms can provide the patient and family with a warning signal that, if reported early, potentially can decrease the chances of a catastrophic episode.

Lidocaine

Actions and Clinical Uses

Lidocaine hydrochloride (Xylocaine) is well recognized as a first-line drug in emergency treatment of simple and complex ventricular dysrhythmias, including those related to digitalis intoxication [11]. Although the specific mechanism of lidocaine's antiarrhythmic effect is not entirely clear, the drug is thought to decrease automaticity by slowing the rate of spontaneous phase 4 diastolic depolarization. Lidocaine has also been shown to reduce conduction velocity and increase refractoriness, which produces a beneficial effect on the suppression of reentrant tachyarrhythmias.

Most recently, lidocaine's ability to reduce the degree of excitability in ischemic tissue has been recognized as a means for evaluating the threshold for developing ventricular fibrillation [33]. Lidocaine prophylaxis is now commonly used in the period following acute infarction to reduce the incidence of ventricular fibrillation. Some centers now routinely discharge all patients with a diagnosis of coronary artery disease with a self-injector of lidocaine in the event of a myocardial infarction [68].

More selective use of lidocaine prophylaxis has been recommended, however, in order to reduce the potential for unnecessary complications related to toxic reactions. It has been suggested that younger patients (40 to 50 years old) without prior history of failure or acute myocardial infarction who are seen within 4 to 6 hours of the onset of chest discomfort are at highest risk for the development of ventricular fibrillation, and therefore are the best candidates for prophylaxis. The risk of ventricular fibrillation appears reduced in elderly patients, who may show toxic effects more easily [1].

Generally, lidocaine is not used in the treatment of supraventricular dysrhythmias, although there have been isolated reports both of its effectiveness in the control of paroxysmal atrial tachycardia associated with Wolff-Parkinson-White syndrome and of the conversion of atrial fibrillation to normal sinus rhythm after lidocaine administration [28]. In usual clinical doses, lidocaine does not appear to have any marked effects on myocardial contractility, arterial blood pressure, or atrioventricular or intraventricular conduction.

Dosage and Administration

Lidocaine is usually administered intravenously, although it may be administered by means of intramuscular injection. The intramuscular route is avoided because of the subsequent difficulties in establishing the diagnosis of infarction by means of serum enzyme levels.

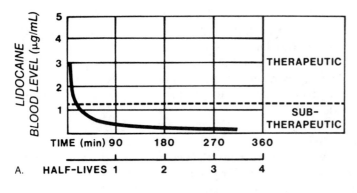

A.

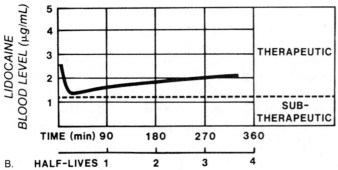

B.

FIGURE 14.1

Effect of lidocaine injection, and timing on estimated blood levels. (A) Estimated blood levels of lidocaine following 100 mg bolus injection (man of average weight). (B) Estimated blood levels of lidocaine following 100 mg bolus injection and 2 mg per minute infusion (man of average weight). (From McIntyre, K. M., and Lewis, A. J. *Textbook of Advanced Cardiac Life Support.* Dallas: American Heart Association, 1983. Used with permission.)

A loading dose of lidocaine (1 mg/kg) is generally administered in a bolus injection of 50 to 100 mg and followed by a continuous infusion of 1 to 4 mg per minute (20 to 50 μg/kg per minute). Lidocaine is commercially prepared in a number of ways, which vary in usefulness according to the particular clinical setting. Prefilled syringes containing 50 mg (5 ml) or 100 mg (10 ml) of 1% lidocaine are available for bolus injection. For the preparation of continuous drip, vials and syringes containing 1 or 2 gm of lidocaine are useful, depending on whether the solution for the admixture is in bottles or bags. Lidocaine drips are also now available in premixed solutions of 250 or 500 ml of D_5W.

The half-life of lidocaine is approximately 8 minutes. A single bolus injection is not considered to be sufficient to maintain a therapeutic blood level and must be followed by a continuous infusion [5] (Figure 14.1). If marked ventricular dysrhythmias occur during this period, an additional 50 mg bolus (0.5 mg/kg) may be administered every 5 minutes if necessary to reach an appropriate therapeutic level up to a total dose not exceeding 225 mg. The continuous drip should be increased by 1 mg per minute following each bolus, with the total infusion not to exceed 4 mg per minute [68]. Lidocaine is metabolized by the liver and excreted in the urine, so that dosage adjustment may be necessary in patients with hepatic or renal failure.

Side Effects

The earliest signs of lidocaine toxicity are central nervous system effects such as drowsiness, disorientation, and slurred speech. Paresthesias and muscle twitching may progress to focal and grand mal seizures and frequently have been related to the rate of administration. Symptomatic treatment and withdrawal of lidocaine are indicated in such situations.

The nature of lidocaine's pharmacological effect warrants caution during its administration to patients with documented conduction system defects. Hypotension and bradycardia may also occur in some patients who are hypersensitive or prone to toxic reactions.

Bretylium Tosylate

Actions and Clinical Uses

Originally introduced as an antihypertensive agent, bretylium (Bretylol) is now considered to be extremely useful for the emergency management of life-threatening ventricular tachycardia and ventricular fibrillation [50]. The exact mechanism of bretylium's antiarrhythmic effect is not entirely understood but is thought to be related to the drug's direct inotropic effect on the heart as well as on the autonomic nervous system.

The suppression of dysrhythmias likely is due to bretylium's effect on the adrenergic nerve terminals rather than to a direct effect on the cell membrane. Experimental models have demonstrated an elevation in the threshold for ventricular fibrillation, however, which occurs independent of any adrenergic effects. Bretylium's effects also involve an increase in the action potential duration and the refractory period.

Dosage and Administration

Bretylium is not considered to be a first-line drug in the emergency management of dysrhythmias and is generally used when lidocaine and procainamide hydrochloride have been ineffective. Its major advantage is its ability to facilitate the conversion of ventricular fibrillation by defibrillation. The initial dose of bretylium is usually a 5 mg/kg bolus administered intravenously, with treatment repeated in doses up to 10 mg/kg if ventricular fibrillation persists in spite of the initial dose followed by countershock. This dosage can be increased to a dose of 30 mg/kg to be repeated at 30-minute intervals.

Maintenance therapy may be administered at 6- to 8-hour intervals by diluting the medication in at least 50 ml of D_5W and infusing the 5 to 10 mg/kg dose over a period of 8 to 10 minutes. If necessary, a continuous drip of bretylium can be prepared with 500 mg (10 ml) in 500 ml of D_5W and infused at a rate of 1 to 2 mg per minute.

Side Effects

The most serious side effects of bretylium are related to its adrenergic effects, which may initially increase the heart rate and blood pressure but later result in postural hypotension because of the peripheral vasodilatation. The hypotension is usually responsive to assumption of the supine or Trendelenburg position and the IV administration of fluids if necessary. Nausea and vomiting may occur during the rapid administration of the drug in conscious patients.

Verapamil

Actions and Clinical Uses

Verapamil hydrochloride (Isoptin, Calan) is a calcium channel or slow channel blocking agent that has been found to be extremely useful in the treatment of supraventricular dysrhythmias. It produces electrophysiological and hemodynamic effects by virtue of its ability to block the influx of calcium into the cell and its contractile mechanism. Verapamil exerts its specific antiarrhythmic action by slowing conduction and enhancing refractoriness in the AV node [40].

Clinically, it is very useful in terminating AV node reentrant tachyarrhythmias as well as slowing atrial fibrillation and atrial flutter. It does not appear to be particularly helpful in patients with Wolff-Parkinson-White syndrome.

Verapamil's ability to relax vascular smooth muscle and thereby produce coronary and peripheral vasodilatation results in beneficial hemodynamic effects that reduce contractility and myocardial O_2 consumption. These effects will be discussed further in the section describing drugs used in the treatment of coronary artery disease.

Dosage and Administration

Verapamil is approved for IV administration only in the treatment of supraventricular dysrhythmias. The initial dose is 0.075 to 0.15 mg/kg, administered as an IV bolus over 1 minute. The peak effect is thought to occur within 3 to 5 minutes. If the dysrhythmia persists, a continuous drip may be infused at a rate of 5 μg/kg per minute.

Side Effects

The intrinsic nature of verapamil's actions warrants careful monitoring initially in order to identify any adverse hypotensive responses. Although the vasodilatation that occurs is thought to compensate for any potential depression of myocardial contractility, the administration of verapamil can exacerbate an episode of congestive heart failure in predisposed patients. The use of verapamil should also be avoided in patients with sick sinus syndrome and AV node dysfunction.

Quinidine

Actions and Clinical Uses

Quinidine (quinidine sulfate, quinidine gluconate; Quinidex, cardioquin) produces a depression of phase 4 in cells, demonstrating automaticity and a reduction in the rate of depolarization and the overshoot during phase 0. Membrane responsiveness is reduced, elevating the threshold for excitability. There is little effect on the action potential duration or the duration of the absolute refractory period at therapeutic concentrations.

Clinically, increases in the QRS duration reflect the conduction slowing that predominates in the atrial, Purkinje, and ventricular muscle fibers and has been correlated with therapeutic levels. Increases in the QT interval demonstrate repolarization changes, which indicate toxicity if markedly prolonged.

Quinidine is used in the treatment of atrial flutter, atrial fibrillation, premature atrial contractions, paroxysmal atrial tachycardia associated with Wolff-Parkinson-White syndrome, and all forms of ventricular ectopy [60]. Anticholinergic and vagolytic effects can also occur with quinidine administration. These effects have their greatest clinical significance in the treatment of atrial flutter and fibrillation, when the ventricular response rate increases because of enhanced conduction across the AV node. For this reason, digitalization is usually required to maintain control of the ventricular rate.

Although quinidine is known to slow the atrial rate in atrial fibrillation, it does not consistently restore normal sinus rhythm. But quinidine can suppress premature atrial contractions thought to trigger the dysrhythmias and can maintain sinus rhythm occurring spontaneously or following cardioversion.

Dosage and Administration

A number of quinidine preparations are available (Table 14.1). Quinidine sulfate is typically administered orally every 6 hours in 200 to 300 mg doses. Loading doses of 200 mg every 2 hours for five doses have been used in attempts to convert atrial fibrillation chemically. Peak plasma levels occur approximately 1 to 2 hours following oral or intramuscular administration. Gastrointestinal absorption is almost complete, whereas intramuscular absorption generally produces lower peak plasma levels. Intravenous administration is rarely used because of the risk of adverse hemodynamic effects.

The plasma half-life of quinidine is 5 to 6 hours. Metabolism occurs primarily in the liver, with most of the drug being excreted in the urine. Concomitant administration of digoxin and quinidine is known to result in elevated serum digoxin levels through possible effects on digoxin absorption and renal clearance [22]. As with most antiarrhythmics, dose adjustment may be necessary in patients with congestive heart failure or hepatic or renal failure.

Side Effects

The most frequent side effects relate to gastrointestinal disturbances. Loose, diarrheal stools, abdominal colic, nausea, vomiting, and anorexia may be severe enough to warrant discontinuation of therapy. Occasionally, a different preparation produces less intense symptoms. Fever, urticaria, rash, and hematological abnormalities, particularly thrombocytopenia, have also been reported.

The most serious side effect has been described as "quinidine syncope," which generally involves QT prolongation disproportionate to the drug level. This finding may be accompanied by an increase in the frequency and severity of ventricular dysrhythmia. Toxic doses produce headaches, visual and auditory disturbances, flushing, confusion, delirium, and exacerbation of gastrointestinal disturbances. QRS and QT duration are prolonged, with all ECG waveforms broadened and flattened (Figure 14.2).

Quinidine also produces a weak alpha-receptor blockage and has a direct relaxant action on vascular smooth muscle. These effects are thought to explain the substantial increase in adrenergic tone and subsequent cardiovascular collapse that occurs with IV quinidine administration.

Procainamide

Actions and Clinical Uses

The electrophysiological actions of procainamide hydrochloride (Pronestyl) are similar to those of quinidine. Automaticity and conductivity are depressed, and the effective refractory period is increased [65]. Anticholinergic effects similar to those of quinidine make it difficult to control the ventricular response

TABLE 14.1
Quinidine Preparations

Agent	Dosage/Administration	Peak Plasma Concentration Time	Therapeutic Plasma Level	Toxic Plasma Level
Quinidine sulfate, USP	200–300 mg PO q. 6–8 hr	60–120 min	2.3–5.0 μg/ml when measured by double extraction method	> 5.0 μg/ml
Long-acting (Quinidine Extentabs)	600 mg PO q. 8–12 hr			
Quinidine gluconate (Quinaglute Duratabs)	1–2 tablets (324 mg each) PO q. 8–12 hr	240 min	As above	As above
Quinidine gluconate injection, USP	IM dose: 600 mg initially followed by 400 mg as often as q. 2 hr IV dose: usually 330 mg or less but occasionally 500–750 mg; dilute 10 ml (80 mg) to 50 ml with D_5W; administer at rate not exceeding 1 ml/minute	Within minutes	As above	As above
Quinidine polygalucturonate (Cardioquin)	275 mg tablets PO loading dose: 1–3 tablets to terminate arrhythmia, repeated in 3–4 hours; if NSR not restored after 3 or 4 equal doses, increase dose by ½–1 tablet administered 3–4 times before any further increase PO maintenance dose: 1 tablet b.i.d.-t.i.d.: usually 1 tablet q. 12 hr	. . .	As above	As above

PO = by mouth; IM = intramuscular; IV = intravenous; NSR = normal sinus rhythm.

Adapted from Underhill, S. L., et al.: *Cardiac Nursing.* Philadelphia: Lippincott, 1982, p. 444. Used with permission.

rate, limiting the usefulness of the drug in the treatment of atrial flutter and fibrillation.

Intravenous procainamide administration is effective in the emergency management of ventricular dysrhythmias that are refractory to lidocaine. It is also the drug of choice for emergency IV therapy during the accessory tract conduction associated with Wolff-Parkinson-White syndrome [38].

Dosage and Administration
Procainamide is administered orally or intravenously. Intramuscular absorption is considered to be less reliable. The usual IV dose is 100 mg every 2 to 5 minutes until the dysrhythmia is suppressed or 1 gm is administered. This dose is followed by a continuous infusion of 2 gm per 500 cc of D_5W at 1 to 4 mg per minute (20 to 80 μg/kg per minute).

Continued control of the dysrhythmia may require 2 to 4 gm orally in six divided doses daily. The peak plasma concentration after oral ingestion

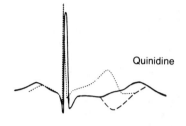

Quinidine

FIGURE 14.2
Effect of quinidine on the electrocardiogram. The normal configuration is shown by the dotted line, the quinidine effect by the bold line, and an alternate expression of the quinidine effect on the ST-T segment by the dashed line. Note the widening of the P wave and QRS intervals resulting from reduced conduction velocity. Prolongation of the QT interval occurs with variation in the form of the ST-T segment, which resembles that in severe ischemia or hypokalemia. (From Braunwald, E. B. *Heart Disease: Textbook of Cardiovascular Medicine.* Philadelphia: Saunders, 1980. Used with permission.)

occurs at 1 hour. The drug half-life is relatively short, between 2.2 and 4 hours. Procan SR is a sustained-action preparation that allows the period between doses to be extended to 6 hours. Procainamide is metabolized by the liver and excreted in the urine.

Side Effects

Negative inotropy and peripheral vasodilatation can produce hypotension following administration of procainamide. This effect is frequently associated with rapid IV administration of the drug and occurs relatively infrequently with oral use. The ECG reflects QRS widening with therapeutic drug effect and QT interval prolongation with drug toxicity.

Gastrointestinal symptoms such as nausea, vomiting, and diarrhea are common side effects. The most serious side effect of procainamide therapy is a syndrome resembling systemic lupus erythematosus, including polyarthralgia, fever, skin rash, and hepatomegaly. These symptoms occur in association with serological abnormalities such as a positive antinuclear antibody test result or agranulocytosis, necessitating close attention to baseline and follow-up hematological studies. Drug withdrawal generally results in the resolution of symptoms.

Disopyramide Phosphate

Actions and Clinical Uses

Disopyramide (Norpace) has been approved for clinical use in the United States since 1977. The drug primarily decreases the upstroke velocity and the rate of diastolic depolarization during phase 4 of of the action potential. The duration of the action potential is somewhat prolonged, with increased atrial and ventricular refractoriness [43].

Disopyramide has been shown to be useful in the treatment of atrial and ventricular dysrhythmias. In patients with atrial flutter, the improvement in AV node conduction may lead to 1:1 conduction with a rapid ventricular rate. This result is similar to the effect of quinidine and procainamide that necessitates pretreatment with digoxin or propranolol. Disopyramide also appears to be useful in the depression of bypass tract conduction for the treatment of Wolff-Parkinson-White syndrome.

Dosage and Administration

Disopyramide is available as an oral or IV preparation, although it is approved only for oral administration in this country. A loading dose of 200 to 300 mg may be administered initially to produce the desired therapeutic effect. The usual maintenance dose is 100 to 200 mg every 6 hours up to a total daily dose of 400 mg to 2.4 gm.

Peak blood levels are achieved within 2 to 3 hours following ingestion, with an elimination half-life of 6 to 8 hours. Therapeutic plasma levels are achieved at 2 to 5 μg/ml. Excretion of the drug occurs primarily through the kidney.

Side Effects

The most common side effects of disopyramide therapy have been attributed to its anticholinergic effects. Among the most common are urinary retention, dryness of the mouth, and blurred vision. These are likely to cause particular problems for those patients with benign prostatic hypertrophy or glaucoma.

Gastrointestinal effects of nausea, vomiting, constipation, and diarrhea are less commonly described. Other symptoms that have been reported incude skin rash, dizziness, weakness, fatigue, nervousness, and insomnia. Agranulocytosis, which clears with the discontinuation of therapy, has also been reported. Hypotension, increasing congestive heart failure, QRS widening or QT prolongation of more than 25%, bradycardia, and new conduction disturbances may serve as warning signs of drug toxicity [31].

Phenytoin

Actions and Clinical Uses

Although well recognized as an anticonvulsant, phenytoin (Dilantin, DPH) possesses electrophysiological properties similar to those of lidocaine, making it a useful alternative in the management of ventricular dysrhythmias. It is known to be particularly effective in the control of digitalis-toxic ventricular dysrhythmias [67].

Dosage and Administration

Phenytoin is available as an oral or parenteral preparation; the intramuscular route is not recommended, however, because of local tissue inflammation and unpredictable absorption. The dosage range is similar for the oral and IV routes. The loading dose is usually 1 gm in the first 24 hours, followed by maintenance doses of 300 to 400 mg daily. The IV dose is administered by direct injection, slowly, at approximately 50 to 100 mg per minute.

Peak plasma levels are noted approximately 4 to 6 hours after oral ingestion. The drug may be administered in one dose or divided doses according to patient preferences. Plasma levels are closely monitored because of the drug's long half-life and its unpredictable absorption in the small bowel. Metabolism occurs primarily in the liver.

Side Effects

Intravenous administration is known to cause a variety of serious side effects, such as bradycardia, hypotension, heart block, ventricular fibrillation, and respiratory arrest. These have been related primarily to the rate of administration.

Gingival hyperplasia has been most frequently associated with long-term treatment. Central nervous system side effects such as nystagmus, diplopia, blurred vision, dysarthria, ataxia, and dizziness are often dose related. Idiosyncratic reactions include the development of toxic hepatitis, systemic lupus erythematosus, and pseudolymphoma, as well as skin rash, depigmentation, and hirsutism. Megaloblastic anemia associated with low blood folate levels have also been attributed to phenytoin therapy.

TRENDS IN ANTIARRHYTHMIC THERAPY

Recently attention has been focused on the development of new antiarrhythmic drugs because of their potential to reduce the incidence of sudden cardiac death. The following drugs have been undergoing trials in the United States and are likely to be marketed extensively in the near future.

Amiodarone

Actions and Clinical Uses

The electrophysiological effects of amiodarone (Cordarone) involve a prolongation of the action potential in atrial, ventricular, and Purkinje tissue without significant alteration of the resting membrane potential or automaticity. In the sinus node the action potential duration is prolonged and there is a decrease in the slope of phase 4 depolarization. Electrophysiological studies have demonstrated a slowing of the sinus node discharge rate, a lengthening of AV node conduction time, and an increase in atrial and ventricular refractoriness. This drug is extremely useful in the treatment of all tachyarrhythmias, including Wolff-Parkinson-White syndrome, as well as other atrial and ventricular dysrhythmias. Initially developed in Europe as an antianginal agent, amiodarone also produces some beneficial hemodynamic effects related to a decrease in vascular resistance, a decrease in blood pressure, and an increase in coronary blood flow [51].

Clinically, a prolonged PR interval may occur as a result of increased AV conduction time. The QRS complex is generally unchanged, although T wave abnormalities, QT prolongation, and U waves may be noted. Because of these effects, amiodarone may be relatively contraindicated in patients with sinus bradyarrhythmias or atrioventricular or intraventricular block.

Dosage and Administration

The usual oral dose ranges from 200 mg to as much as 1200 mg daily. Intravenously 5 to 10 mg/kg may be given in a single loading dose of up to 300 mg over 3 to 5 minutes. The dosage varies depending on the type of dysrhythmia; ventricular dysrhythmias usually require a higher dose. The oral loading dose ranges from 600 to 1200 mg per day for 1 to 2 weeks.

The onset of action is thought to occur within 6 hours after oral administration. A long half-life has been reported, ranging from 20 to 60 days, with 3 to 5 days usually required initially to achieve a therapeutic level. As a result, the exact timing of each daily dose is not important. The details of metabolism and excretion are unclear and continue to be investigated.

Side Effects

Patients may experience nausea, vomiting, and occasionally constipation as a result of amiodarone therapy. One of the most undesirable effects is the occurrence of corneal microdeposits, which appear as yellow-brown granular pigmentations of the cornea. As a result, patients will experience a feeling of sand in the eye, which is usually reversible with the cessation of treatment and can be prevented, usually, by the use of methylcellulose eye drops. Amiodarone is also known to cause thyroid dysfunction (both hypothyroidism and hyperthyroidism), photosensitivity, dermatitis, and, less commonly, bluish-gray skin discoloration [23]. An interaction with warfarin sodium necessitates that attention be paid to abnormally elevated prothrombin times. Reports of the development of pulmonary infiltrates and drug interactions with digoxin have also been concerns with amiodarone therapy. Careful attention must be paid to guidelines for follow-up, which is to include baseline and periodic chest roentgenograms, ophthalmic examinations, and close monitoring of thyroid functions, prothrombin times, and digoxin levels.

Ethmozin

Actions and Clinical Uses
Ethmozin was developed in the Soviet Union during the late 1960s [44]. It is similar to quinidine in its electrophysiological action and is used in the treatment of atrial and ventricular tachycardia. It is known to decrease the maximal rate of phase 0 and especially to depress the Purkinje fiber action potential duration and amplitude. Increased refractoriness has also been noted. Clinically, the PR interval or QRS segment may be prolonged, without marked effect on the QT interval.

Dosage and Administration
The total daily dosage usually ranges from 600 to 900 mg orally, administered in three divided doses. The peak action occurs within approximately 1 hour, with the maximum plasma levels noted anywhere from 2 to 6 hours after the initiation of therapy. The elimination half-life ranges from 4 to 13 hours. Ethmozin is thought to be metabolized by the liver and excreted by the urine [54].

Side Effects
The most common side effects include nausea, vomiting, and heartburn. Central nervous system symptoms include vertigo, mild headaches, and twitching. Occasionally, a pruritic drug rash as been reported. Although studies have shown ethmozin to be effective in dysrhythmia suppression, continued investigation is needed to determine the proper place of this agent in the treatment of dysrhythmias.

Mexiletine

Actions and Clinical Uses
Mexiletine is a new antiarrhythmic agent whose chemical structure and electrophysiological properties are similar to those of lidocaine [35]. There is a shortened action potential duration and a decreased rate of phase 0 rise. Mexiletine results in little change in the sinus node discharge rate or intra-atrial conduction or refractoriness. In patients with sinus node disease and intraventricular conduction disturbances, however, severe bradycardia and abnormal sinus node recovery times have been noted. Mexiletine effectively suppresses acute and chronic ventricular dysrhythmias, including those resulting from digitalis intoxication.

Dosage and Administration

The initial loading dose is 400 to 600 mg orally, followed by a daily dose ranging from 400 to 1,200 mg. The daily prescription may be administered in divided doses every 6 to 8 hours, depending on the individual patient's needs and tolerance. An IV dose of 200 mg can be administered over 3 to 5 minutes and followed by a 1 to 1.5 mg per minute drip.

Mexiletine is well absorbed following oral administration. The onset of action has been noted within an hour, with peak plasma levels occurring 2 to 4 hours after ingestion. The mean plasma half-life is approximately 11 hours. Delayed absorption and prolonged elimination have been noted in patients after myocardial infarction [52]. Mexiletine is metabolized predominantly by the liver and excreted by the kidneys, and thus may be contraindicated in patients with hepatic or renal failure.

Side Effects

Side effects have been related to dosage and plasma levels. Gastrointestinal upset, nausea, vomiting, and dyspepsia have been severe enough to require withdrawal of the drug. Taking the drug with a snack or meals minimizes this side effect. Mild side effects involving the central nervous system include tremors and nystagmus. Other central nervous system side effects include light-headedness, blurred vision, paresthesias, ataxia, confusion, and drowsiness. Rarely, hypotension, bradycardia reversible with atropine administration, and aggravation of rhythm disturbances have been noted. Thrombocytopenia with a positive antinuclear antibody test result has also been associated with mexiletine therapy. As with all these antiarrhythmic agents, the need for close follow-up of patients necessitates monitoring of the results of laboratory tests, including serum drug levels, to permit titration of dosage.

Tocainide

Actions and Clinical Uses

Lidocaine is well known for its efficacy as an antiarrhythmic agent, yet it is available only in parenteral form. Tocainide (Tonocard), commonly referred to as oral lidocaine, has been shown to be effective in controlling both acute and chronic ventricular dysrhythmias. An individual's response to lidocaine is helpful but not conclusive in predicting the response to tocainide. Generally, when lidocaine is ineffective, it is unlikely that tocainide will be beneficial. A patient's response to lidocaine, however, does not guarantee a similar effect with tocainide [53]. This drug decreases the rate of phase 0 rise and the slope of phase 4 spontaneous depolarization. The total duration of the action potential is also decreased.

Dosage and Administration

The total daily dosage ranges from 600 to 2,400 mg orally, which may be given in 200 to 800 mg doses every 6 to 8 hours. When the IV form is used, a 50 to 200 mg loading dose may be followed by a 1 to 4 mg per minute continuous drip, a dosage similar to that recommended for lidocaine therapy.

The peak action after initial oral administration usually occurs at 60 to 90 minutes. The half-life is reported to be approximately 14 hours, with reports in the literature ranging from 10 to 15 hours. Tocainide is metabolized by the liver and excreted by the kidney, so that dosage adjustment may be required in patients with hepatic or renal failure. Dosage change may also be necessary in patients with left ventricular dysfunction [59].

Side Effects

The side effects of tocainide use involve the gastrointestinal and central nervous systems. Nausea, vomiting, anorexia, constipation, and abdominal pain have been reported. The drug affects the central nervous system much as lidocaine does, producing tremor, twitching, light-headedness, and mental and sensory changes. These effects appear to be very much related to dose and drug level.

DRUGS USED IN THE TREATMENT OF CORONARY ARTERY DISEASE

The treatment of coronary artery disease (CAD) is directed toward the reduction of myocardial O_2 demands and the improvement of myocardial O_2 supply. Pharmacologically, demands can be reduced with beta-adrenergic blocking agents, nitrates, and calcium channel blockers. Nitrates and calcium channel blockers can also be employed to increase myocardial O_2 supply.

Nursing Responsibilities

Antianginal therapy necessitates close monitoring of heart rate and blood pressure changes prior to the administration of the medications, during the onset of action, and at the approximate time of peak effect. Dosage generally begins at the low end of the range and increases in small increments to achieve the desired therapeutic effect, that is, relief of symptoms. As medications are titrated, these variables will provide an index of patient tolerance as well as drug effect. Most reactions are dose related, although serious idiosyncratic reactions such as hypotension and fainting may necessitate the use of lower than usual doses or alternate preparations.

During the initiation of therapy for angina, one must be attentive to the patient's description of the angina, which will guide prescription of treatment. Angina can have a variety of presentations, which makes it imperative that a distinction be made between such terms as chest pain, stable angina, unstable angina, and heart attack. Any changes in the frequency or severity of angina should be promptly reported to the physician, because drug modifications may be necessary to prevent ongoing ischemia.

Difficulties with patient recall will interfere with optimal management. Angina diaries are useful tools that help patients initially identify patterns that warrant nitroglycerin prophylaxis or the attention of a physician (Exhibit 14.2). Patients require realistic reassurance that increases in the frequency of anginal episodes may be related to a variety of factors that do not necessarily indicate a worsening of the underlying condition. Reinforcing the nature of the patient's control over risk factors, activity progression, symptom reporting, and knowledge of emergency management promotes the development of a healthier and more realistic perspective.

EXHIBIT 14.2
Angina Diary

Date	Time Episode Began	Time Episode Relieved	Severity of Discomfort Mild (1–3) Moderate (4–6) Severe (7–10)

Nitrates

Actions and Clinical Uses

Nitrates are the most frequently prescribed medications for the treatment of angina. First used in the nineteenth century for a variety of disorders, nitroglycerin is now widely accepted as the prototype for many compounds used to relieve angina pectoris.

Nitrates reduce myocardial O_2 demands and improve coronary blood flow through a series of actions. As potent vasodilators, their primary effect is the reduction of venous tone in the capacitance vessels, which decreases the return of blood to the heart (preload). This, in turn, reduces wall tension, thereby minimizing myocardial O_2 consumption to relieve or prevent an episode of angina.

Nitrates have a lesser effect on the arterial circulation (resistance vessels). This effect is demonstrated in the slight drop in arterial blood pressure following the administration of nitrates, reflecting the decreased resistance to flow and the reduction in myocardial work. This is additional evidence suggesting that nitrates dilate the coronary arteries even in the presence of diffuse CAD [16].

These effects make nitrates very useful in the treatment of coronary insufficiency and congestive heart failure, when the reduction in preload and afterload is most beneficial.

No. of Nitroglycerin Tablets Taken	Cause of Episode (emotion, exercise, no obvious cause)	Activity when Episode Occurred (walking, lifting, running, eating, sleeping, relaxing, arguing, worrying, other)

Dosage and Administration

The various available preparations differ primarily in terms of their speed of onset of action and duration of effect (Tables 14.2 and 14.3). Nitroglycerin for sublingual use is routinely prescribed because of its rapid onset of action and its ability to alleviate and prevent acute anginal episodes. Prescription of the longer-acting preparations is considered to maximize the patient's exercise capacity and adherence to a long-term treatment regimen. For this reason, timing of the doses should consider the patient's usual activity schedule.

Oral administration. Initially, the oral use of nitrates was questioned because of concerns about the rapid metabolism of the drug and the difficulty in achieving adequate serum drug levels [61]. The potential for tolerance development raised the issue of long-term efficacy. Ongoing experience, however, has demonstrated a clear relationship between the increasing dose of nitrates and the relief of symptoms.

Cutaneous administration. The administration of nitroglycerin paste requires a fairly consistent approach in order to avoid adverse hemodynamic effects or skin irritation. Studies have demonstrated that the rate of absorption is affected by the size of the area used for application, the cutaneous blood flow at the

TABLE 14.2
Dosage and Actions of Long-Acting Nitrates for Anginal Therapy

Name		Effects[a]	
Generic	Trade	Physiological	Therapeutic
Isosorbide dinitrate	Isordil; Sorbitrate	Relaxes vascular smooth muscle	Decreases venous return
Pentaerythritol tetranitrate	Peritrate	Dilates arterioles; reduces peripheral vascular resistance	Decreases blood pressure; decreases net myocardial O_2 consumption
Erythrityl tetranitrate	Cardilate	Reflex tachycardia	

[a]These effects refer to all long-acting nitrates.
[b]Also available as "sustained action" tablets; efficacy not well documented.

TABLE 14.3
Dosage and Actions of Nitroglycerin for Anginal Therapy

Name		Effects[a]	
Generic	Trade	Physiological	Therapeutic
Glyceryl trinitrate (nitroglycerin)	Nitrostat	Relaxes vascular smooth muscle	Decreases venous return
	Nitrobid	Dilates arterioles	Decreases blood pressure
	Nitroglyn	Reduces peripheral vascular resistance	Decreases net myocardial O_2 consumption
	Nitrospan	Reduces mean arterial pressure	
	Nitro-SA	Reflex tachycardia	
	Nitrong		
	Nitrol ointment		

[a]These effects refer to all formulations of nitroglycerin.

Dosage

Beginning	Usual	Maximal	Formulation	Route	Supplied	Side Effects
5 mg q. 2–3 hr	5–10 mg q. 3 hr	20 mg	Sublingual[b] tablets	SL	2.5, 5, 10, 20 mg	Headache; flushing; tachycardia
5 mg q.i.d. or 40 mg b.i.d.	5–30 mg q.i.d. or 40 mg b.i.d.	30 mg q.i.d. or 40 mg t.i.d.	Tablets and capsules	PO	5, 10 mg	Dizziness
10 mg q.i.d.	10–20 mg q.i.d. or 80 mg b.i.d.	60 mg q. 4 hr	Oral[b]	PO	10, 20 mg	Postural hypotension
5 mg q.i.d.	5–15 mg q.i.d.	45 mg q. 2 hr	Oral, sublingual, and chewable tablets	SL or PO	5, 10, 15 mg; 10 mg chewable	Possibly causes tachyphylaxis to nitroglycerin with prolonged use

Adapted from Wolfson, S., and Costin, J. C. Medical therapy in angina pectoris. In Donoso, E., and Gorlin, S. (eds.), *Angina Pectoris,* vol. 3. New York: Stratton Intercontinental Medical Book Corp., 1977, p. 121. Used with permission.

Dosage

Beginning	Average	Maximal	Formulation	Route	Supplied	Side Effects
0.3 mg	0.6 mg	p.r.n.	Sublingual tablets	SL	0.3, 0.4, 0.6 mg	Headaches; flushing; tachycardia
2.5 mg b.i.d.	2.5 mg t.i.d. 6.5 mg b.i.d.	6.5 mg t.i.d.	Sustained release capsules	PO	2.5, 6.5 mg	Dizziness; postural hypotension
1.3 mg b.i.d.	1.3 mg t.i.d. 6.5 mg b.i.d.	6.5 mg t.i.d.	Sustained action tablets	PO	1.3, 2.6, 6.5 mg	
2.5 mg before breakfast and at h.s.			Sustained release microdialysis cells	PO	2.5 mg	
2.5 mg b.i.d.	2.5 mg b.i.d.	2.5 mg t.i.d.	Sustained release capsules	PO	2.5 mg	
	2.6 mg t.i.d.		Controlled release tablets	PO	2.6 mg	
1–2 in h.s.	2 in h.s.	6 in h.s.	Lanolin, petrolatum	Topically	1 and 2 oz tubes 2% nitroglycerine	

Adapted from Wolfson, S., and Costin, J. C. Medical therapy in angina pectoris. In Donoso, E., and Gorlin, S. (eds.), *Angina Pectoris,* vol. 3. New York: Stratton Intercontinental Medical Book Corp., 1977, p. 121. Used with permission.

site, and the rate of evaporation [30]. It has been recommended that the ointment be spread evenly over a 6 × 6 inch area without rubbing the ointment immediately into the skin. The use of plastic wrap or a nonocclusive dressing is determined by the nurse or patient preference. The advent of nitroglycerin patches provides a convenient way of establishing consistent dosage and application (Table 14.4).

Intravenous administration. The availability of an IV preparation now permits a continuous infusion for the emergency treatment of unstable angina, coronary artery spasm, systemic and pulmonary hypertension, and left ventricular failure [24]. Close observation of the patient usually involves hemodynamic monitoring and careful titration of the drip according to the patient's symptoms. A significant reduction in the actual concentration of drug infused has been noted with plastic IV bags and certain administration sets [3]. Consequently, glass bottles and special tubing are recommended for continuous IV infusions.

Side Effects

The use of any nitrate preparation is accompanied by the possibility of an unpredictable hypotensive episode. It is generally advisable to give initial sublingual doses of nitroglycerin in a supervised situation because of the rapid onset of effect and the intensity of the response. Nitrate headaches, postural hypotension, and fainting sufficiently frighten patients into avoiding the use of nitroglycerin and other nitrate preparations. These side effects can be minimized by adjusting the dosage. Headaches may be relieved by routinely administering a mild analgesic during the initial days of therapy.

Beta Blockers

Over the last 25 years, several beta blockers have been introduced for the treatment of cardiovascular disorders such as angina, hypertension, and dysrhythmias. Most recently, their efficacy in reducing the incidence of recurrent myocardial infarction and sudden cardiac death following myocardial infarction has been appreciated [47].

Actions and Clinical Uses

Beta-blocking drugs inhibit the effects of catecholamines at the beta-adrenergic receptor sites. Their primary therapeutic effect involves the reduction of the resting heart rate and heart rate response to exercise. Additionally, beta blockers decrease sympathetic tone, limiting the increase in O_2 consumption associated with exercise and emotion. The beneficial effect in reducing blood pressure and contractility may also exacerbate heart failure and increasing heart size by blocking the effects of catecholamines.

Certain pharmacological properties contribute to the variable effects of the different beta blockers [13, 17]. Beta-blocking potency is determined by the degree of inhibition of a tachycardia produced by isoproterenol. That is, the strength of the beta blocker is determined by the degree to which a tachycardia produced by isoproterenol can be reduced. Pindolol and timolol maleate are considered to be the most potent agents in this regard.

TABLE 14.4
Transdermal Nitroglycerin Preparations[a]

Product (Mfr)	Product Surface Area (cm²)	NTG Content (mg)	NTG Delivered over 24 Hr (mg)
Transderm-Nitro 5 (Ciba)	10	25	5.0
Transderm-Nitro 10 (Ciba)	20	50	10.0
Nitro-Dur 5 (Key)	5	26	2.5
Nitro-Dur 10 (Key)	10	51	5.0
Nitro-Dur 15 (Key)	15	77	7.5
Nitro-Dur 20 (Key)	20	104	10.0
Nitrodisc 16 (Searle)	8	16	5.0
Nitrodisc 32 (Searle)	16	32	10.0

[a]The differences in composition of each manufacturer's unit do not alter the mechanism of drug delivery. The potency of the units does vary according to manufacturer, however.

Mfr = manufacturer; NTG = nitroglycerin.

Adapted from Black, C. D. Transdermal drug delivery systems. *US Pharmacist,* Nov. 1982, p. 73. Used with permission.

Cardioselectivity refers to the ability to block beta 1 receptors selectively without affecting the non-cardiac tissue. When a certain critical dose is exceeded, the drug appears to affect both beta 1 and beta 2 receptors with the same intensity. This characteristic varies widely and does not necessarily imply that there is an effect only on cardiac tissue (cardiospecificity).

Intrinsic sympathomimetic activity is a partial agonist activity that allows a certain degree of beta stimulation at the same doses that produce beta blockade. It is thought that drugs with this property are less likely to produce adverse bradycardic responses and myocardial depression. The rebound effect associated with discontinuation of beta blockers is also thought to be lessened.

The solubility of beta blockers varies, influencing the distribution of these drugs in the body. Higher degrees of lipid solubility suggest a greater penetration of the drug into the central nervous system, resulting in side effects such as depression and sleep disturbances. Drugs that are more water soluble are thought to equilibrate to a lesser extent across the blood-brain barrier and therefore produce fewer central nervous system side effects. Metoprolol tartrate, atenolol, nadolol, and timolol are considered to have a low degree of lipid solubility.

Beta blockade reduces renin secretion by the kidneys. Renin stimulates the production of aldosterone, which promotes sodium and water retention and thereby increases both blood volume and blood pressure. Renin also stimulates the production of angiotensin 1, which is converted to angiotensin 2, a potent vasoconstrictor. The increased vascular tone and systemic resistance that contribute to high blood pressure are inhibited by beta blockade.

Beta blockers are also known to have a membrane-stabilizing or local anesthetic effect similar to that of quinidine. With usual doses, this effect does not appear to be marked. Beta blockers are not considered to be first-line antiarrhythmic agents but do produce beneficial effects when used in conjunction with other antiarrhythmic therapy.

Dosage and Administration

Propranolol hydrochloride is the prototype for this classification of drugs and is the most frequently prescribed beta blocker in the United States. In the last few years, a number of new beta blockers have been marketed in this country; they differ primarily in the pharmacological actions we have described (Table 14.5).

The metabolism of beta blockers varies somewhat in relation to their solubility. Drugs that have a greater degree of lipid solubility are metabolized primarily by the liver, whereas the kidneys play a more important role in the metabolism of those drugs that are more water soluble. Generally, beta blockers have an elimination half-life of 2 to 4 hours and are excreted via the kidneys.

Beta blockers are usually administered orally; the IV administration of propranolol has been useful, however, in the emergency treatment of supraventricular tachyarrhythmias. Ampules containing 1 ml or 1 mg are available for direct injection.

Side Effects

A variety of effects have been associated with beta blocker therapy [27]. The most serious effects, including hypotension, bradycardia, heart block, congestive heart failure, and bronchospasm, generally result from the direct action of the drug. Symptoms of claudication are likely to be increased during beta blocker therapy because of the increased peripheral vascular resistance. An increased risk of hypoglycemic reactions without the sympathetic nervous system warning signs also appears to exist.

Side effects such as nightmares, lethargy, and depression result from the degree of lipid solubility. These may subside with the use of an alternate preparation or dose schedule. For example, long-acting beta blockers may be taken at night without markedly interfering with the drug's therapeutic effect, thereby minimizing the drowsiness that may be experienced at midday. Efforts to alleviate disturbing side effects will greatly decrease the likelihood that the patient will abruptly stop drug administration without supervision. Avoiding such an event is particularly important in light of the rebound effects that can produce an exacerbation of ischemic pain and myocardial infarction.

Calcium Channel Blockers

The most recent advance in the pharmacological management of CAD is the development of calcium channel blockers. Although their use was not approved by the Food and Drug Administration until 1983, these drugs have been widely investigated and prescribed throughout the United States and Europe for over 20 years. The introduction of these drugs is having a major impact on the treatment of a number of cardiovascular disorders, including cardiac dysrhythmias, hypertension, and hypertrophic cardiomyopathy as well as myocardial ischemia.

TABLE 14.5
Dosages and Pharmacological Characteristics of Beta Blockers

Generic (Trade) Name	Comparative Beta-blocking Activity	Cardioselectivity	Average IV Dose (mg/kg body weight)	Average Oral Dose (mg/day)	Half-Life (hr)
Propranolol (Inderal)	1.0	−	0.15	80–320	2–3
Pindolol (Visken)	4.0	−	0.15	20–40	3–4
Metoprolol (Lopressor)	0.8	+	0.15	100–450	3–4
Atenolol (Tenormin)	0.5	+	. . .	100–300	5–7
Nadolol (Corgard)	1.0	−	. . .	40–240	16–18
Timolol (Blocadren)	6.0	−	. . .	20–60	4

IV = intravenous.

Actions and Clinical Uses

Calcium channel blocking agents inhibit the flux of calcium ions across the cell membrane during phase 2 of the action potential. This is the plateau phase of the action potential, when the cell is less permeable to sodium entry through the fast channel and more permeable to calcium entry through the slow channel. All of the drugs share this same basic mechanism of action; they produce different effects, however, depending on the specific cardiac cells affected and the extent to which these cells depend on an influx of calcium.

Calcium channel blockade produces electrophysiological effects that are most evident in the sinoatrial and AV nodes. In doses employed clinically, verapamil and diltiazem hydrochloride depress the rate of sinus node discharge and reduce the conduction velocity through the AV node. The resultant negative chronotropic (slowing of sinus node discharge) and negative dromotropic (slowing of AV conduction) effects depend on the dose, route of administration, and concomitant therapy. Generally, diltiazem and verapamil produce slowing of AV conduction that results in a prolongation of the PR interval on the ECG. Nifedipine, in contrast, does not appear to have any direct effect on AV node conduction [2].

Each calcium channel blocking agent relaxes vascular smooth muscle, decreasing resistance and increasing blood flow in the coronary arteries and the peripheral circulation. Verapamil and diltiazem additionally reduce myocardial work by slowing the heart rate. The net effects vary according to the degree of myocardial ischemia, the patient's ventricular function and sympathetic nervous system tone, and the specific calcium channel blocker being used [63].

Dosage and Administration

The available calcium channel blockers are listed in Table 14.6. Verapamil is the only drug that is available as an IV preparation. As mentioned earlier in the chapter, it is approved for the treatment of supraventricular dysrhythmias.

Combination therapy with beta blockers and nitrates produces beneficial effects by virtue of the complementary actions of these agents. Special caution

TABLE 14.6
Doses and Pharmacological Characteristics of Calcium Channel Blockers

Generic (Trade) Name	Clinical Dose[b]	Onset of Action	Peak Effect	Common Side Effects
Nifedipine (Procardia)	10–30 mg PO q. 4–8 hr; 10 mg SL	< 20 min PO; < 3 min SL	1–2 hr PO	Headache; hypotension; flushing; pedal edema; dysesthesias
Verapamil[a] (Calan, Isoptin)	60–80 mg PO q. 8 hr; 75–150 µg/kg IV; 0.005 mg/kg/min (for continuous infusion in selected patients)	< 2 hr PO; < 2 min IV	5 hr PO; 10–15 min IV	Headache; hypotension; AV block; constipation; vertigo
Diltiazem (Cardizem)	60–90 mg PO q. 8 hr; 75–150 µg/kg IV	< 15 min PO	30 min PO	Headache; hypotension; flushing; AV block

[a]Intravenous preparation approved for supraventricular tachycardia; IV nifedipine and diltiazem are still investigational.
[b]Vital signs should be monitored during and after administration of the initial dose to assess patient tolerance. Doses are started at the low end and increased in small increments until symptoms are relieved.

AV = atrioventricular.

From Rossi, L. P., and Antman, E. M. Calcium channel blockers; new treatment for cardiovascular disease. *Am. J. Nurs.* 83: 383, 1983. Used with permission.

is warranted, however, in using verapamil with beta blockers, particularly if any underlying conduction disturbances are suspected.

Side Effects
In the management of CAD, diltiazem appears to have the fewest side effects. The most serious side effects include hypotension and bradyarrhythmias, which actually result from the desired effect of the drugs [57]. Other side effects include dizziness, headaches, and flushing. Complaints of constipation are common with verapamil and may be alleviated with early dietary intervention, stool softeners, or both. Pedal edema is commonly associated with nifedipine and generally necessitates leg elevation during the day and the use of support stockings.

DRUGS USED IN THE TREATMENT OF CONGESTIVE HEART FAILURE

Congestive heart failure presents a challenge because of the difficulties that the disease and its treatment impose on the patient. With long-standing failure, there is an extremely fine line between adequate control and exacerbation of symptoms.

The primary goals of treatment are the reduction of myocardial O_2 demands and consumption and the enhancement of myocardial contractility. In order for these goals to be achieved, it is important that the nurse be familiar with the somewhat opposing yet complementary nature of the required interventions.

**Nursing
Responsibilities**

The nurse assumes a key role in the care of patients with congestive heart failure by closely monitoring the patient's response to drugs and reinforcing the necessary lifestyle adaptations. Regimens are frequently complex, with many medications required several times a day.

The disease progression necessitates an increasingly complex regimen and affects virtually every functional pattern. Sodium and fluid restrictions as well as potassium replacements are critical adjuncts to maximize the effectiveness of pharmacological therapy. Elimination may be delayed because of hepatic or renal failure; such changes alert one to the early and subtle signs of drug toxicity.

Close monitoring of all vital signs during the initiation of therapy provides a concrete index of the patient's response to medications. Records of intake and output as well as daily weighings are often difficult to maintain, for reasons ranging from the priorities of the nurse to the nonadherence of the patient. Nevertheless, the value of these measures cannot be underestimated.

Gradual activity progression is particularly important during the titration of therapy, which frequently requires an extended period. Efficacy is often judged by the patient's improvement in activity tolerance and decrease in symptoms as well as by more objective measures of myocardial working capacity.

Treatment often produces a major stress for the patient, who is also confronted with the need to adjust his self-image from one of independence to one of dependence on others for the simplest of tasks. Coping is compromised because of the chronicity and poor prognosis in spite of what may be described as optimal therapy. Conflicts regarding adherence frequently arise as patients question the value of therapy in relation to their desired quality of living.

*INOTROPIC
AGENTS*

Inotropic agents are known for their ability to improve the strength of myocardial contraction. Among the pharmacological agents used to create this effect are the beta-adrenergic agonists. To date, the cardiac glycosides are the agents most commonly prescribed in the treatment of congestive heart failure; investigations of new inotropic agents have yielded impressive results, however [4].

Digitalis

Actions and Clinical Uses
Digitalis preparations (digoxin, digitoxin) have been widely recognized for their usefulness in the treatment of congestive heart failure and supraventricular dysrhythmias, particularly atrial fibrillation. A major effect of digitalis therapy is the improvement in the force and velocity of myocardial contraction. This positive inotropic effect is not dependent on catecholamine stimulation and therefore is essentially unaffected by beta-adrenergic receptor blockade. The exact mechanism by which the inotropic effect is accomplished is not clear, but the effect is thought to occur because of inhibition of the sodium–potassium pump and an increase in the intracellular pool of calcium ions available for excitation–contraction coupling [5].

Digitalis produces important antiarrhythmic effects by prolonging atrial, ventricular, and AV node refractoriness and conduction time. These electrophysiological effects make digitalis particularly effective in controlling the fast ventricular rates that occur with atrial fibrillation and flutter. During digitalis

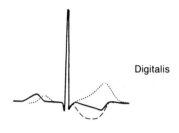

Digitalis

FIGURE 14.3
Effect of digitalis on the electrocardiogram. The normal configuration is shown by the dotted line, the digitalis effect (nontoxic) by the bold line, and the digitalis toxicity pattern by the dashed line. The digitalis effect includes PR segment prolongation, a ramplike descent of the ST segment, and shortening of the QT interval. With toxicity there is further depression of the ST segment; atrioventricular block and rhythm disturbances are common associated manifestations. (From Braunwald, E. B. *Heart Disease: Textbook of Cardiovascular Medicine*. Philadelphia: Saunders, 1980. Used with permission.)

therapy, the ECG will typically demonstrate diffuse ST-T wave changes in all leads (Figure 14.3).

Concern about the use of digoxin in the acute period following myocardial infarction is related to the increased potential for toxicity and the differential effects in patients with normal hearts versus patients with diseased hearts. In normal hearts there is an increase in the myocardial O_2 consumption, whereas in the failing heart, the net effects produce a decrease in ventricular size and wall tension. The direct vagal effect of digitalis additionally reduces myocardial work.

The nature of the increased myocardial O_2 consumption makes the use of digoxin contraindicated in the treatment of congestive cardiomyopathy unless absolutely necessary for ventricular rate control.

Dosage and Administration

Although a variety of preparations are available, digoxin is by far the most commonly used. A loading or digitalizing dose is generally administered every 4 to 6 hours over a 24- to 48-hour period, depending on the patient's clinical response. Increments of 0.25 mg orally or intravenously are generally used to initiate therapy.

Adequacy of digitalization is judged more by the degree of heart rate control and the overall improvement in patient's status than by the total dose used, which may vary according to the individual.

Side Effects

Of critical importance in the management of the patient receiving digitalis therapy is the observation of signs and symptoms that indicate toxicity. Noncardiac symptoms such as anorexia, nausea, vomiting, diarrhea, and visual disturbances (photophobia, blurred or dimmed vision) are among the earliest and frequently most subtle patient complaints.

Cardiac dysrhythmias of any kind can be associated with digitalis excess, although the most common rhythm disturbances include ventricular bigeminy or tachycardia, atrial tachycardia, and nonparoxysmal AV node tachycardia with or without AV block.

Because of the high incidence of serious complications associated with digitalis intoxication, serum levels are used to evaluate the presence of toxicity. One should be alert to the factors that have been associated with elevated serum levels and an increased level of responsiveness to digoxin, such as hy-

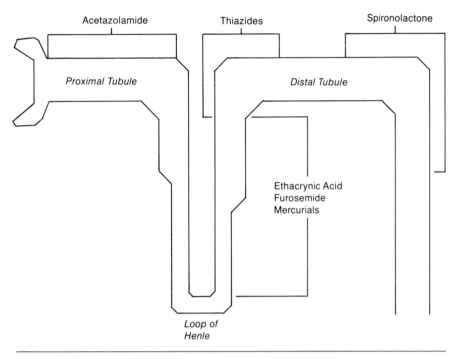

FIGURE 14.4
Major sites of action of commonly used diuretics. (From Taormina-Paplanus, L. M., Strebel, C. A. and Michaelson, C. R. Drug therapy for congestive heart failure. In C. R. Michaelson, ed., *Congestive Heart Failure*. St. Louis: Mosby, 1983. Adapted from Augus, A., and Goldberg, M. Renal functions in congestive heart failure. In H. J. Levine, ed., *Clinical Cardiovascular Physiology*. New York: Grune & Stratton, 1976. Used with permission.)

pokalemia, concomitant administration of quinidine, pulmonary disease, and hypothyroidism [32].

DIURETICS

Diuretics are given to promote the excretion of sodium and water through the kidneys. Different categories have been defined according to their specific physiological effects [6, 42, 64] (Figure 14.4).

Proximally Active Diuretics

Actions and Clinical Uses
Carbonic anhydrase inhibitors such as acetazolamide (Diamox) produce their diuretic effect by acting at the proximal tubule. Carbonic anhydrase is an enzyme responsible for hydrogen secretion. Inhibition of this enzyme interferes with the reabsorption of sodium in exchange for hydrogen ions produced within the tubules.

Osmotic agents such as mannitol introduce a higher concentration of solute into the renal tubule. This increase interferes with the usual reabsorption of sodium and water that occurs at the proximal tubule. These agents also decrease renal vascular resistance and improve renal blood flow. They are not commonly used in the treatment of congestive failure but may be useful in potentiating the action of other, distally active diuretics.

Dosage and Administration
Acetazolamide may be administered orally or intravenously; it is given less commonly intramuscularly because of the pain of injection. The parenteral preparation is available in a 500 mg vial that is reconstituted with sterile water. The daily dose ranges from 250 mg to 1 gm in divided doses given every 12 hours. Mannitol is administered intravenously as a 5%, 10%, 15%, or 20% solution.

Side Effects
Reactions to acetazolamide are similar to those associated with sulfonamide therapy and include fever, rash, crystalluria, renal calculi, and a variety of blood dyscrasias. Paresthesias, drowsiness, and confusion may also be noted.

Drug tolerance is the major concern with the administration of carbonic anhydrase inhibitors after two to three days. The decreased reabsorption of sodium, chloride, and bicarbonate is also accompanied by a potassium loss that may result in the development of metabolic acidosis.

The major concern with the administration of mannitol is the increased plasma volume contributing to circulatory overload prior to the diuresis.

Loop Diuretics

Actions and Clinical Uses
Furosemide and ethacrynic acid are the most commonly used diuretics for the emergency relief of pulmonary edema or volume overload. They are referred to as loop diuretics because they produce their effect through the reabsorption of sodium in the proximal and distal tubule as well as the loop of Henle.

Dosage and Administration
A direct IV push injection improves the therapeutic effect of these agents which may be lost with prolonged exposure to light. The IV injection of these drugs should be performed slowly to avoid any acute hypotensive response. Loss of hearing has also been associated with the rapid administration of large doses of furosemide. Furosemide is available as an oral preparation in 40 to 80 mg white tablets. The manufacturers provide IV preparations in 2 ml, 10 ml, and 100 mg (10 mg/ml) ampules as well as prefilled syringes. Ethacrynic acid is available in IV form and must be reconstituted with 50 ml of D_5W or normal saline to provide a 50 mg dose. An oral preparation is also available.

Side Effects
Dehydration and electrolyte depletion, particularly potassium loss, are the most serious side effects of therapy with these diuretics. Hyperosmolality and metabolic alkalosis may also occur. Sulfonamide sensitivity is associated with a preexisting hypersensitivity to furosemide.

Thiazides

Actions and Clinical Uses
Thiazides produce their diuretic effect by acting at the ascending loop of Henle and the distal convoluted tubule to inhibit the reabsorption of sodium. This action results in the renal excretion of sodium, potassium, chloride, and water.

TABLE 14.7
Pharmacological Characteristics of Selected Diuretic Agents

Generic (Trade) Name	Usual Dosage and Administration	Effect		
		Onset	Peak	Duration
Chlorothiazide (Diuril)	500–1,000 mg OD	1 hr	4 hr	6–12 hr
	500 mg IV, OD	15 min	30 min	2 hr
Hydrochlorothiazide (HydroDIURIL)	50–100 mg OD	2 hr	4 hr	12 hr or more
Chlorthalidone (Hygroton)	100 mg OD	2 hr	6 hr	24 hr or more
Metolazone (Zaroxolyn)	5–10 mg OD	1 hr	2–4 hr	24–48 hr
Acetazolamide (Diamox)	250–375 mg OD	1 hr	2–4 hr	8 hr
	250–375 mg IV, OD	2 min	15 min	4–5 hr
Spironolactone (Aldactone)	25 mg q.i.d.	24–48 hr	3–5 days after start of therapy	Up to 14 days after cessation of therapy
Triamterene (Dyrenium)	100–300 mg OD	2 hr	6–8 hr	12–16 hr
Amiloride (Midamor)	5–10 mg OD	2 hr	6–10 hr	24 hr
Furosemide (Lasix)	40–120 mg OD, PO, or IV	PO: 1 hr	PO: 1–2 hr	PO: 6 hr
		IV: 5 min	IV: 30 min	IV: 2 hr
Ethacrynic acid (Edecrin)	50–100 mg OD, PO, or IV	PO: 30 min	PO: 2 hr	PO: 6–8 hr
		IV: 15 min	IV: 45 min	IV: 3 hr
Mannitol (Osmitrol)	5–10–20–25% concentration p.r.n. IV infusion	1–3 hr	Duration of the diuresis	Dependent on medullary tonicity

Adapted from Michaelson, C. R. *Congestive Heart Failure*. St. Louis: Mosby, 1983, p. 288. Used with permission.

These agents are likely to be used for the prompt alleviation of symptoms related to right ventricular and mild left ventricular failure. Thiazides are less effective in the treatment of severe heart failure, when glomerular filtration may be compromised.

Dosage and Administration
A number of different preparations are available for oral administration (Table 14.7). These drugs are well absorbed from the gastrointestinal tract and produce an effect within 1 to 2 hours of ingestion. The peak action occurs in 3 to 6 hours and lasts for up to 24 hours, depending on the specific agent.

Side Effects
The most serious side effects of thiazides are attributed to the hypokalemia that results, increasing the possibility of digitalis toxicity and its associated dysrhythmias. Other signs of hypokalemia include the development of leg cramps, muscle weakness, and fatigue.

Potassium-sparing Diuretics

Actions and Clinical Uses

Potassium-sparing diuretics inhibit the exchange of sodium and potassium in the distal tubule. Spironolactone is the most well known of these agents and acts as a competitive antagonist of aldosterone. Triamterene and amiloride produce this effect directly, irrespective of the influence of aldosterone. These agents are generally reserved for the treatment of long-standing failure that has been unresponsive to other diuretics. They are commonly used in combination with another agent.

Dosage and Administration

These drugs are usually given in four divided doses except for amiloride, which may be given once daily. Spironolactone produces its beneficial effects after about two days of continuous therapy. Triamterene and amiloride produce diuresis more rapidly, within 2 hours, and the effects last for up to 12 or 24 hours, respectively.

Side Effects

Unlike the other commonly used diuretics, the most serious side effect of the potassium-sparing agents is the potential for hyperkalemia and a resultant metabolic alkalosis. Other common side effects are associated with gastrointestinal symptoms. Large doses of spironolactone are associated with the development of gynecomastia in men and menstrual difficulties in women.

VASODILATORS

In the treatment of congestive heart failure, vasodilators are generally used to optimize cardiac performance by altering peripheral vascular tone [10]. Venous dilators increase venous capacitance and reduce cardiac filling pressures (preload); arteriolar dilators improve cardiac output by reducing the resistance to blood flow (afterload). Certain agents, such as hydralazine and Prazosin hydrochloride, produce combined effects.

Nitroprusside

Actions and Clinical Uses

Nitroprusside is a potent vasodilator that produces an equivalent effect on the arterioles and venules, thereby reducing both preload and afterload. There is no direct inotropic or chronotropic effect. Considerable increases in heart rate have been attributed to a reflex-mediated response to excessive hypotension or inadequate left ventricular filling pressure.

Perhaps the primary indication for the use of nitroprusside relates to its effectiveness in reducing arterial blood pressure in an acute hypertensive crisis. Its use in the treatment of an acute myocardial infarction has produced mixed results depending on the timing in the post-infarction period from onset of infarction to initiation of therapy and the degree of left ventricular failure [10, 14, 49].

Nitroprusside can also be used to stabilize chronic congestive heart failure during the titration of appropriate oral therapy.

Dosage and Administration

Nitroprusside is commercially available in a 50 mg vial, which may be reconstituted only in 2 to 3 ml of D_5W. A continuous infusion, 50 mg per 250 ml of D_5W, is usually started at a low dosage of 10 μg per minute. The initial dose may range from 0.5 to 8.0 μg/kg per minute. The solution must be wrapped in the aluminum foil that accompanies the vial to prevent the deterioration that occurs with exposure to light. The manufacturer recommends that the solution not be used beyond 24 hours from the time of reconstitution.

The action of nitroprusside begins almost immediately and terminates abruptly with the initiation and discontinuance, respectively, of the infusion. For this reason, therapy is usually guided by the use of intra-arterial monitoring and an infusion pump.

Side Effects

The most common adverse effect of nitroprusside is hypotension, which is generally related to the rate of infusion. Vigilant monitoring during the initiation of therapy and when changing solution bags and IV tubing is extremely important in order to evaluate the patient's response and minimize the chance of an adverse effect.

The metabolism of nitroprusside to thiocyanate also warrants close monitoring of serum thiocyanate levels after the drug has been infusing for 48 hours. Blood levels of less than 10 mg per 100 ml are considered to be safe for continued use. Such symptoms of thiocyanate toxicity as fatigue, nausea, tinnitus, blurred vision, and delirium have been reported [41].

Hydralazine

Actions and Clinical Uses

Originally used widely as an antihypertensive agent, hydralazine is known primarily for its ability to relax the vascular smooth muscle and dilate the arterioles. A lesser effect of relaxing the veins produces an additional benefit in lowering left ventricular filling pressure [36]. Hydralazine is also thought to produce a small degree of positive inotropy. Systemic vascular resistance decreases with an improvement in renal, splanchnic, and hepatic blood flow. Hydralazine has also been found to enhance myocardial O_2 supply despite any related increases in myocardial O_2 consumption. Increases in heart rate have been attributed to the direct effect of the drug, although a reflex-mediated response has also been implicated [37].

Dosage and Administration

The usual oral dose of hydralazine ranges from 25 to 100 mg administered three or four times a day. The IV route is generally reserved for selected situations requiring immediate interventions. Doses of 20 to 40 mg may be diluted in 50 ml of D_5W and infused over a 30-minute period.

The onset of action with oral administration occurs within 30 minutes, with a half-life ranging from 2 to 8 hours. Metabolism and excretion occur in the liver and the kidneys, respectively, which may warrant dose adjustment for patients in hepatic or renal failure.

Side Effects

The most common side effects involve headaches, nausea, and vomiting. Taking the drug with meals or snacks has been suggested as a means for reducing the gastrointestinal effects. Long-term treatment with higher doses has been associated with toxicity and adverse effects, such as drug fever and rash and a syndrome of systemic lupus erythematosus.

Prazosin

Actions and Clinical Uses
Prazosin hydrochloride (Minipress) is an alpha-adrenergic blocking agent that blocks alpha 1 adrenergic receptors and thereby reduces peripheral vascular resistance. The selective adrenergic blockade is thought to be the mechanism for preventing the reflex tachycardia that occurs as a consequence with most vasodilators. Prazosin exerts a combined and equivalent vasodilating effect on the arterioles and veins, thus resembling nitroprusside in action. Although prazosin may be very effective in the treatment of hypertension and congestive heart failure, the desired effect is not always maintained during long-term therapy [42].

Dosage and Administration
The initial oral dose is 1 mg. This may gradually be increased to a total daily dose of 20 mg, given in divided doses. A peak effect is observed within 45 minutes and lasts for approximately 6 hours. The elimination half-life may be prolonged with advanced degrees of failure.

Side Effects
Postural hypotension accompanied by faintness and palpitation is commonly noted following the initial dose. Other reported side effects include transient headaches, drowsiness, nausea, lethargy, dry mouth, mental depression, fluid retention, skin rash, urinary incontinence, and polyarthralgias.

Captopril

Actions and Clinical Uses
As renin–angiotensin activity in congestive heart failure is explored, new pharmacological approaches evolve [41]. Captopril is known as a converting-enzyme inhibitor that blocks the action of the converting enzyme kininase in the degradation of the potent vasodilator bradykinin and the conversion of angiotensin I to angiotensin II. A reduction in the release of aldosterone is another important effect, particularly in the treatment of congestive heart failure.

Clinical improvements are related to a decreased peripheral resistance, an increased cardiac index, and a decreased left ventricular end-diastolic pressure, effects similar to those of other vasodilators. Captopril is not generally considered to be a first-line agent but may be used when progressive heart failure is unresponsive to more conventional agents.

Dosage and Administration
Patients usually start at a very low dose of captopril, 2.5 to 5 mg, because of the potential for an extreme hypotensive response. The dose may be increased slowly to as much as 150 mg daily given in divided doses every 6 to 8 hours [42].

Side Effects

The most serious of the side effects include leukopenia and glomerulonephritis-related proteinuria that appears within 3 to 6 months from the initiation of treatment but is reversible with the cessation of therapy. Pruritic rash and loss of taste have also been reported and attributed to a dose-related response.

SUMMARY

The nurse's knowledge of cardiovascular pharmacology should include a sound physiological basis and clinically relevant information about dosage, administration, and side effects.

With the increasing complexity of medical therapy, it is important to anticipate cardiovascular responses. In the critical care unit, physiological variables are likely to be the major determinant of therapy. As patients progress, however, an accurate functional pattern assessment will yield useful cues to promote adherence.

STUDY QUESTIONS

1. List Gordon's functional patterns, and comment on the effects of drug therapy.
2. List three general guidelines for preparing IV admixtures.
3. Define *therapeutic* and *pharmaceutical incompatibilities.*
4. Describe the common complications associated with the administration of sodium bicarbonate.
5. In the event that a patient is unresponsive to atropine, which drug is likely to be prescribed next?
6. Identify the different adrenergic receptors according to their location, physiological action, and responsiveness to catecholamines.
7. Explain the rationale for cautious administration of isoproterenol in the setting of an acute myocardial infarction.
8. Differentiate the effects and indications for high- and low-dose dopamine administration.
9. When is lidocaine prophylaxis indicated?
10. What measures should be taken if a patient has received a 75 mg bolus of lidocaine intravenously followed by a 2 mg per minute drip yet demonstrates ventricular tachycardia within 10 minutes of its initiation?
11. What ECG changes require special attention during the administration of antiarrhythmic therapy? Explain.
12. What is the major hazard associated with antiarrhythmic therapy?
13. List the pharmacological properties of beta blockers, and define their clinical significance.
14. Describe the various nitrate preparations and the indications for their use.
15. What would you teach a patient about proper use of nitroglycerin?
16. How do the different calcium channel blockers produce their beneficial effects?

17. What ECG changes occur normally as a result of the administration of digitalis preparations?

18. Which key factor determines the adequacy of digitalization?

19. What are the most common manifestations of digitalis intoxication?

20. What factors contribute to the development of digitalis intoxication?

21. Why is it necessary to give digitalis to patients receiving quinidine for the treatment of atrial flutter?

22. What is the most common complication of diuretic therapy?

23. Explain the usefulness of vasodilators in the treatment of congestive heart failure.

24. When should thiocyanate levels be monitored?

25. Explain the concern related to the administration of nitroprusside in the setting of an acute myocardial infarction.

REFERENCES

1. Antman, E. M. Acute myocardial infarction. In R. Rakel (ed.), *Current Therapy,* Philadelphia: Saunders, 1984.

2. Antman, E. M., et al. Calcium channel blocking agents in the treatment of cardiovascular disorders. I. Basic and clinical electrophysiologic effects. *Ann. Intern. Med.* 93:875, 1980.

3. Baaske, D. M., et al. Nitroglycerin compatibility with intravenous fluid filters, containers, and administration sets. *Am. J. Hosp. Pharmacol.* 37:201, 1980.

4. Baim, B. S., et al. Evaluation of a new bipyridine inotropic agent — Milrinone — in patients with severe congestive heart failure. *N. Engl. J. Med.* 309:748, 1983.

5. Braunwald, E. *Heart Disease: Textbook of Cardiovascular Medicine* (2nd ed.). Philadelphia: Saunders, 1984.

6. Brest, A. N. Diuretic drug management of heart failure. *Primary Cardiol.* (Suppl.) 2:134, 1983.

7. Cantwell, R., Hollis, R., and Rogers, M. P. Think fast — what do you know about cardiac drugs for a code? *Nurs. '82* 12(10):34, 1982.

8. Chatterjee, K. Long-term vasodilator therapy for chronic heart failure. *Primary Cardiol.* (Suppl.) 2:126, 1983.

9. Chidsey, C. A. Calcium metabolism in the normal and failing heart. *Hosp. Pract.* 8:65, 1972.

10. Cohn, J. N., et al. Effect of short-term infusion of sodium nitroprusside on mortality rate in acute myocardial infarction complicated by left ventricular dysfunction. *N. Engl. J. Med.* 306:1129, 1983.

11. Collinsworth, K. A. The clinical pharmacology of lidocaine as an antiarrhythmic drug. *Circulation* 50:1217, 1974.

12. Dauchot, P., and Gravenstein, J. S. Bradycardia after myocardial ischemia and its treatment with atropine. *Anesthesiology* 44:501, 1976.

13. de Soyza, N. The role of beta-blocking drugs. *Primary Cardiol.* 5:43, 1979.

14. Durrer, J. D., et al. Effect of sodium nitroprusside on mortality in acute myocardial infarction. *N. Engl. J. Med.* 306:1121, 1982.

15. Elkayam, U. Marked early attenuation of hemodynamic effects of oral prazosin in chronic congestive heart failure. *Am. J. Cardiol.* 44:540, 1979.

16. Feldman, R., and Conti, R. Relief of myocardial ischemia: what is the mechanism? *Circulation* 64:1098, 1981.

17. Frishman, W. Clinical pharmacology of the new beta-adrenergic blocking agents. I. Pharmacodynamic and pharmacokinetic properties. *Am. Heart J.* 97:663, 1979.

18. Gillespie, T. A. Effects of dobutamine in patients with acute myocardial infarction. *Am. J. Cardiol.* 39:588, 1977.

19. Gilman, A. G. *Goodman and Gilman's The Pharmacological Basis of Therapeutics* (6th ed.). New York: Macmillan, 1980.

20. Gong, H. Inadequate drug mixing: a potential hazard in continuous intravenous administration. *Heart Lung* 12:528, 1983.

21. Gordon, M. *Nursing Diagnosis: Process and Application.* New York: McGraw-Hill, 1982.

22. Hager, W. D., et al. Digoxin-quinidine interaction: pharmacokinetic evaluation. *N. Engl. J. Med.* 300:1238, 1979.

23. Harris, L., McKenna, W., Rowland, E., et al. Side effects of long-term amiodarone therapy. *Circulation* 67:45, 1983.

24. Hill, N. S., et al. Intravenous nitroglycerin: a review of pharmacology, indications, therapeutic effects, and complications. *Chest* 79:69, 1981.

25. Hollenberg, N. K., and Williams, G. H. The renin–angiotensin system in congestive heart failure. *J. Cardiovasc. Med.* 6:359, 1981.

26. Huss, P., et al. The new inotropic drug, dobutamine. *Heart Lung* 10:121, 1981.

27. Johnson, G. P., and Johanson, B. C. Beta-blockers. *Am. J. Nurs.* 83:1034, 1983.

28. Josephson, M. E., Kasto, J. A., and Kitchen, J. G. Lidocaine in Wolff-Parkinson-White syndrome. *Ann. Intern. Med.* 84:44, 1976.

29. Kerber, R. E., and Sarnat, W. Factors influencing successful defibrillation in man. *Circulation* 60:226, 1979.

30. Kirby, J. A., and Woods, S. A. A study of variation in measurement of doses of nitroglycerin ointment. *Heart Lung* 10:814, 1981.

31. Koch-Weser, J. Disopyramide, *New Engl. J. Med.* 300:957, 1979.

32. Lee, T. H., and Smith, T. W. Serum digoxin concentration and diagnosis of digitalis toxicity current concepts. *Clin. Pharmcokinet.* 8:279, 1983.

33. Lie, K. I., Wellens, N. J., and van Capelle, F. J. Lidocaine in the prevention of primary ventricular fibrillation: a double-blind, randomized study of 212 consecutive patients. *N. Engl. J. Med.* 291:1624, 1974.

34. Livesay, J. J., et al. Optimizing myocardial supply/demand balance with alpha-adrenergic drugs during cardiopulmonary resuscitation. *J. Thorac. Cardiovasc. Surg.* 76:244, 1978.

35. Lown, B., Podrid, P. J., DeSilva, R. A., and Graboys, T. B. Sudden cardiac death: management of the patient at risk. In *Current Problems in Cardiology.* Chicago: Year Book, 1980.

36. Magorien, R. D., et al. Prazosin and hydralazine in congestive heart failure. *Ann. Intern. Med.* 95:5, 1981.

37. Magorien, R. D., et al. Dobutamine and hydralazine: comparative influences of positive inotropy and vasodilation on coronary blood flow and myocardial energetics in non-ischemic congestive heart failure. *J. Am. Coll. Cardiol.* 1:499, 1983.

38. Mandel, W. J., et al. The Wolff-Parkinson-White syndrome: pharmacologic effects of procainamide. *Am. Heart J.* 90:744, 1975.

39. Massumi, R. A., et al. Ventricular fibrillation and tachycardia after intravenous administration of atropine for the treatment of bradycardias. *N. Engl. J. Med.* 287:336, 1972.

40. McGoon, M. D., et al. Clinical use of verapamil. *Mayo Clin. Proc.* 57:495, 1982.

41. McIntyre, K. M., and Lewis, A. J. *Textbook of Advanced Cardiac Life Support.* Dallas: American Heart Association, 1983.

42. Michaelson, C. R. *Congestive Heart Failure.* St. Louis: Mosby, 1983.

43. Morady, F., Scheinman, M. M., and Desai, J. Disopyramide. *Ann. Intern. Med.* 96:337, 1982.

44. Morganroth, J., Pearlman, A., Dunkman, W. B., et al. Ethmozin: a new antiarrhythmic developed in the USSR: efficacy and tolerance. *Am. Heart J.* 98:621, 1979.

45. Morris, M. E. Intravenous drug incompatibilities. *Am. J. Nurs.* 79:1288, 1979.

46. Mueller, H. S., Evans, R., and Ayers, S. Effect of dopamine on hemodynamics and myocardial metabolism in shock following acute myocardial infarction in man. *Circulation* 57:36l, 1978.

47. Norwegian Multicenter Study Group. Timolol-induced reduction in mortality and reinfarction in patients surviving acute myocardial infarction. *N. Engl. J. Med.* 304:801, 1981.

48. Opie, L. H. *Drugs for the Heart.* Orlando: Grune & Stratton, 1984.

49. Passamani, E. Nitroprusside in myocardial infarction. *N. Engl. J. Med.* 306:1168, 1982.

50. Patterson, E., and Lucchesi, B. R. Bretylium: a prototype for the future development of antidysrhythmic agents. *Am. Heart J.* 106:426, 1983.

51. Podrid, P. J., and Lown, B. Amiodarone therapy in symptomatic sustained refractory atrial and ventricular tachyarrhythmias. *Am. Heart J.* 101:374, 1981.

52. Podrid, P. J., and Lown, B. Mexiletine for ventricular arrhythmias. *Am. J. Cardiol.* 47:895, 1981.

53. Podrid, P. J., and Lown, B. Tocainide for refractory symptomatic ventricular arrhythmias. *Am. J. Cardiol.* 49:1279, 1982.

54. Podrid, P. J., Lyakishev, A., Lown, B. et al. Ethmozin, a new antiarrhythmic drug for suppressing ventricular premature complexes. *Circulation* 61:450, 1980.

55. Richman, S. Adverse effect of atropine during myocardial infarction: enhancement of ischemia following intravenously administered atropine. *J.A.M.A.* 228:1414, 1974.

56. Roberts, J. R., et al. Blood levels following intravenous and endotracheal epinephrine administration. *Journal of American College of Emergency Physicians*, 8:53, 1979.

57. Rossi, L. P., and Antman, E. M. Calcium channel blockers: new treatment for cardiovascular disease. *Am. J. Nurs.* 83:382, 1983.

58. Ruskin, J., et al. Antiarrhythmic drugs: a possible cause of out-of-hospital cardiac arrest. *N. Engl. J. Med.* 309:1302, 1983.

59. Ryan, W., Engler, R., Dewinter, M., et al. Efficacy of a new oral agent (tocainide) in the acute treatment of refractory ventricular arrhythmias. *Am. J. Cardiol.* 43:285, 1979.

60. Selzer, A. Quinidine in perspective: the rise and fall of quinidine. *Heart Lung* 11:20, 1982.

61. Somberg, J. C., et al. Pharmacology of nitrates and other drugs in the treatment of ischemic heart disease. *Cardiovasc. Rev. Rep.* 3:1450, 1982.

62. Steen, P. A., et al. Efficacy of dopamine, dobutamine, and epinephrine during emergence from cardiopulmonary bypass in man. *Circulation* 57:378, 1978.

63. Stone, P. H., et al. Calcium channel blocking agents in the treatment of cardiovascular disorders. II. Hemodynamic effects and clinical applications. *Ann. Intern. Med.* 93:886, 1980.

64. Underhill, S. L., et al. *Cardiac Nursing.* Philadelphia: Lippincott, 1982.

65. Weily, H. S., and Genton, E. Pharmacokinetics of procainamide. *Arch. Intern. Med.* 130:366, 1972.

66. White, R. D., et al. Plasma ionic calcium levels following injection of chloride, gluconate, and gluceptate salts of calcium. *J. Thorac. Cardiovasc. Surg.* 71:609, 1976.

67. Wit, A. L., Rosen, M. R., and Hoffman, B. F. Electrophysiology and pharmacology of cardiac arrhythmias: cardiac effects of diphenylhydantoin. *Am. Heart J.* 90:397, 1975.

68. Wyman, M. G., et al. Multiple bolus technique for lidocaine administration during the first hours of an acute myocardial infarction. *Am. J. Cardiol.* 41:313, 1978.

69. Wyman, M. G., and Gore, S. Lidocaine prophylaxis in myocardial infarction: a concept whose time has come. *Heart Lung* 12:358, 1983.

70. Yakaitis, R. W., Otto, C. W., and Blitt, C. D. Relative importance of alpha and beta adrenergic receptors during resuscitation. *Crit. Care* 7:293, 1979.

CHAPTER 15

Cardiac Rehabilitation

Alyce Souden Lanoue

INTRODUCTION

The American Heart Association (AHA) estimates that more than 4 million people in this country have a history of acute myocardial infarction (MI), angina pectoris (AP), or both. Approximately 550,000 survivors of MI are discharged from hospitals each year [3]. Improved medical care, including coronary care units, emergency care, and the availability of coronary artery surgery, as well as secondary prevention through cardiac risk factor modification, has increased the number of survivors of acute MI [38]. In 1982, 170,000 myocardial revascularization procedures were done [3]. The concept that many of these patients can return to active and productive lives is the basis of cardiac rehabilitation [31].

Interest in the rehabilitation of persons with cardiovascular disease has been generated by many factors, including advances in diagnosis and treatment of cardiac diseases, an appreciation of the deleterious effects of prolonged bed rest, and the realization that merely surviving a critical illness may not be enough. A definition of rehabilitation was given by the European Office of the World Health Organization (WHO) in 1969 and is still valid today [44].

> The rehabilitation of cardiac patients can be defined as the sum of activities required to ensure them the best possible physical, mental, and social conditions so that they may, by their own efforts, resume as normal a place as possible in the community.

Provision of this care has become an accepted and necessary part of the intervention for patients with coronary artery disease.

Historically, cardiac patients were treated with prolonged bed rest (minimum of six to eight weeks) and were cautioned against strenuous activity. It is not surprising, therefore, that many cardiac patients became invalids after the onset of their disease. Studies that challenged the provision of prolonged bed rest for cardiac patients found no differences in morbidity or mortality with decreased periods of bed rest.

With the demonstration that no ill effects followed early mobilization came the hope that cardiac patients could eventually be restored to full working lives. Concepts from vocational rehabilitation and exercise were initially emphasized in the 1960s and 1970s. Today, several disciplines are considered essential parts of a system designed to treat this multifactorial disease. Once the apparently healthy person becomes a victim of MI, he and his family are confronted with a potentially fatal, chronic illness with physiological, psychological, and socioeconomic consequences [37]. A comprehensive approach to those affected includes observation and treatment of complications, rehabilitation, and secondary prevention [31]. Patient rehabilitation after MI includes disease prevention; diagnosis; medical and surgical care; assessment of physical, emotional, and educational function; and the provision of medical services, education, training, and other means of enhancing function [41]. Secondary prevention is a part of rehabilitation, although the efficacy of rehabilitation in preventing new cardiac events has not been proved.

International acceptance of cardiac rehabilitation has grown, as has the research that is being conducted on this topic. In spite of interest and research, some aspects of cardiac rehabilitation remain controversial. Patient selection, effects on morbidity and mortality, and effects on vocational, psychological, and sexual status are in the process of being studied. Cost justification and reimbursement by third-party payers are issues that must be resolved [34].

This chapter presents the current rationale for the various components in cardiac rehabilitation programming and the focus of the multidisciplinary team. Specific emphasis is placed on the role of the critical care and progressive care unit nurse in the cardiac rehabilitation process.

MANAGEMENT OF CARDIAC REHABILITATION

Components

Cardiac rehabilitation programming should offer a comprehensive approach with multifactorial management to the patient with coronary artery disease [5, 26, 28]. Programs, in fact, vary widely in scope, intent, type, and delivery of services. Sivarajan [36] attributes this variety to problems finding qualified personnel, cost, and the lack of research regarding effectiveness of existing methods and programs. Several components, however, generally are included in cardiac rehabilitation programs: patient and family education, progressive ambulation, and psychosocial support and counseling. Because there may be many differences among individual programs, principles rather than specifics are stressed in this chapter.

Delineation of the stages of cardiac rehabilitation into phases is a convenient way to describe the process. At least two different labeling systems exist in the literature, however.

The AHA utilizes the following classifications [2]. Representative lengths of each phase are listed.

Phase I: coronary care unit (CCU) (1 to 4 days)

Phase II: remainder of hospital stay (8 to 14 days)

Phase III: convalescence—outpatient (6 to 10 weeks)

Phase IV: recovery/maintenance (post-healing MI/coronary artery bypass [CABG] surgery)

Another system is used by the American College of Sports Medicine (ACSM) [1]:

Phase I: hospitalization (10 to 14 days)

Phase II: convalescence—outpatient (6 to 10 weeks)

Phase III: recovery/maintenance (post-healing MI/CABG)

Either is adequate as long as the reader understands which classification system is being used. For the purposes of this chapter, the ACSM classification will be employed.

Candidates for Rehabilitation

Organized cardiac rehabilitation programs have gained wide acceptance within the medical community for patients recovering from an MI or a CABG. Inpatient candidates (phase I) consist mostly of MI and CABG patients. Patients with angina and patients with other indications of high risk for cardiac disease may be included, however. Certain components of the program, such as mobilization, are delayed if the patient is not physiologically stable, but other components, including education and support, can be initiated. Age of the individual is not by itself a contraindication, although program modification is often necessary for persons over 70 years of age. Patients with coexisting diseases such as severe pulmonary disease may not respond well to exercise, even with supplemental oxygen and a modified program. The mental status of the patient should be such that he or she demonstrates the capacity to understand and cooperate with the program.

The rationale for the inclusion of patients following CABG is that because myocardial revascularization does not treat the underlying atherosclerosis, the patient must still modify his lifestyle, reduce risk factors, and participate in cardiac conditioning [49].

Candidates for a phase II (outpatient) program include discharged MI patients, recovering surgical patients, and patients with stable angina. A low-level exercise test done before discharge is useful in identifying the exercise prescription as well as those patients who are not good candidates for continued rehabilitation. Generally, patients should be able to perform exercise up to a level of two and a half to three times resting without untoward signs. The availability of monitoring capability is taken into account when referring certain patients to a program.

Two to four months after the MI or surgery, patients may be referred for phase III. Phase III programs are also offered with various monitoring options. The need for monitoring in the particular case must be considered in selecting a program for the patient.

Ideally, patients will be referred for all three phases of rehabilitation in sequence. Eligible patients may be referred for entry into rehabilitation at any stage, however. Counseling and education, therefore, should be offered through all three phases.

Multidisciplinary Team Members and Role Functions

The concept of cardiovascular disease as a multifactorial problem requires that interventions be implemented in several areas, such as psychosocial activity, nutrition, and smoking cessation. Although some of these problems may be more significant for a particular patient and family, most patients have needs across this whole spectrum. Members of the cardiac rehabilitation team may vary, depending on the institution or program and also on the stage of the patient's illness. Most often, nurses, physicians, physical or occupational therapists, dieticians, and social workers form the core of the team for the inpatient. Other professionals, such as a psychiatric nurse specialist, psychiatrists, psychologists, a chaplain, and a vocational rehabilitation counselor, are used for consultation to the team as the need arises. Communication among the team members is crucial. Regularly scheduled team conferences, as well as concise documentation, are important.

Nursing Coordinator

A nurse coordinator with particular expertise in cardiovascular nursing may formally or informally coordinate the team effort, either in phase I (inpatient) or through all phases. In some institutions this coordinator is a cardiovascular clinical specialist or a member of nursing management, such as the head nurse for progressive care or the patient care supervisor. Functions of this role may include orientation of new hospital personnel to the cardiac rehabilitation program, continuing professional education, and direct implementation and evaluation of the program. Serving as spokesperson for cardiac rehabilitation in the community, consulting within the organization, and initiating, implementing, and evaluating nursing research projects related to rehabilitation are also important facets of the coordinator's role.

Nursing Staff (Inpatient)

Nurses in critical care and medical units participate in cardiac rehabilitation by collecting the initial nursing data, monitoring patients for physiological changes, and directly implementing parts of the program. For example, coronary care unit (CCU) nurses may complete the initial exercise steps while patients are in the CCU. The initiation of patient education is also a major nursing function. The nurse is in an ideal position to teach as well as to observe patient understanding and compliance. Staff nurses may also participate in research regarding cardiac rehabilitation by initiating their own studies or by collecting data for a study in progress.

Nursing Staff (Outpatient)

Nurses are also involved in phases II and III of hospital-based cardiac rehabilitation (outpatient). Their role functions (along with other team members) include implementation and evaluation of patient and family education, implementation of appropriate exercise, participation in groups in which patients and families discuss their feelings and reactions to coronary artery disease, and documentation of the interventions and patient response in the medical record. Nurses may also participate in professional education and research.

Community health nurses may get involved in cardiac rehabilitation for selected patients by coordinating community resources and supervising patients maintained on complicated treatment regimens. Nurse practitioners in the community manage patients with chronic illnesses and therefore may become involved in cardiac rehabilitation. Nurses in the community also serve as a source of referral to the program. It is therefore important that the availability and scope of cardiac rehabilitation be communicated to those nurses working with physicians in clinics, in schools, and in industry.

Physicians

A physician is usually designated as the medical director of cardiac rehabilitation and serves as a consultant to the team on a daily basis. The patient's primary physician is responsible for initiating referral to a cardiac rehabilitation program, however. The physician also manages the medical therapy of the patient and modifies the rehabilitation plan to meet the individual's needs. Physicians may participate in hospital-based phase III exercise programs, particularly if the exercise site is off the hospital grounds.

Physical Therapist

The physical therapist participates in the identification of candidates for rehabilitation and gathers initial data related to previous exercise habits and any contraindications to activity. The therapist may also supervise the implementation of the exercise program for patients in all three phases of rehabilitation, modifying the program for persons with specific and limiting musculoskeletal problems. Patient and family education specifically related to exercise and activity is important. The physical therapist may also become involved in community teaching about cardiac rehabilitation.

Dietician

The dietician coordinates the nutritional care of patients in all three phases of rehabilitation. After completing an initial assessment of usual dietary habits with particular reference to sodium, fat, calorie, and caffeine intake, the dietician makes recommendations to the physician about dietary modification. Another important responsibility is patient and family education. Instruction of the patient and family individually and in groups about general nutrition principles and the prescribed diet should be completed before discharge. The dietician may also become involved in community teaching about cardiac rehabilitation.

Social Worker

The social worker participates in the rehabilitation effort by completing initial psychosocial assessments of patients referred to the program, and by providing intervention and counseling for patients and families. Specific areas of concern may relate to emotional responses to the illness, return to work, financial concerns and resources, and family adjustment, including sexuality. The social worker also participates in patient and family education in the areas of normal reactions to the illness, stress and personality factors, and adjustments during convalescence. Group settings designed to meet educational and support needs of outpatients and their families may be facilitated by a social worker.

Other Personnel

As stated previously, a need may exist for the expertise of other professionals, such as a vocational counselor or a chaplain. The focus of additional consultants is to meet individual needs of patients and families that have been identified by the core multidisciplinary team.

PHASE I

The goals of phase I include education of the patient and family, progressive mobilization, and preservation of the patient's self-image and family relationships. Although the entire hospitalization is considered phase I, specific concerns relating to critical care are discussed separately, because critical care nursing is the focus of this book. Patient problems and nursing interventions, however, overlap from the critical care area to the progressive and/or medical unit.

Cardiac Intensive Care Unit

Initial nursing and medical intervention in the acute phase for patients after MI or CABG is directed toward alleviation of physiological problems, rapid identification and management of existing problems, and prevention and detection of complications [48]. After the patient's physiological condition has stabilized, cardiac rehabilitation can begin. This may occur within 24 hours of admission for the patient who has had an uncomplicated MI. Rehabilitation and preparation for discharge for the patient who has undergone CABG should begin shortly after transfer from the critical care unit [49].

Nursing Data Base

An initial nursing history and assessment are obtained to create a data base from which interventions can be planned. A nursing data base includes the patient's biopsychosocial history, physical examination findings, and results from laboratory tests [13]. Information from an assessment of the functional health patterns is also added to the data base. Specific assessment of those areas that affect cardiac rehabilitation individualizes the nursing intervention. Table 15.1 delineates areas of assessment and their relationship to rehabilitation.

Nursing diagnoses commonly identified in the initial stages of cardiac rehabilitation (in the CICU) may include, but are not limited to, those listed in Table 15.2. In stating potential causes, the words "related to" are recommended rather than "due to" for legal reasons; cause and effect have not yet been established for most nursing diagnoses.

Nursing intervention for the identified patient problems is directed toward certain outcomes (see Table 15.2). Elements of the three major components of cardiac rehabilitation (education, exercise, psychological support) are integrated to meet beginning needs of patients in critical care settings.

TABLE 15.1
Nursing History

Assessment Factor	Rationale for Assessing Prior to Cardiac Rehabilitation
I. Perception of illness	
a. Knowledge of diagnosis (what told vs. what understood)	a. Erroneous information re diagnosis and cause of MI can be corrected in educational sessions; patient's misunderstanding may provide clues to his behavior, i.e., anxiety, depression
b. Perception of cardiac rehabilitation/changes in lifestyle expected	b. Concepts of rehabilitation can be introduced; teaching is individualized
II. Medical data	
a. Previous unresolved medical problems	a. Presence of problems: orthopedic, respiratory, renal, neurological, etc., may increase MVO_2 and create imbalance in myocardial O_2 supply and demand, and ischemia
b. Occupation — physical/emotional demands, other factors, e.g., commuting, overnight travel	b. Return to work is realistic goal for most patients, but demands of job and other factors may necessitate longer convalescence, job modification, and/or retraining

TABLE 15.1 *(continued)*

Assessment Factor	Rationale for Assessing Prior to Cardiac Rehabilitation
c. Living arrangements — stairs, home responsibilities/housework/maintenance	c. Baseline established; counseling for return to activities individualized; women especially may have difficult time avoiding housework after discharge
d. Health insurance arrangements/financial concerns	d. Financial concerns may increase the patient's anxiety, may indicate need for immediate social service consult
e. Mental and emotional responses/presence of expected reactions and their resolution/maladaptive coping mechanisms	e. Cardiac patients commonly express anxiety, denial, depression, anger, and sexual aggressiveness in response to illness

III. Functional patterns and changes secondary to hospitalization

Assessment Factor	Rationale for Assessing Prior to Cardiac Rehabilitation
a. Comfort/discomfort — before hospitalization, treatment, and response; since hospitalization, why patient believes discomfort occurs	a. Many patients experience warning symptoms, i.e., angina before MI; discomfort since hospitalization may be extension of MI, angina, other complications, i.e., pericarditis or unrelated problems; baseline useful
b. Rest/sleep — usual pattern; hours and length, sleep routine, sleep meds, naps, number of pillows and why, problems since hospitalization	b. Sleep problems common after MI; sleep disruption common in critical care units; emotional responses may affect sleep; number of pillows may be related to increasing respiratory distress or simply to patient preference; scheduled meds in CCU, vital signs, etc., may continually disrupt sleep; some meds disrupt REM sleep
c. Hygiene — usual patterns, i.e., bath, shower; care of nails, hair	c. Assessment of usual pattern individualizes patient goals; also predicts patient satisfaction/reaction to alternate methods, i.e., bed bath vs. shower
d. Mobility, activity pattern, ROM; usual exercise level: type, duration, intensity, compliance, limitations due to other problems, e.g., prior back injury; understanding of when return to activity is possible; presence of claudication symptoms: distance and grade patient can comfortably walk, number of stairs and at what speed	d. One of the major components of rehab concerns exercise; knowing previous level, interest, and limitations allows logical and individualized progression; i.e., previously sedentary person will generally progress at a slower rate than an athlete; assessing knowledge of when patient expects to return to certain activity is also helpful; symptoms of claudication may require program modification and may be exacerbated by beta blockers
e. Cognitive, perceptual — patient's major language, ability to read and hear at a level that allows patient to participate in education; how does patient feel he learns best; any changes since patient hospitalized	e. Educational methods may require modification, i.e., alternate language, large print, individual vs. group instruction; particular need may exist for family involvement, community resources, e.g., VNA
f. Nutrition — usual pattern at home and changes since hospitalization; who cooks and shops; examples of usual meal pattern at home, and when dining out, with particular emphasis on salt, calories, caffeine, and fats; frequency of dining out; number of meals per day; usual mealtime atmosphere; present weight and "ideal weight"; limitations in diet related to other medical problems, likes/dislikes, ethnic foods, finances, transportation, etc.; any problems since hospitalization	f. Dietary changes are likely to be permanent lifestyle modifications; therefore, people who shop and prepare food should also receive instruction; extensive travel (with job or for pleasure) may impede patient's attempts to modify diet; other limitations, financial constraint, likes, etc., in diet may not be compatible with prescribed diet; note cholesterol, HDL, and triglyceride levels, if available; eating under stress increases demand on myocardium

TABLE 15.1   *(continued)*

Assessment Factor	Rationale for Assessing Prior to Cardiac Rehabilitation
g. Elimination — usual pattern of bowel and bladder elimination; laxative use and effect; any changes in elimination since hospitalization	g. Combination of inactivity, diet changes, meds, and need to use commode/bedpan frequently causes constipation; straining causes Valsalva effect on heart and should be avoided; preexisting urinary tract problems, e.g., BPH, may require early intervention, e.g., standing to void even while confined to bed
h. Respiratory/breathing — any problems at home, i.e., dyspnea, SOB; distance and number of flights of stairs patient can comfortably manage, number of pillows, any recent change in that pattern; smoking history — what, how long, how patient feels about quitting, previous attempts at quitting, and results	h. Patient may experience SOB related to deconditioning, pulmonary congestion, or other medical problems; cigarette smoking is a major risk factor for CAD; patient should be strongly encouraged to quit smoking
i. Sexuality — usual patterns, i.e., availability of partner, frequency (times per week or month), average duration of coitus, usual time, favored positions, past experience with chest pain during intercourse, history of any sexual difficulty prior to MI, understanding of when return to sexual activity is possible	i. Goal is to return patient to previous level; assessment of baseline indicates if need for sexual counseling or therapy at later time; chest pain during intercourse is not uncommon; fear is common with MI; physician may prescribe prophylactic nitroglycerin; expectations of resumption of intercourse may be incorrect — many post-MI patients and partners are fearful and choose abstinence; patient may be more likely to verbalize questions if the subject has already been brought up by the nurse
j. Interpersonal relationships, social supports — closest person to patient; coping styles with any past illnesses; "stresses" in life; usual coping styles, e.g., Type A or Type B behavior	j. CV response to stress increases MVO_2, stress is likely a precipitating factor in CAD and affects long-term rehab; MI patients typically go through stages of adaptation to illness — however effective, coping mechanisms used in past may be used again; giving information to patient re potential changes is especially important since the anticipation of a stress may diminish the response associated with the event, i.e., preparation for transfer; manipulation of environment and promotion of sleep also help
k. Medications — meds taken prior to admission; patient's knowledge of action, side effects; self-report of compliance; feelings about taking meds; other problems, e.g., transportation to get meds, expense, inconvenience; understanding of present med regimen and possibility of prescribed meds after discharge	k. Patient's previous experience with meds, compliance, etc., may predict his behavior relative to medication after discharge; patient may not expect present meds to be continued after discharge or may be planning to resume old med schedule after discharge, especially if taking antihypertensives (indicates need for education)
l. Allergies — note known allergies, any problems suspected to be related to meds, etc.; determine presence of asthma, hay fever, etc., especially if patient is taking beta blockers	l. Patient may discontinue prescribed meds if he suspects allergies; respiratory allergies may be contraindication to beta blockers
m. Cardiac risk factors — list as + or −	m. Risk factor modification is major goal in cardiac rehabilitation; sharing list with patient is important teaching tool

MI = myocardial infarction; MVO_2 = myocardial oxygen consumption; CCU = coronary care unit;
REM = rapid eye movement; ROM = range of motion; VNA = Visiting Nurses Association;
HDL = high-density lipoprotein; BPH = benign prostatic hypertrophy; SOB = shortness of breath;
CAD = coronary artery disease; CV = cardiovascular.

TABLE 15.2
Nursing Diagnoses

Nursing Diagnosis	Probable Nursing Orders/ Intervention	Outcomes: Patient Goal
Activity intolerance, related to physical inactivity/MI	Monitor vital signs, ECG, symptoms before, during, and after activity; document responses and deviations	Maintain an activity pattern compatible with therapeutic and personal goals
Cardiac output, alteration in, reduction in, related to myocardial muscle damage, potential dysrhythmias	Provide rest periods between activity periods (including meals)	Demonstrate adequate cardiopulmonary function
Breathing patterns ineffective, related to cardiac effects on respiratory system, smoking history	Initiate rehabilitation steps according to protocol	Be free of chest discomfort
Sleep pattern, disturbance in, related to CICU, physical symptoms, emotional responses	Before beginning activity, assess the patient's sleep pattern; organize activity to allow rest/sleep	Demonstrate a sleep pattern of at least 4 consecutive hr per night after physical condition stabilizes
Bowel elimination, alteration in, constipation, related to inactivity, diet, environmental changes, medications	Provide adequate fluid and roughage in diet; document/use prescribed medications as necessary; provide privacy for commode; discourage straining	Maintain normal bowel pattern
Anxiety, related to diagnosis/CICU	Monitor/document behavioral responses of patient/family; support them and answer questions	Demonstrate expected behavioral responses to MI, i.e., anxiety or denial
Self-concept, disturbance in, related to diagnosis, need for period of time away from occupation, adjustment in family responsibilities	Encourage verbalization of feelings/ concerns related to diagnosis, adjustments, environment	Begin to acknowledge feelings about expected lifestyle adjustment and loss
Coping, ineffective, individual, related to life-threatening illness, sudden hospitalization	Support and encourage patient to verbalize fears and concerns	Acknowledge concerns and feelings regarding hospitalization, CICU, diagnosis
Grieving, anticipatory, related to potential lifestyle modifications, e.g., smoking cessation, dietary changes		
Knowledge deficit, related to new diagnosis, hospitalization, first admission to a CICU	Provide simple/repeated explanations regarding CICU and routine; provide transfer preparation; reinforce usual temporary nature of restrictions	Verbalize understanding of CICU routine and eventual transfer
	Answer questions regarding diagnosis; provide reading material regarding CAD, if appropriate	Know what symptoms to report and when (i.e., chest pain)

MI = myocardial infarction; ECG = electrocardiogram; CICU = coronary intensive care unit;
CAD = coronary artery disease.

Reassessment and evaluation of the effectiveness of the intervention is a continuous process based on patient responses. The plan, therefore, undergoes constant revision.

Activity and Exercise

Physical activity and progressive ambulation constitute one of the major components of cardiac rehabilitation. Initial progessive activity for the patient with an acute ischemic event is designed to decrease the deconditioning effects associated with prolonged bed rest [47]. Activity and exercise after hospital discharge are directed toward improving functional capacity.

It is important that nurses and others involved in cardiac rehabilitation have a basic understanding of the physiology of exercise. The physiological response to exercise involves rapid adjustments to deliver increased blood flow to exercising muscles. This flow is necessary to supply O_2 and nutrients and to remove accumulated waste products of metabolism. Maximal physical activity is limited by factors related to the ability of the cardiovascular system to supply O_2 to working muscles, the functional capabilities of the respiratory system, and the metabolic capabilities of skeletal muscle.

Types of exercise.   There are basically two types of exercise: static (isometric) and aerobic (isotonic) exercise. Static exercise involves sustained muscle tension that produces little or no change in muscle length or joint movement [11]. Examples of this type of exercise include lifting, carrying, and maintaining a sustained hand grip. Aerobic exercise involves rhythmic, repetitive isotonic muscle relaxation and contraction, and joint movement [11]. Examples of this type of exercise include activities that use large muscle groups simultaneously, such as walking, jogging, swimming, and bicycling.

The physiological responses of the cardiovascular system to these two types of exercise differ widely. Most exercises people engage in, however, involve elements of both isometric and isotonic exercise; the proportion of isometric to isotonic work determines the amount of myocardial work [46]. Isometric work causes marked increases in heart rate, systemic vascular resistance, and blood pressure and contributes little to cardiovascular conditioning. Stroke volume remains unchanged in normal people and may fall in people with left ventricular dysfunction. Cardiac output increases slightly in normal people and minimally in persons with heart disease. In addition, strong muscular contractions that reduce the blood supply to the muscles may cause a shift to anaerobic metabolism and limit the duration of exercise. The increase in myocardial afterload increases myocardial O_2 consumption (MVO_2). Thus, isometric exercise may be poorly tolerated by persons with coronary artery disease, especially if left ventricular dysfunction exists. Isotonic (aerobic) activity, on the other hand, increases aerobic metabolism and contributes to cardiovascular conditioning or training [11]. Cardiac output increases, with a rise in heart rate and stroke volume. Ventilation increases, and the arteriovenous O_2 difference becomes greater. Blood flow is redistributed to areas of greatest need, such as exercising muscles. Trained muscles eventually extract a greater amount of O_2 from the blood. Systolic blood pressure during maximal dynamic exercise normally increases 60 to 100 mm Hg in males and 30 to 60 mm in females. Diastolic blood pressure decreases up to 50 mm Hg for both sexes [11].

Different physiological responses are also noted for arm and leg exercise. Arm exercise results in higher heart rates and systolic blood pressure value than does a comparable amount of leg exercise, a fact that must be considered when advising patients about various activities of daily living.

Maximum oxygen uptake (VO_2 max), or aerobic capacity, is a measure of the maximal transport of O_2 (circulation) from the lungs to the tissues. Endurance-type exercise enhances aerobic capacity, which is the major objective of intervention in normal subjects and in those participating in cardiac rehabilitation [12]. VO_2 max is the best measure of fitness and in addition can be used to prescribe exercise. To produce a training effect, the intensity of the workload should be at 75% of the person's VO_2 max. Clinically, 85% of maximum heart rate attained on a stress test correlates to 75% of the VO_2 max [11]. A trained person would have a higher VO_2 max and be able to perform a given amount of work at a lower heart rate and blood pressure than would a deconditioned person doing the same amount of work.

Because MVO_2 depends on heart rate, blood pressure, and the contractile state of the ventricle, activities that are performed at a lower heart rate and systolic blood pressure may be tolerated better by persons with coronary artery disease. The rate pressure product (RPP), or heart rate multiplied by systolic blood pressure, may be used to determine the point clinically below which a person should exercise to avoid an imbalance in myocardial O_2 supply and demand. An imbalance between myocardial O_2 supply and demand results in ischemia, manifested in symptoms such as angina and electrocardiographic changes in the ST segment.

Exercise response in persons with cardiovascular disease correlates to some extent with the degree of impairment from the disease. The inability to increase stroke volume in order to increase cardiac output is the major factor that limits exercise capacity in cardiac patients. Greater increases in heart rate at lower workloads may occur to compensate. These further increase MVO_2 in cardiac patients and may cause ischemic symptoms sooner.

Protective effect of exercise.   The role of physical activity in secondary prevention continues to be studied. A definitive demonstration that conditioning exercise among coronary patients reduces the likelihood of sudden death and recurrent MI would be of tremendous importance in clarifying recommendations for patient management. Debate and research continue, however, over both the role of physical inactivity in the genesis of coronary artery disease (CAD) and the role of exercise as part of primary prevention.

Physical activity on a regular basis is thought to be involved in the control and prevention of elevations in certain cardiovascular risk factors [6]. The relationship of habitual physical inactivity to obesity, hypertension, and elevated blood lipid levels has been studied in numerous clinical trials, with exercise usually prescribed as part of the intervention. Although a cause-and-effect relationship has not been established, inferences can be made about the control of coronary risk factors and regular physical activity [6]. The studies also demonstrate that at a given submaximal workload, some post-MI patients can improve endurance and work performance, lower their RPP, reduce electrocardiographic manifestations of ischemia, and develop less angina with exercise that is gradually increased and that is supervised by trained personnel. Although it can be stated that such exercise is not harmful, problems with study designs preclude a definitive statement about any specific protective effect of exercise on survival.

Effects of prolonged inactivity.   The rationale for the inclusion of progressive activity and early mobilization for cardiac patients is related to research evaluating the effects of prolonged inactivity on normal subjects.

Studies on weightlessness done primarily for the space program indicate that prolonged inactivity causes decreases in plasma volume, decreased circulating blood volume, decreased red cell mass, loss of muscle mass, decreased subcutaneous skin turgor, abnormal heart rate responses to effort, and orthostatic intolerance [21]. The hazards of bed rest were dramatically demonstrated when five normal college students were confined to bed for 20 days [30]. Maximal O_2 uptake decreased 20% to 40%, indicating a rapid loss of physical work capacity from bed rest alone. A vigorous eight-week period of training after bed rest increased the VO_2 max, but a substantial period of time was required for the subjects to return to prior levels (28 and 43 days for athletic subjects). The higher the degree of physical fitness prior to bed rest, the longer the training required to return to the prior functional level. Heart rate increased significantly, from a mean of 125 bpm before bed rest to 164 bpm after bed rest, and decreased again after training. It can be seen that the more vigorous person deconditions more rapidly when subjected to bed rest.

Early mobilization.   Earlier mobilization of patients with CAD has meant that clinical problems related to the effects of prolonged bed rest, such as venous stasis and pulmonary embolization, are reduced. Another benefit of early mobilization is a more positive psychological outlook. Hackett [14] describes a "homecoming depression" triggered by weakness and fatigue. An early mobilization program while the patient is hospitalized may decrease this depression.

Specific intervention to mobilize the patient gradually may be introduced when no physiological alterations, such as uncontrolled anginal pain, unstable dysrhythmias, heart failure, uncontrolled hypertension, pulmonary emboli, severe physical or emotional impairments, and uncompensated valve diseases, exist [46]. Activity at this stage of the illness is designed to minimize the hazards of bed rest, instill confidence in patients that they are not permanently disabled, and reduce the length of hospital stay [46]. Early mobilization is justified on the basis of preventing the complications of immobility, rather than for its own therapeutic value, because no therapeutic value has been proven [43].

A variety of structured programs exist (Tables 15.3 and 15.4) that involve progressing activity according to the patient's tolerance. Activities of daily living such as bathing and feeding are integrated with progressive passive and active activity. Patients generally advance one activity level per day; however,

TABLE 15.3
Inpatient Rehabilitation: Seven-Step Myocardial Infarction Program

Step	Date	M.D. Initials	Nurse/PT Notes	Supervised Exercise	CCU/Ward Activity	Educational-Recreational Activity
CCU						
1	—			Active and passive ROM all extremities, in bed Teach patient ankle plantar and dorsiflexion — repeat hourly when awake	Partial self-care Feed self Dangle legs on side of bed Use bedside commode Sit in chair 15 min 1–2 times/day	Orientation to CCU Personal emergencies, social service aid as needed
2	—			Active ROM all extremities, sitting on side of bed	Sit in chair 15–30 min 2–3 times/day Complete self-care in bed	Orientation to rehabilitation team, program Smoking cessation Educational literature if requested Planning transfer from CCU
Ward						
3	—			Warm-up exercises, 2 METs: Stretching Calisthenics Walk 50 ft and back at slow pace	Sit in chair ad lib To ward class in wheelchair Walk in room	Normal cardiac anatomy and function Development of atherosclerosis What happens with myocardial infarction 1–2 METs craft activity
4	—			ROM and calisthenics, 2.5 METs Walk length of hall (75 ft) and back, average pace Teach pulse counting	OOB as tolerated Walk to bathroom Walk to ward class, with supervision	Coronary risk factors and their control
5	—			ROM and calisthenics, 3 METs Check pulse counting Practice walking few stairsteps Walk 300 ft b.i.d.	Walk to waiting room or telephone Walk in ward corridor p.r.n.	Diet Energy conservation Work simplification techniques (as needed) 2–3 METs craft activity
6	—			Continue above activities Walk down flight of steps (return by elevator) Walk 500 ft b.i.d. Instruct on home exercise	Tepid shower or tub bath, with supervision To OT, cardiac clinic teaching room, with supervision	Heart attack management Medications Exercise Surgery Response to symptoms Family, community adjustments on return home Craft activity p.r.n.

TABLE 15.3 (continued)

Step	Date	M.D. Initials	Nurse/PT Notes	Supervised Exercise	CICU/Ward Activity	Educational-Recreational Activity
7	—			Continue above activities Walk up flight of steps Walk 500 ft b.i.d. Continue home exercise instruction; present information regarding outpatient exercise program	Continue all previous ward activities	Discharge planning: Medications, diet, activity Return appointments Scheduled tests Return to work Community resources Educational literature Medication cards Craft activity p.r.n.

PT = physical therapist; CCU = coronary care unit; ROM = range of motion; OOB = out of bed; OT = occupational therapy.

Adapted from Wenger, N. K. Rehabilitation of the patient with symptomatic coronary disease. In J. W. Hurst (ed): *The Heart,* 5th ed. New York, McGraw-Hill, 1982, p. 1151. Used with permission.

TABLE 15.4
Inpatient Rehabilitation: Postsurgical Patient

Exercise[a]	Ward Activity	Educational Activity[a]
Step 1 (Day of Surgery)		
1. None	1. Complete with assistance: side–back–side	Introduction to Riley special care unit
Step 2		
1. Active ROM to all extremities while lying down — shoulder/elbow flexion and extension, hip/knee flexion and extension; each motion 5×, 4× daily 2. Instruct in active foot circling to be done every 2 hr while awake	1. Complete bed bath by nurse; if patient is able, allow to wash face and genital area, do oral hygiene 2. Self-turning 3. Use of bedside commode 4. Feed self 12 hr after extubation 5. Sitting up in chair, 2× daily for 20 min 6. May take a couple of steps with assistance	Introduction to cardiac rehabilitation
Step 3		
1. Active ROM to all extremities with the bed at 45°, using mild resistance — shoulder/elbow flexion and extension, hip/knee flexion and extension; each motion 5×, 4× daily 2. Encourage foot circles	1. Complete bed bath by nurse; allow patient to wash face and genital area, do oral hygiene 2. Sitting in chair, 20 min for meals and at bedtime 3. Walk 25 ft with assistance 2× daily	Anatomy and physiology/healing process

TABLE 15.4 *(continued)*

Exercise[a]	Ward Activity	Educational Activity[a]
Step 4		
1. Active ROM to arms, while sitting on side of bed, using mild resistance — shoulder/elbow flexion and extension; each motion 5×, 4× daily 2. Encourage foot circles	1. Partial bed bath by nurse; allow patient to wash front of upper torso, do oral hygiene 2. Walk 50 ft with assistance 2× daily	Discussion of medications/diet restrictions
Step 5		
1. Active ROM to arms, while sitting on one side of bed; using moderate resistance — shoulder/elbow flexion and extension, hip/knee flexion and extension; each motion 5×, 4× daily 2. Walk 50 ft 3. Encourage foot circles	1. Partial bed bath by nurse; allow patient to wash front of upper torso, do oral hygiene 2. May sit 20 min for meals, 1× in between and at bedtime 3. Walk to bathroom with assistance	Risk factors in coronary artery disease
Step 6		
1. Standing warm-up exercises: (a) full shoulder abduction, (b) arms straight out from shoulder; simultaneously rotate arms in big circles; (c) leg abduction while leaning against wall, 5× each leg; each motion 5×, 4× daily	1. Walk 50 ft with assistance, 3× daily 2. Bathroom privileges 3. Shower if no chest wires; may walk to shower	Introduction to new unit
Step 7		
1. Standing warm-up exercises: (a) arms straight out from shoulders; simultaneously rotate arms in big circle, 5× each direction; (b) lateral side bends, 5× each side; (c) bend at waist and touch fingers to knees, 10×; each to be done 4× daily	1. Sitting ad lib 2. Walk to solarium 2× daily; may stay ½ hr if tolerated	Group sessions available: Psychosocial adjustments to coronary heart disease[a] Exercise and coronary heart disease[a] Diet and coronary heart disease[a] Smoking and health Hypertension[a] Modification of lifestyle[a]
Step 8		
1. Standing warm-up exercises: (a) full shoulder abduction with 1 lb weights (5×); (b) slight knee bends with hands on hips, 10× (discontinue if reported pain in any leg incisions); (c) 4-way body	1. Walk to solarium, 2× daily; may stay 1 hr if tolerated	Individual sessions: Include but not limited to the following: Sexuality and coronary heart disease[a]

TABLE 15.4 *(continued)*

Exercise[a]	Ward Activity	Educational Activity[a]
bends (bend forward, then erect; to the right, then erect; to the left, then erect); this completes one time; should be done 5×; each of the above to be done 4× daily 2. Walk 2 lengths of the corridor and down 1 flight of stairs; take elevator up		Pulse taking[a] Medications Adjustment in lifestyle

Step 9

1. Standing warm-up exercises: (a) touch knees, 1 lb weight in each hand, 10×; (b) full shoulder abduction with 1 lb weights, 10×; do each 4× daily 2. Walk 2 lengths of the corridor and down 2 flights of stairs; take elevator up	1. Dress with assistance after bath; remain dressed 4 hr	

Step 10

1. Standing warm-up exercises: (a) bend and touch knees, 2 lb weight in each hand, 10×; (b) full shoulder abduction with 2 lb weights, 10×; (c) stand and face wall, 1 arm's length away; place palms on wall; bend elbows and touch nose to wall; straighten elbows and push away (wall push-ups), 10×; do each 4× daily 2. Walk 2 lengths of the corridor, down 2 flights of stairs, and take elevator up	1. Dress tolerated; no girdles 2. Solarium ad lib 3. Sitting ad lib	Cardiac rehabilitation program

Step 11

1. Standing warm-up exercises: (a) bend and touch knees with 2 lb weight in each hand, 10×; (b) full shoulder abduction with 2 lb weights, 10×; (c) wall push-ups, 10×; do each 4× daily 2. Walk 2 lengths of the corridor, up 1 flight of stairs, and then down 1 flight of stairs	1. Up ad lib on floor 2. Dressed ad lib 3. Sitting ad lib	Physician authorization Date _____

[a]Exercises and educational sessions adapted from La Crosse exercise program, La Crosse, Wisconsin.

ROM = range of motion.

the treatment of CABG patients is often more aggressive. Because the average length of stay for a patient following an uncomplicated MI or CABG is 7 to 10 days, structured programs require periodic revision to remain congruent with changes in current practice.

Physical activity in the CICU involves progressive self-care, supervised active and passive extremity movements, and progressive activity from bed rest to chair rest to minimal ambulation. The concept of METS is useful in recommending activity to patients. One MET is defined as approximately the energy expended per minute while sitting quietly in a chair, which correlates with an O_2 consumption of 3.5 ml/kg per minute of O_2. MET charts of common activities are published and readily available. The energy expenditure of activity in the acute phase is approximately 1.5 to 2.0 METS and should be closely supervised by CICU nurses or physical therapists who have expertise in treating patients with cardiac problems [46]. Particular attention is paid to arm work versus leg work, rest periods, and the relationship of physical activity to other activities that increase MVO_2, such as eating, emotional stress, and extremes of temperature.

The patient is monitored for untoward responses to physical activity by objective and subjective means. Vital signs, symptom responses, and electrocardiogram (ECG) are monitored before, during, and after exercise. Documentation in the record by the nurse of the extent of the activity and the patient's response to it should be specified in relation to cardiovascular values (vital signs, ECG), central nervous system (changes in alertness; confusion), respiratory characteristics (unusual increase in respiratory rate or shortness of breath), skin temperature and color (changes), and miscellaneous data (ischemic symptoms) [25]. The nurse also arranges and enforces rest periods between activities to avoid excessive increases in myocardial O_2 demand and to enhance the patient's ability to tolerate increased activity. It is important that the patient and family be given repeated explanations about the objectives and procedures of the progressive activity program to alleviate any possible misconceptions. Some patients and families display alarm when informed about activity progression, whereas others view increased activity as a sign that "no damage to the heart occurred — if it had, I wouldn't be allowed out of bed like this."

A detrimental response to exercise indicates that the patient's level of physical activity should be decreased [40, 43]. Such responses include:

Chest pain, dyspnea, palpitations

An increase in heart rate to over 120 bpm or 20 bpm over baseline

Fall in systolic blood pressure of more than 15 to 20 mm Hg

Occurrence of significant dysrhythmias

Increased ST segment displacement (over 1 mm up or down during exercise)

Exercise-induced hypertension (over 180 mm Hg systolic)

Adjustments in the exercise regimen are individualized according to the patient's response to activity.

Patient Education

It has been well documented in the literature that patient and family education is a major component of cardiac rehabilitation. Teaching is an activity that involves the intention to produce learning but not necessarily success [30]. Learning is a change in human behavior that persists over long periods of time. Patients have the right to know what has happened to them and the ways that they can help themselves. Helping them reach this goal is a major responsibility and an independent function of nurses.

A patient education component is included in cardiac rehabilitation partially because of the fact that, although return to a normal life after an MI is an expected outcome for most patients, they need support and information to do this. The adequacy of the patient's knowledge depends partly on the information made available, as well as on his ability to assimilate that information. Any patient who must make life modifications has a need and right to know the rationale for the recommendations and the potential effects of changing or not changing. Patients with CAD, as victims of a chronic illness, should learn to modify life habits that are believed to affect the progression of atherosclerosis. Maintenance of health and control of disease, not cure, become the focus of health care when the disease is chronic [20].

Accepting the professional responsibility for patient education and implementing it are two very different activities. Providing patient education takes planning, skill, and time. Content, the readiness of the patient to learn, different methodologies, evaluation and compliance, and the effective use of the principles of teaching and learning are all important concerns related to patient and family education. Using a multidisciplinary team approach is an effective way to enhance learning, because each team member lends individual expertise. A variety of teaching approaches may both motivate and stimulate the patient and family to learn.

Adherence to the principles of teaching and learning is recommended in the implementation of patient education, because many factors already complicate the acutely ill patient's ability to learn [27]. Nurses can implement these principles by teaching patients what they want to learn, by taking the patient's emotional reactions, physical condition, age, and preexisting knowledge into account, and by providing education via a variety of methods. Nurses should also teach by example. MI patients are asked to make significant modifications in their lifestyle. Nurses who "practice what they preach" by demonstrating interest in healthful living, avoidance of smoking, and proper diet emphasize their acceptance of the ideas they are teaching patients [27].

Planning for teaching in clinical situations must take the following factors into account [27]:

1. Nurse–patient relationship

2. Effectiveness of communication

3. Patient's learning needs

4. Realistic objectives for teaching

5. Planning for time for teaching

6. Control of environment

7. Appropriate application of learning principles

8. Teaching skill of teacher

9. Evaluation of teaching

Assessment of the patient's knowledge base precedes instruction. The typical psychological reactions to MI that can affect readiness to learn (anxiety, denial, depression) must be considered. Teaching involving formal or structured learning about specific information has been shown to be more effective and is preferred, although informal teaching is done in many settings [20].

The content of teaching should be disease specific, with emphasis on lifestyle modification. The readiness of the patient to learn, as well as the immediate concerns in the situation, dictate what content is emphasized. For instance, patients need one kind of information at the time of transfer from the critical care unit and another type prior to returning to work. Information initially taught must often be reinforced because of the crisis atmosphere brought about by the illness. Patient education includes information about the illness, self-care, warning symptoms, risk factors, and resources. Advice about self-care, including the progressive return to normal living activities, enhances successful adjustment to MI and eventual return to work.

Both group and individual instruction has been shown to be useful for patients with chronic diseases, including cardiovascular ones. Group classes generally are more efficient, because more patients are taught at once and patients can learn from one another as well as from the instructor. The obvious disadvantage is the lack of individualization. One-to-one instruction must supplement the group approach so that patients and families gain an understanding of information that is specific to them. Individual teaching also allows the nurse to assess the effectiveness of the teaching for that patient, specifically, the knowledge gained. Individual instruction is more appropriate while the patient is in the critical care unit, because not only is he physically unable to tolerate a group setting, but psychologically he is less able to tolerate listening to the concerns of other patients at that time in his own illness.

Teaching methods that use several senses and written instructions are often the most successful. Behavior modification concepts may be useful in helping patients make long-term changes in lifestyle but probably have more applicability to the outpatient than to the inpatient setting [37].

Various visual aids enhance learning by using many senses. Some of the advantages of using visual aids are consistency in content, potential for multiple viewings by patients, documentation of content for quality assurance and legal purposes, availability of the teaching when the patient is ready, and the opportunity for nurses to use teaching time more effectively. Again, the lack of individualization and the lack of immediate feedback from the patient are disadvantages. Combinations of teaching strategies offer the best hope for meeting the educational needs of cardiac patients.

Documentation of education is important, both for legal reasons and for continuity of care. A variety of forms have been devised for this purpose. Equally important, however, is the documentation of effectiveness of teaching. Most nurses who practice within the hospital setting do not have the opportunity to follow patients closely after discharge; several appropriate methods exist to continue and/or reinforce education begun during the inpatient phase, however. Among these methods are telephone contact, referral to community agencies, and outpatient cardiac rehabilitation programs. Such follow-up is important, because many patients are unable to recall information given during the acute phase of the illness.

The effectiveness of patient education is examined in terms of both knowledge acquisition and compliance to the treatment plan. Studies on the effectiveness of teaching have demonstrated varying amounts of knowledge gained after intervention [31, 37]. Although measuring knowledge gained is useful, even more important is determining whether the patient can be motivated to act on the basis of information and whether the patient will indeed learn to comply with a regimen that is developed for him. Noncompliance with the medical regimen, unfortunately, is an important problem, with a hiatus often existing between knowledge and action. Patient education has a positive effect on compliance but is clearly not the only influence.

In general, factors such as extent of knowledge, gender, level of education, and socioeconomic status are not useful in predicting compliance. Becker, [4] using the Health Belief Model, has identified three variables of value in predicting compliance. They are the patient's perception of his susceptibility to the condition, his perception of the severity of the condition, and his perception of the value of taking action (the perceived efficacy and safety of the action). Although knowledge does not guarantee compliance, lack of knowledge increases the likelihood of noncompliance [47].

Education of the patient and family in the acute phase is limited to explaining procedures and policies of the CICU, reinforcing initial explanations, and answering questions about the diagnosis. The goals of teaching and learning should be short term, with concrete objectives [7]. The major focus is reduction of the patient's and the family's anxiety rather than in-depth education at this stage. In-depth education has not been found to be effective in critical care units, because of a variety of barriers [22].

Barriers may be present in the CICU that discourage or prevent nurses from teaching patients [22, 27]. Lack of time for teaching continues to be a major problem. Incorporating explanations while providing care — for example, teaching about medications while administering them — not only is time efficient but may be more educationally sound as well. Teaching must be seen as a priority in clinical practice and as a behavior expected of the staff if it is to be accomplished. Physician interference remains an obstacle to teaching in some units. Working cooperatively with physicians, enlisting support of nursing management, and inviting input from all health providers involved may be useful. Finally, lack of teaching preparation among nurses may be a barrier to providing education. Increasing the skill of nurses who teach patients will improve the quality of patient education.

Barriers to learning may be psychological, physiological, environmental, sociocultural, or iatrogenic. Psychological barriers involve the emotional and behavioral responses to MI. Anxiety enhances learning in some settings but may be too high in the CICU to facilitate learning in either patients or families. Anxiety may also involve other behavioral expressions that hamper learning. Denial, a defense mechanism used to decrease anxiety, may decrease the patient's perception of the MI and, therefore, of its seriousness. The patient is therefore less motivated to learn while in a state of denial. Denial is an extremely common early coping mechanism in MI, but it may persist for days to months, having serious implications for learning later in the convalescence. Depression also impedes learning and is a natural reaction that occurs three to four days after the MI [32].

Physiological barriers include factors related to the seriousness of the illness, pain and discomfort, restlessness, age, prognosis, and disruption in biorhythms. Teaching sessions should take individual factors such as age, physical symptoms, and alertness into account.

Environmental factors include continuous disruptions, excessive stimuli, loss of privacy, lack of sleep, and restrictions on family visiting. Repeated explanations about procedures, routines, and equipment, and attention to problems of lack of privacy and sleep, reduce the impact of the environmental factors. Development of a trusting nurse–patient relationship is also helpful [22].

Sociocultural factors such as language barriers, educational level, religion, and degree of family support also affect learning. The family's reactions, particularly those of the spouse, affect the patient's ability to learn. Spouses strive to find a cause for the illness, often expressing guilt at their possible contribution. Spouses and significant others should be included in the explanations given to the patient in the CICU.

Iatrogenic barriers include those barriers consciously or unconsciously set up by nurses in the CICU. These include giving information in a manner that is too hurried, fragmented, or complex for the patient to understand, and ignoring such cues from patients as questions and nonverbal behavior that indicate that the patient is uncomfortable or tired.

As noted earlier, individual instruction is the appropriate teaching method in critical care settings, because patients are not physically or emotionally able to participate in group instruction. Answering specific questions or referring them to the appropriate multidisciplinary team member may decrease anxiety, although no in-depth learning should be expected at this time.

In addition to providing explanations about the CICU and the diagnosis, preparing the patient for transfer from the CICU is important. Studies have demonstrated an increased level of anxiety at transfer and, therefore, an increased susceptibility of the patient to the effects of increased circulating catecholamines. Several approaches are suggested in the literature to help the patient and his family view the transfer as a positive step.

Because the goal of education in the CICU is to decrease anxiety rather than to provide in-depth knowledge, it is neither surprising nor disturbing that studies in the critical care unit have revealed poor knowledge retention. Most clinicians still support the effort, because the provision of information to patients and families reduces anxiety and encourages the asking of questions [31, 47].

Psychological Support and Counseling

The rationale for including interventions for the psychosocial concerns of cardiac patients and their families in cardiac rehabilitation is related to well-documented reactions to cardiac disease, as well as the need for patients and families to adapt psychologically and socially to the illness. Goals for nursing include restoring and maintaining normal behaviors and helping patients to adjust to their situation [9].

In addition to passing through several phases of adaptation — shock and disbelief, developing awareness, resolution, reorganization, and identity — patients exhibit typical behavioral responses to cardiac disease. These may include anxiety, denial, depression, anger, guilt, and sexual aggressiveness [32]. Patients may be referred for cardiac rehabilitation at any stage of their illness, from 24 hours to several months after MI or surgery. The range of behavioral responses may, therefore, include all those stages just described and may influence the rehabilitation process. Programs that emphasize systematic progression of activity have demonstrated beneficial physical and emotional effects, particularly the effect on depression. The reactions of the family are also important; evidence suggests that the attitudes of the spouse influence patient participation in a rehabilitation program and the degree of compliance to medical regimens [33].

Interventions for patients exhibiting these behavioral responses are best handled by a multidisciplinary team, because various approaches may be indicated. The expertise of a social worker or psychiatric nurse familiar with cardiovascular problems and reactions should be available to patients in the CICU who exhibit exaggerated or prolonged emotional reactions to acute MI or CABG. Also, patients may verbalize immediate concerns related to home management while hospitalized; for example, the patient may have been responsible for the care of children or an elderly parent at home. The social worker is generally the best member of the team to obtain information for patients about community resources and financial and other concerns.

Utilization of the expertise of members of the multidisciplinary team should be coordinated by the CICU nurse to avoid unnecessary disruptions and duplications in patient care and to facilitate effective communication among team members. Documentation of assessments, goals, and interventions planned by any health professional should be in the patient's record so that this information is readily available to all involved in the patient's care.

Transfer from Critical Care to Hospital Discharge

After the patient is transferred from the critical care unit, the focus of care is directed toward preparation for discharge. As noted earlier, most patients after an uncomplicated MI or CABG are discharged within one to two weeks after admission. Therefore, less time is available to accomplish more in terms of patient adjustment, education, and mobilization. Common nursing diagnoses identified during this period (in addition to those listed for the CICU) include:

Knowledge deficit, related to need for lifestyle modifications, self-care, self-monitoring/action for reportable symptoms

Coping, ineffective, patient and/or family, related to imminent discharge

Home maintenance management, impaired, related to restricted activity, need to stay out of work at least temporarily

Nutrition, alteration in: potential for more than body requirements, related to decreased physical activity, boredom, anxiety, restricted diet

Sexual dysfunction, related to emotional factors, decreased physical capacity, medications that decrease libido

Interventions involving the multidisciplinary team are directed toward helping the patient achieve certain outcomes by discharge (Exhibit 15.1).

Mobilization

Supervised mobilization by nurses or physical or occupational therapists is continued progressively yet cautiously with variables similar to those employed in the CICU used to guide progression. Most programs include supervised stair climbing before discharge. Activity tolerance is carefully assessed and documented, because activities added at this stage may significantly increase myocardial O_2 demand.

Most patients with uncomplicated conditions at discharge can tolerate activities at peak levels of about 3.5 to 4.0 METS for short durations [36]. Some patients may be formally stress tested at a low level (3.5 METS) to prescribe activity further after discharge. The highest heart rate attained without adverse effects is the heart rate under which activities may be done after discharge. The patient should be instructed not only about resuming activities after discharge but also about exercise-related variables and warning signs. Sexual activity, in particular, should be either discussed with the patient by the nurse or referred to another health team member who is able to discuss with the patient and the sexual partner resumption of sexual activity with precautions. Education relative to activity is included as part of the formal teaching for cardiac patients but should also be emphasized during exercise treatments.

Exercise guidelines for the CABG patient are less well developed than those for post-MI patients [46]. Use of similar, but modified, physiological variables has been suggested to monitor response to exercise in CABG patients. Criteria for hypotension, in particular, may be different in these patients, because many of them exhibit either orthostatic or exercise-induced hypotension. Any symptomatic hypotension or an asymptomatic drop of 20 mm Hg or more is considered a contraindication to exercise. Stair climbing may be more likely to result in hypotension than exercise on the treadmill. Therefore, CABG patients should be monitored carefully as they progress to stair climbing.

Education

A major nursing focus during the remainder of the hospitalization is patient education in preparation for discharge for both post-MI and CABG patients. At this stage, education is designed to provide adequate information about CAD and its management to enable the patient to assume some responsibility for subsequent health care and lifestyle changes.

Although multiple studies have been conducted evaluating patient education, little information is available about the "survival skills" required by patients at discharge. Patients must have a knowledge level at discharge adequate for beginning self-care, including diet and risk factor modification, with particular emphasis on activity guidelines and prescribed medication. In addi-

EXHIBIT 15.1
Patient Outcomes at Discharge

1. Describe the signs and symptoms that necessitate medical advice.
2. Accurately describe own planned action if any of the signs appear.
3. Describe acute myocardial infarction and approximate healing period.
4. Describe angina.
5. Identify own cardiac risk factors.
6. Describe factors that increase the work of the heart: weather, stress, digestion of food, exercise, sexual activity.
7. State name, dose, schedule, adverse reactions, and action of prescribed medications.
8. State own planned action if an adverse rreaction to any medication occurs.
9. Discuss plan to decrease/eliminate cigarette smoking.
10. Describe own dietary restrictions.
11. Complete phase I activity/exercise component.
12. State intention to comply with prescribed treatment plan.

tion, patients must be knowledgeable about reportable symptoms and ways to access the emergency medical system. Although further study is needed to determine the knowledge that patients should demonstrate at discharge from the hospital, content is presently directed toward helping patients acquire the knowledge for adequate self-care. Various methods are used, depending on the patient's assessed needs. Generally, group instruction using a multidisciplinary team is appropriate at this stage, with individual follow-up to ensure that specific questions of the patient and family are answered. Take-home material in the form of AHA literature and other commercially available pamphlets, and in-house printed materials relating to nutrition, stress, and community resources, are important provisions for reinforcement.

Even though patients probably have greater retention of material taught just prior to discharge, long-term retention has been shown to be poor. Referral for follow-up teaching in the outpatient setting is an appropriate nursing intervention. Continuity in rehabilitation programs from phase I through Phase III is the ideal and should be used if such programs exist. Other community resources for referral are the Visiting Nurses Association, nurses employed in physicians' offices and industry, clinics, and nurse practitioners. Adequate documentation of the patient's degree of goal attainment at discharge should accompany the referral.

Psychological Support

Patients and families should be prepared for the possibility of emotional reactions to the MI or surgery after discharge. Discussing these as normal reactions may decrease the patients' and families' concern, should they occur. Continued counseling by the social worker on the team may be necessary after discharge. Some institutions make group discussions available to families while patients are still hospitalized. The focus of these discussions, which are often led by nurses, is to share information about the physical and emotional aspects of heart disease. Spouses and families will play an integral part in the patient's care after discharge, as well as in the degree of compliance to the treatment plan. Family needs must be dealt with, as well as those of the patient.

Rehabilitation of the Patient after Complicated MI

Post-MI patients who demonstrate continuing evidence of ischemia, heart failure, or electrical instability pose problems in cardiac rehabilitation [8]. Components of the inpatient program are still made available to these patients and their families. Mobilization should be postponed, however, until a reasonable certainty exists that the infarction is completed. Other contraindications to early ambulation include cardiogenic shock, hypotension, and dysrhythmias.

Rehabilitation of such a patient in the CCU should consist of early use of the bedside commode and chair, with activity progressing according to assessment of the clinical status [8]. The in-chair position may be beneficial for the patient with congestive heart failure, because preload and, therefore, myocardial work is decreased with the legs down. Clinical guidelines used in assessing whether the activity exceeds the cardiac reserve are fatigue, dyspnea, and lowered blood pressure. Use of a bedpan is to be avoided because of the increased energy expenditure and psychological stress.

After transfer from the CCU, similar guidelines apply for mobilization, with ambulation and exercise prescribed only within the patient's physical limits. A portable ECG is a useful and necessary tool for assessment during increased activity.

The need for explanations, both in the CCU and after transfer, cannot be overemphasized, because increased anxiety produces an increased heart rate and myocardial O_2 demand. If these changes occur in a patient who is already unstable, the MVO_2 may exceed the O_2 supply and cause extension of the area of necrosis. Patients who experience postinfarction angina either in the CICU or after transfer may be especially fearful of having another MI. Explanations of the difference between angina and MI become vital to alleviating their fears.

OUTPATIENT CARDIAC REHABILITATION

Phases II and III constitute outpatient cardiac rehabilitation and include exercise, education, and psychological support.

During phase II, the cardiac patient returns home to continue recovery. Although involvement of critical care and progressive care unit nurses ends at discharge from the hospital, it is important that nurses working in these areas understand the goals and interventions that take place during this phase of the illness. The goals during phase I are coordinated with goals of the acute care period. Individualized follow-up is facilitated if adequate documentation of the progress of the patient is available from phase I. Involvement of the same health care team members facilitates continuity of care for the patient and family.

Nursing goals for phase II include assisting the patient to resume usual daily activities, to reestablish his usual relationships, and to restore self-esteem. In addition, intervention is directed toward reinforcing knowledge, skills, and attitudes necessary to achieve lifestyle adjustment. Nursing diagnoses commonly observed during outpatient rehabilitation include alteration in cardiac output, knowledge deficit, activity intolerance, maladaptive coping (individual and family), grieving, alteration in home maintenance, sexual dysfunction, and noncompliance (potential). Interventions require a multidisciplinary team approach, incorporating elements of exercise, support, and education into a structured outpatient program.

Exercise: Phase II   Exercise and activity should be prescribed, as are other interventions. The specific exercise prescription should delineate the target heart rate and the intensity, duration, and frequency of the activity. The prescription should be revised periodically according to the responses of the patient and the status of the healing myocardium.

Exercise during phase II may be supervised or unsupervised. Progressive walking or activity on a stationary bicycle are examples of appropriate activity [45].

The patient should be instructed carefully about the intensity, duration, frequency, and type of activity to be done during the convalescent period. Patients may be given guidelines defined in terms of METS or in terms of usual household activities allowed. The MET concept is more specific but is limited by the fact that values on a MET chart are average estimates of energy expended. Performing the activity at a different speed or with a different skill level may make the estimate inaccurate. Giving patients permission to return to their "usual activity," or providing guidelines that tell patients to "take it easy," can often be misinterpreted, creating a potentially dangerous workload on the myocardium. In addition, conflict can occur between the patient and spouse when the patient's activity exceeds the spouse's interpretation of the instructions.

A combination of activity lists and more specific physiological measures is beneficial. Some patients will have had a low-level exercise test prior to discharge or in the immediate discharge period. In addition to identifying patients who are at increased risk for recurrent cardiac events and serving as a guide for future medical or surgical therapy, this low-level stress test can serve as the basis for the exercise prescription. The heart rate at which ischemic symptoms appeared (objective and/or subjective) is the heart rate below which activity is prescribed.

Phase II is ended by a symptom-limited, full-scale exercise test. The results of this test are useful in writing the exercise prescription as well as in assessing myocardial functional impairment. The information derived may influence future therapy in addition to defining the amount of exercise that can safely be performed. Tests should be conducted according to specified standards, using one of various protocols and types of equipment available. A complete discussion of this topic is beyond the scope of this chapter. Several comprehensive documents are available for this purpose [2].

Exercise: Phase III   Participants enter phase III exercise programs two to six months after MI or CABG, when healing is complete. These programs may be hospital or community based. The type of exercise used in phase III is designed to increase cardiovascular fitness. Aerobic exercise, performed three to four times weekly for 20 to 30 minutes at an intensity high enough to maintain the heart rate at

75% to 85% of maximum (training range), is appropriate in supervised programs [46]. Patients exercising without supervision should exercise at an intensity that raises the heart rate to at least 60% but not more than 80% of the maximum heart rate [36]. Adequate warm-up and cool-down periods should be included. Some cardiac patients may benefit from a prolonged warm-up period as well as from prophylactic nitroglycerin administration before starting the actual training exercise. Commonly prescribed cardiovascular drugs are a matter of concern, because they can significantly alter the exercise capacity of cardiac patients [42]. The effects of these drugs must be considered when prescribing and assessing the response to exercise. Of particular concern are beta blockers, nitrates, digitalis, diuretics, and calcium blockers.

Because the prescription of conditioning exercise includes the intensity at which exercise is to be performed and is usually guided by heart rate, patients should be stress tested on their medical regimens and the prescription written from that information rather than from tables of age-predicted heart rates.

Education: Phases II and III

The goal of education in phases II and III is helping the patient and family understand the nature of the disease process and the prescribed treatment. It is hoped that this knowledge will increase motivation to modify risk factors, maximize physical potential, and increase compliance with the prescribed regimen. As stated earlier, however, lack of knowledge is only one of several factors involved in noncompliance.

Despite the demonstration of an increased knowledge level on tests at discharge, most patients require education in the outpatient phase if they are to deal with ongoing health status changes and meet the goals stated. Studies [31, 50] have repeatedly recommended continuation of education and support for the patient and family after discharge. Lack of information or misinformation on the part of the family members with whom the patient lives may create conflict in the home situation as the patient attempts to comply with the treatment regimen. The family and others can have a direct effect not only on the patient's acceptance of his illness, but also on his adaptation and modification of risk factors. Education, behavior modification, and positive reinforcement are long-term concerns. Further study is indicated to define strategies that facilitate the long-term behavior changes necessary for cardiovascular health.

Psychological Support: Phases II and III

Patients and families may continue to display the same emotional and behavioral responses to MI that were evident during hospitalization. Other adjustments are often required, however.

Discharge from the hospital may necessitate a period of role adjustment. Additionally, if patients have not been accustomed to spending prolonged periods of time at home, they may find continual contact with young children stressful when coupled with their own feelings of frustration and boredom. Insomnia, irritability, and exaggerated dependency may lead to tension in the family. The family should be encouraged to be supportive and should be helped to understand personality changes that the patient may exhibit upon return home.

Support groups for patients and spouses, possibly including separate groups for each, are helpful in encouraging the free expression of emotions during this time. Support and understanding are emphasized in groups, rather than confrontation or encounter techniques. Social workers and nurses with cardiovascular expertise may co-lead a group for outpatients. Topics are opened for discussion by the participants, with guidance from the co-leaders. Common topics of discussion include reactions to the hospitalization and the illness, family reactions, preparation for return to work or independent living, and sexual activity. Although the major focus of the group is support, it is often a forum for answering medical questions. Spending a portion of the group time answering general questions is helpful.

Issues may also surface in the later part of the rehabilitation period. Anxiety can exist in the individual for several years after the cardiac illness and may be exacerbated by certain events. Uncertainty about physical activity and the existence of physical symptoms related to deconditioning may be associated with anxiety and depression. A comprehensive rehabilitation program that facilitates lifestyle adjustments as well as physical conditioning will, it is hoped, also assist the individual and family in making adjustments to the cardiovascular event.

SUMMARY

This chapter has presented concepts of cardiac rehabilitation applicable to the cardiovascular patient, including those with angina, uncomplicated MI, and CABG. In addition, particular concerns relating to complicated conditions or patients with other medical problems are discussed.

A description of the components of activity and exercise, patient and family education, and psychosocial support was presented, with emphasis on the three phases of the rehabilitative process and the multidisciplinary team.

Further research is required to determine the effectiveness of rehabilitation for cardiovascular patients. Additionally, further validation of the nurse's role in relation to the commonly identified nursing diagnoses and interventions is a potential focus for future research.

STUDY QUESTIONS

1. List three necessary components of cardiac rehabilitation programming.
2. The critical care nurse's role in cardiac rehabilitation includes (indicate all that apply):
   a. physiological monitoring during initial mobilization
   b. delivery of comprehensive, in-depth patient and family education in preparation for discharge
   c. provision of information to the patient and family about transfer from the critical care unit
   d. composition of the activity prescription prior to discharge
3. List four multidisciplinary team members central to a phase I cardiac rehabilitation program.

4. Interest was originally generated in mobilizing cardiac patients when (indicate all that apply):
   a. the hazards of prolonged bed rest were documented on normal individuals
   b. it was appreciated that simply surviving a critical illness is not indicative of comprehensive treatment
   c. advances in diagnosis and treatment resulted in more survivors
   d. chair rest was shown not to be harmful

5. Indicate which of the following patients are candidates for progressive ambulation at this time (indicate all to whom category applies):
   a. Mr. X: 40 years old, s/p acute inferior MI two days ago, stable vital signs and ECG.
   b. Ms. P: 56 years old, had uncomplicated CABG five days ago, transferred from surgical intensive care unit two days ago.
   c. Mr. V: 56 years old, s/p acute anterior MI six days ago, still markedly short of breath on minimal exertion, blood pressure 92 mm Hg systolic, apical pulse—sinus tachycardia at 110, no dysrhythmia except sinus tachycardia.
   d. Mr. Q: 43 years old, had angina pectoris diagnosed three months ago, now admitted to hospital for evaluation and treatment of increasingly frequent chest pain.

6. List four potential role functions of the cardiac rehabilitation nurse coordinator.

7. True or False: Initial mobilization after the ischemic event is designed to decrease the deconditioning effects associated with prolonged bed rest.

8. State the two types of exercise, and give two examples of each.

9. A clinical correlate to 75% of VO_2 max is _____ .

10. Name a class of drugs that blunts the normal blood pressure and heart rate response to exercise.

11. State three characteristics of the patient-learner that must be considered before implementing comprehensive post-MI education.

12. True or False: Group education is equally applicable to all patients during hospitalization for acute MI.

13. List three advantages to using audiovisual aids in patient and family education.

14. Which of the following factors have been found to affect compliance with a therapeutic regimen? (Check all that apply.)
    a. Educational level
    b. Self-perceived susceptibility
    c. Socioeconomic status
    d. Knowledge level

15. True or False: Cardiac rehabilitation that includes activity progression has been found to have an impact on depression.

16. Name three common emotional responses of the patient who is faced with an unexpected cardiac event.

17. State the goals of phase I cardiac rehabilitation.

18. What is the rationale for determining the baseline level of the patient's knowledge, perception, and functional patterns early in the hospitalization?

19. List three nursing diagnoses potentially observed in phase I.

20. Select one diagnosis and discuss possible cause, desired patient outcome, and nursing intervention.

21. True or False: Early mobilization is justified because it prevents the complications of immobility, rather than because of its own therapeutic value.

22. Specify three pertinent assessments that indicate an untoward response to increased activity in the early phase of the illness.

23. Identify two useful resources for the continued follow-up of post-MI and CABG patients after discharge.

24. Discuss the rationale for the inclusion of patient and family education in outpatient cardiac rehabilitation.

CASE STUDIES

CASE 1

A 52-year-old man is referred for cardiac rehabilitation. The medical diagnosis is uncomplicated inferior MI three days prior. The patient is awaiting transfer to the progressive coronary care unit.

The initial assessment is as follows: Patient is a young-appearing, middle-aged man, seated in a bedside chair. He is continuously monitored and is in normal sinus rhythm, and vital signs are stable (blood pressure, 92/70 mm Hg; apical pulse, 62 bpm; respiration rate, 14 per minute; breath sounds clear). Skin is tanned and warm to touch; urine output has been satisfactory. Medications include Inderal 20 mg. every six hours; nifedipine, 10 mg every 6 hours; nitroglycerine sublingually gr 1/150 as needed for chest discomfort. Chart review reveals that this is the first MI. Patient is employed as a middle manager for a local manufacturing company. As the nurse enters the room, he asks, "When can I get out of here and go home? My doctor said I would be leaving today."

1. What additional assessments should be done to complete the nursing data base on this patient?

2. Discuss the patient's apparent misinterpretation of his transfer—not discharge. What behavioral elements and knowledge deficits are apparent here? Outline appropriate nursing interventions.

3. Discuss initial plans for mobilization. What amount, duration, and intensity of activity is appropriate?

4. Discuss documentation of physical activity for the patient. What assessments should be included?

5. What are the educational needs of the patient at this point? What outcomes are reasonable at this stage of the illness?

CASE 2

A 48-year-old man was diagnosed as having significant left main CAD after a routine stress test. He has undergone subsequent catheterization and CABG x 4, four days prior, and is transferred to your unit from the SICU. His course has been stable, and he is expected to be discharged within five days. Initial assessment by the CICU nurses indicated a knowledge deficit because this is the patient's first hospitalization for coronary disease. Risk factors include cigarette smoking (two packs per day, filtered) for thirty years, sedentary lifestyle, Type A personality, very stressful occupation, and a father who died at age 46 of MI. The medical plan of care includes progressive ambulation according to cardiac rehabilitation protocol; low-sodium, low-saturated-fat diet; routine monitoring of vital signs and weights. No cardiac medications.

1. What additional assessments are indicated before formal education is implemented?

2. What knowledge outcomes are appropriate at discharge for this patient?

3. Determine appropriate content for the educational sessions, including resources.

4. Discuss the involvement of the multidisciplinary team in the education of this patient.

5. What factors are involved in predicting compliance? What enhances compliance with a treatment plan that requires lifestyle modification for a patient such as this?

REFERENCES

1. American College of Sports Medicine. *Guidelines for Graded Exercise Testing and Exercise Prescription* (2nd ed.). Philadelphia: Lea & Febiger, 1980.

2. American Heart Association. *Exercise Standards Book*. Dallas: American Heart Association, 1979.

3. American Heart Association. *Heart Facts 1985*. Dallas: American Heart Association, 1985.

4. Becker, M. H. *The Health Belief Model and Personal Health Behavior*. Thorofare, N. J.: Charles B. Slack, 1974.

5. Bille, D. A study of patients' knowledge in relation to teaching format and compliance. *Superv. Nurs.* 8:55, 1977.

6. Blackburn, H. Physical activity and CHD: a brief update and population view. *J. Cardiac Rehab.* 3:101, 1983.

7. Burke, L. Learning and retention in the acute care setting. *Crit. Care Q.* 4:67, 1981.

8. Cohen, N. Cardiac rehabilitation in the CCU. II. *Heart Lung* 7:861, 1978.

9. Cook, R. Psychosocial responses to myocardial infarction. *Heart Lung* 8:130, 1979.

10. Cosmoss, P. M., et al. *Cardiac Rehabilitation: A Comprehensive Nursing Approach*. Philadelphia: Lippincott, 1979.

11. Dehn, M. The effects of exercise. *Am. J. Nurs.* 80:435, 1980.

12. Fardy, P. Exercise physiology for cardiac rehabilitation. In P. Fardy (ed.), *Cardiac Rehabilitation*. St. Louis: Mosby, 1982.

13. Guzzetta, C., and Dossey, B. Nursing diagnosis: framework, process and problems. *Heart Lung* 12:281, 1983.

14. Hackett, T. P., and Cassem, N. H. The psychological adaptation of myocardial infarction patients to convalescence. *Heart Lung* 2:382, 1973.

15. Hartley, L. H. Devising an exercise program for the cardiac patient. *J. Cardiovasc. Med.* 7:1307, 1982.

16. Haskell, W. L. Cardiovascular complications during exercise training of cardiac patients. *Circulation* 57:920, 1979.

17. Kallio, V., et al. Reduction in sudden death by a multifactorial intervention programme after acute myocardial infarction. *Lancet* 2:1091, 1979.

18. Kavanagh, T., et al. Prognostic indexes for patients with ischemic heart disease enrolled in an exercise centered rehabilitation program *Am. J. Cardiol.* 44:1230, 1979.

19. Lindskog, B. D., et al. A method of evaluation of activity and exercise in a controlled study of early cardiac rehabilitation. *J. Cardiac Rehab.* 2:156, 1982.

20. Milazzo, V. A study of the difference in health knowledge gained through formal and informal teaching. *Heart Lung* 9:1079, 1980.

21. Miller, P. B., et al. Effects of moderate physical exercise during four weeks of bedrest on circulatory functions in man. *Aerospace Med.* 36:1077, 1965.

22. Murdaugh, C. Barriers to patient education in the CCU. *Cardiovasc. Nurs.* 18:31, 1982.

23. National Hospital Discharge Survey. Unpublished data, Washington, D. C., Division of Health Resources Utilization, National Center for Health Statistics, August 1980.

24. Naughton, J. The national exercise and heart disease project: report number 2. *Cardiology.* 62:352, 1978.

25. O'Brien, M. K. Assessing activity tolerance in critical care settings. *Focus* 9:11, 1983.

26. Owens, J., et al. Cardiac rehabilitation: a patient education program. *Nurs. Res.* 27:148, 1978.

27. Pohl, M. L. *Teaching Function of the Nurse Practitioner.* Dubuque, Iowa: William Brown, 1968.

28. Rahe, R., et al. A teaching evaluation questionnaire for post-MI patients. *Heart Lung* 4:759, 1975.

29. Rechnitzer, P. A. The effect of exercise prescription on the recurrence rate of myocardial infarction in men. *Am. J. Cardiol.* 47:419, 1981.

30. Saltin, B., et al. Response to exercise after bedrest and training. *Circulation* (Suppl.) 38:1, 1968.

31. Scalzi, C. Evaluation of an inpatient educational program for coronary patients and families. *Heart Lung* 9:846, 1980.

32. Scalzi, C., and Burke, L. E. MI: behavioral responses of patient and spouse. In S. Underhill et al. (eds.), *Cardiac Nursing.* Philadelphia: Lippincott, 1982.

33. Scalzi, C., and Burke, L. E. Patient and family education. In S. Underhill et al. (eds.), *Cardiac Nursing.* Philadelphia: Lippincott, 1982.

34. Shaw, L. W. Effects of a prescribed supervised exercise program on mortality and cardiovascular morbidity in patients after MI. *Am. J. Cardiol.* 48:39, 1981.

35. Silvidi, G. E., et al. Hemodynamic responses and medical problems associated with early exercise and ambulation in CABG patients. *J. Cardiac Rehab.* 2:355, 1982.

36. Sivarajan, E. Cardiac rehabilitation: activity and exercise program. In S. Underhill et al. (eds.), *Cardiac Nursing* Philadelphia: Lippincott, 1982.

37. Sivarajan, E. Limited effects of outpatient teaching and counseling after MI: a controlled study. *Heart Lung* 12:65, 1983.

38. Stern, M. The recent decline in ischemic heart disease mortality. *Ann. Intern. Med.* 91:630, 1979.

39. Stoner, M. Cardiac rehabilitation: state of the art. *J. Cardiac Rehab.* 3:165, 1983.

40. Velasco, J. A., et al. Complications during early ambulation and patient selection. *Adv. Cardiol.* 31:142, 1982.

41. Wenger, N. K. *Rehabilitation after Myocardial Infarction.* Dallas: American Heart Association, 1973.

42. Wenger N. K. The coronary patient: interactions of cardiovascular drugs and exercise. *Drug Ther.* 12:59, 1982.

43. Wenger, N. K. Early ambulation: the physiologic basis revisited. *Adv. Cardiol.* 31:138, 1982.

44. WHO, Regional Office for Europe: The rehabilitation of patients with cardiovascular disease: report of a seminar. EURP 0381 (1969).

45. Williams, R. S., et al. Guidelines for unsupervised exercise in patients with ischemic heart disease. *J. Cardiac Rehab.* 1:213, 1981.

46. Wilson, P., et al. *Cardiac Rehabilitation, Adult Fitness, and Exercise Testing.* Philadelphia: Lea & Febiger, 1981.

47. Winslow, E. Progressive exercise to combat the hazards of bedrest. *Am. J. Nurs.* 80:440, 1980.

48. Woods, S. Diagnosis and treatment of the patient with an uncomplicated MI. In S. Underhill et al. (eds.), *Cardiac Nursing.* Philadelphia: Lippincott, 1982.

49. Wulff, K., and Hong, P. Surgical intervention for coronary artery disease. In S. Underhill et al. (eds.), *Cardiac Nursing.* Philadelphia, Lippincott, 1982.

50. Young, D., et al. A prospective controlled study on inpatient hospital myocardial infarction rehabilitation. *J. Cardiac Rehab.* 2:32, 1982.

Index